Sensual Reading

Sensual Reading

New Approaches to Reading in Its Relations to the Senses

Edited by
Michael Syrotinski
and Ian Maclachlan

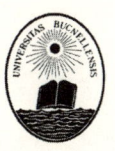

Lewisburg
Bucknell University Press
London: Associated University Presses

© 2001 by Associated University Presses, Inc.

All rights reserved. Authorization to photocopy items for internal or personal use, or the internal or personal use of specific clients, is granted by the copyright owner, provided that a base fee of $10.00, plus eight cents per page, per copy is paid directly to the Copyright Clearance Center, 222 Rosewood Drive, Danvers, Massachusetts 01923. [0-8387-5471-6/01 $10.00 + 8¢ pp, pc.]

Associated University Presses
440 Forsgate Drive
Cranbury, NJ 08512

Associated University Presses
16 Barter Street
London WC1A 2AH, England

Associated University Presses
P.O. Box 338, Port Credit
Mississauga, Ontario
Canada L5G 4L8

The paper used in this publication meets the requirements of the American National Standard for Permanence of Paper for Printed Library Materials Z39.48-1984.

Library of Congress Cataloging-in-Publication Data

Sensual reading : new approaches to reading in its relations to the senses / edited by Michael Syrotinski and Ian Maclachlan.
   p. cm.
   Includes bibliographical references and index.
   ISBN 0-8387-5471-6 (alk. paper)
   1. Senses and sensation in literature.   I. Syrotinski, Michael, 1957–
   II. Maclachlan, Ian, 1960–

PN56.S47 S46   2001
418'.4'019—dc21   00-062091

PRINTED IN THE UNITED STATES OF AMERICA

Contents

Introduction: Hors d'œuvre   7
MICHAEL SYROTINSKI

Part I: Touch

"L'échange de deux fantaisies et le contact de deux épidermes": Skin and Desire   17
NAOMI SEGAL

The Touch of the Other on the Threshold of Sex; or The Skin between Levinas and Irigaray   39
DAVE BOOTHROYD

Long Distance Love: On Remote Sensing in Shakespeare's Sonnet 109   57
IAN MACLACHLAN

Part II: Ears

*Tintern*abulation: Poetry Ringing in the Ears   69
SCOTT BREWSTER

Bodies of Resonance   83
RACHEL JONES

From the Ear to the Eye: Perceptions of Language in the Fictions of Laurence Sterne   106
ALEXIS TADIÉ

Part III: Eyes

Language, Color, and the Enigma of Everydayness   127
MICHAEL SHERINGHAM

Reading *La Lectrice*   153
PAUL SUTTON

The Metamorphosis of Vision in the Surrealist Text: José María Hinojosa's "Granadas de fuego"   166
JACQUELINE RATTRAY

Part IV: Textual Feasts

"Promnesia" (Remembering Forward) in *Midnight's Children*; or Rushdie's Chutney versus Proust's Madeleine   179
    LAURENT MILESI

"Go hang yourself, you who have never been comfortably seated and eating an olive": The Taste and Defiance of an Adolescent Body   213
    JO CROFT

Part V: Synaesthetics / Anaesthetics

Sight, Sound, and Synaesthesia: Reading the Senses in Victor Segalen   229
    CHARLES FORSDICK

The Anaesthesia of Charles Baudelaire's "Le goût du néant"   248
    KNUT OVE ELIASSEN

Reading (in) Proust: With the Senses, beyond the Senses   271
    JANE WALLING

Part VI: Telesensualities

Andy's Wedding: Reading Warhol   295
    PETER KRAPP

Singular Sense, Second Hand   311
    PEGGY KAMUF

Back   327
    NICHOLAS ROYLE

List of Contributors   341
Index   345

Introduction: Hors d'œuvre
MICHAEL SYROTINSKI

*S*ENSUAL READING WAS CONCEIVED OUT OF A SENSE THAT MUCH CONtemporary theory and critical practice has coalesced into increasingly homogenized discourses of the "body" and the "subject." The impetus for the volume was thus a desire to move beyond this homogenization, to break out of this mold, by rethinking traditional aesthetic or phenomenological approaches to the question of "sensing," in order to rearticulate the relationship between reading and the different senses. This initially took the form of an international conference organized by the Aberdeen Critical Theory Seminar (acts), and its success convinced us that we could profitably select a number of papers and ask the authors to expand them into a collection of essays, which could then be made available to a wider public.

Linking reading and the senses is not a particularly new critical maneuver, and indeed there are a number of traditions and historical moments where this conjunction is explicitly foregrounded. (One might think most immediately of the whole empiricist tradition: the "sensualist" philosophers of the Enlightenment—Berkeley, Hume, Locke—and the almost obsessive concern in French literature and philosophy of the eighteenth century, when writers such as Condillac, Diderot, Rousseau, and Batteux endeavoured to theorize the relationship between language and the sensual apprehension of the natural world.) In fact, there are any number of possible takes on the question of the relationship between reading and the senses, once one starts to open the borders of the usual frames of reference and to allow for a greater degree of intertextual and interdisciplinary infiltration. "Sensual reading" might thus be said to encompass aesthetic theory from Democritus and Aristotle all the way through to the great German idealist tradition: Kant, Hegel, Schiller, and Goethe. (Jane Walling, for example, in her essay uses Goethe's version of the "Book of Nature" as a paradigm for looking at Proust's "sensual reading" of the natural world.) It might refer to the pervasive sweep of phenomenology in the first half of this century, with Husserl, Merleau-Ponty, Heidegger, and the literary criticism it spawned, of which the finest examples remain Georges Poulet's and Jean-Pierre Richard's analyses of the act of poetic creation deriving from a sensual or material imagination. Although it may now appear distant and rather outmoded, in the wake of structuralist, deconstructionist, or other more formalist theoretical models, it is given a rich new lease on life in Laurent Milesi's essay comparing Proust's gustatory sensualism to Rushdie's.

Merleau-Ponty's phenomenological investigations are likewise rehabilitated and reworked in two essays: as Michael Sheringham shows in discussing Merleau-Ponty's meditations on color, while the subject's absorption in color suggests an unmediated prelinguistic apprehension of the world, a closer reading reveals that it in fact opens up a complex interplay between color as a "pure" and stable phenomenon, and color as a kind of language system that would be subject to constant mutability. The cinematic experience as described by Paul Sutton likewise participates in the immediacy of sensual experience, to the extent that "all cinematic readings are sensual readings," but it is again the problematization of this experience as a *reading*, through his reading of a film about reading, which raises doubts about any phenomenologically grounded theory of vision. In another context, Dave Boothroyd takes Merleau-Ponty's essay "The Intertwining—The Chiasm" as a basis for looking at Irigaray's "readerly embrace" of Levinas, in order to rethink the category of the ethical in its relation to the experience of sexual difference. In a reformulation of Merleau-Ponty's chiasm, according to Boothroyd, "sexual difference and ethics cross over one another."

To approach the notion of "sensual reading" from another, more scientifically informed angle, one might think about tracing the history of medical understanding of the functioning of the senses. This would encompass Galen's famous treatises on the senses, through Medieval theories of humours, Foucault's theses on Enlightenment rationalism and codification of sensuality, to the birth of psychoanalysis, and modern-day knowledge about how the human body senses, and how the human mind perceives, the complex science of neurophysiology or "psychophysics." All of these are to a greater or lesser extent represented or echoed in the various pieces in this volume, but it should be stated at the outset that this collection in no way pretends to be an exhaustive anthologization. The critical engagement with the traditions that inform the concept of "sensual reading" is itself an important feature of the essays; indeed, it is perhaps their dominant trait. "Sensual reading" denotes various modes of re-reading, a critical fare of second sights and doubletakes, a listening that is attentive to echoes and stuttering, a savoring of foretastes and aftertastes.

It is thus the disaggregating effect of *reading* that is emphasized here, particularly the ways in which language seems to interfere with the immediacy one normally associates with sense experience. Peggy Kamuf, in her narrative of a telling moment in her childhood, mishears the phrase "second hand," or rather hears a hyphen which is not there, an imperceptible, yet irreparably painful difference. Similarly Peter Krapp, in his essay on Andy Warhol's manic experiments in teletechnology, marks out the disturbing effects of mechanical repetition on the senses, and on sense, which would not be so unnerving were it not for the fact that the senselessness of modes of technological reproduction also reveals a senselessness at the heart of language itself. It all gets very confusing, the senses are confused, but not in the Romantic mode of synaesthetic harmony.

This re-evaluation is a way of thinking about the senses that goes beyond seeing them as part of a totalized system, Aristotle's *sensus communis*, the common sense integrating the activity of several senses, or as the various "political allegories" of the senses. (We are thinking, for example, of Diderot's anthropomorphized version of the warring senses, which even in conflict are none the less conceived of as functionally equivalent.) It is rather a world in which sight is no longer just sight, but also touch (as Michael Sheringham points out, again in relation to Merleau-Ponty); or elsewhere (in Rachel Jones's reading of Paula Ludwig's poetry), it is the tactility of sound that comes to the fore. Consequently, the self has to negotiate a whole new range of sensual interrelations, producing, for example, in Ludwig a "self-as-resonance," in Philippe Jaccottet's poetry a color-inflected subjectivity, or in Sterne's *Tristram Shandy* a self that takes shape in the "inky materiality" of his textual experiments. In fact, the senses no longer provide the means to the self-reflexivity of a subject, whether Cartesian, Kantian, or phenomenological. Scott Brewster listens to the English Romantic poets with the "ear of the other" and notes a dissolution of the subject's "punctual integrity" (p. 70), an asymmetrical movement that Ian Maclachlan, in trying to account for the "time" of love in Shakespeare's Sonnet 109, describes succinctly as follows: "the promise of synchrony must be held open by anachrony." (p. 62).

This "ana-" structure is a recurring principle of disarticulation in several essays, from the interplay between anamnesia and promnesia in Laurent Milesi's discussion of the future perfect in Rushdie, through Knut Eliassen's reading of the anaesthetics of Baudelaire's "Le Goût du néant," to Nicholas Royle's exploration of the anasemic, or anasensual, effects of "back." The predominance of what look like neologisms is an essential trait of this rearticulation of the relationship between language and sensing, which involves rethinking or reinventing terms such as "telepathy" (Nicholas Royle) or "consensuality" (Naomi Segal), and giving full weight to connections one might previously have glanced over all too rapidly. Peggy Kamuf's essay on the singular effects of the hyphen, often considered a rather precious affectation of contemporary theoretical prose, is exemplary in this regard, and hyphenation might in fact be taken as the "syncategoremical imperative" (p. 323) of sensual reading itself.

Constance Classen in her book *Worlds of Sense* wonders whether we have lost sight of the subtle nuances and the rich critical potential of the senses, and asks why the postmodern world is so odorless and, by association, so flavorless.[1] This collection is proposed as a step towards addressing and redressing, in a sense, a certain contemporary insensibility. That said, *Sensual Reading* readily confesses the limits of its frames of reference, recognizing that sensing is always to some extent culturally specific and semiotically overdetermined. Indeed, can one talk at all about "a" sense of smell, touch, or taste? Walter Ong has recently suggested that a given culture's particular "sensorium" might provide, almost in the form of a collective genetic encoding, the entire range of its social experience.[2] Taking his cue from this notion, Charles Forsdick, in his reading of Victor Segalen's early medico-literary writings, points to what he sees as the "imperialist hegemony" of the Western sensorium, of which the most symptomatic manifestation has been ethnographic accounts of "primitive" modes of perception (p. 230). Likewise, it seems to us equally impertinent to think in terms of a universal hierarchy of the senses, since this might itself be particular to its cultural place and moment, and would need to take into account factors such as class and gender.

This is reflected in the organization of the volume, which tries to shuffle the sections so as to suspend or rethink the traditional ordering of the senses into "higher" faculties (sight and hearing) and "lower" ones (touch, taste, smell), and to challenge the privileging of sight in particular as coextensive with the highest modes of understanding, what Martin Jay refers to as "ocularcentrism,"[3] as Jacqueline Rattray reminds us in her essay. A rethinking of the hierarchy of the senses is often articulated through the figure of the feminine, or a feminist dislocation and teasing apart of the masculinist sensual mastery of the world and experience, with its supposedly genderless human subject. Several contributors explore this dynamic in a number of ways (see Jones, Brewster, Croft, Segal, and Boothroyd). In displacing the oppositions which derive from this traditional conceptual paradigm (subject/object, noumenal/phenomenal, transcendental/material, mind/body, and so on), the division of the senses into higher and lower faculties is also reconfigured. So, for example, Naomi Segal draws on Didier Anzieu's theory of the *moi-peau* (skin ego) to show how, according to him, it is possible to consider all sensual experience as derived from the sense of touch, which is thereby promoted to the "highest" sense, the one sense that organizes the other senses.

And are we even certain about the number of senses, which has historically been a matter of controversy? This of course raises questions of the sixth sense, telepathy, second sight, and all forms of prescient knowledge. What would it mean to think of modes of sensing that escape or confound the usual categories to which the senses are opposed (the spiritual, the noumenal, the rational, the intellectual, and so on)? Indeed, if telepathy is taken not simply as an additional, supplemental sense, but as one that haunts all the senses, it could be said to be hiding somewhere (anasensually) within each sense. It would have both nothing and everything to do with sensing, the "tele-" or remote control without which none of the senses would work. This is the focus of the last section of the book, entitled "Telesensualities", which addresses the question of this distance that necessarily inhabits the supposed immediacy of sense experience, the very (im)possibility of a singular experience one might be able to call "sensual."

Synaesthesia presents itself as the ideal organizing principle of this collection, both despite, as well as because of, its promise of a unified harmony. We know the most common form of synaesthesia to be "colored hearing," and the early eighteenth-century color organs, which were constructed on the assumption of just such a complementarity between the senses, led to a variety of synaesthetic theories and practices by poets and writers in the nineteenth century, most notably Swedenborg, Baudelaire, Rimbaud, and then Huysmans, with his "taste organ" that played melodies of liqueurs. What the various essays do in their own way is to return to the senses, to their senses, but with the benefit of the refined critical and theoretical language of the last twenty years or so. This entails not only looking at the texts of contemporary writers and theorists, which are well represented here, and not only thinking about how advances in technology—cybernetics, virtual reality, digital image manipulation, and so on—have radically challenged the old certainties about the relationship of the senses to the world (see Peter Krapp's essay on Andy Warhol, for example) but also rereading the pertinent texts of the canonical "sensualist" writers—Proust, Baudelaire, and the English Romantic poets, for example—with a renewed critical vigilance. Indeed, it might be argued that it is precisely the incursions of "reading," in the strong theoretical sense of the term, into "sensual experience," that disarticulate the categories to which the senses have traditionally been assigned. The deliberately open nature of the collection will hopefully allow it to function in a way that is properly (that is to say, problematically) synaesthetic, the various contributions echoing each other as do Baudelaire's perfumes, colors, and sounds in his famous poem "Correspondances," an echoing that will now, following Paul de Man, always have to negotiate the unsettling effects of a reading.[4]

Notes

1. Constance Classen, *Worlds of Sense: Exploring the Senses in History and across Cultures* (London: Routledge, 1993).
2. "The Shifting Sensorium," in *The Varieties of Sensory Experience. A Sourcebook in the Anthropology of the Senses*, ed. David Howes (Toronto: University of Toronto Press, 1991), 25–30.
3. Martin Jay, *Downcast Eyes* (Berkeley: University of California Press, 1993), 173.
4. See in particular "Anthropomorphism and Trope in the Lyric," in *The Rhetoric of Romanticism* (New York: Columbia University Press, 1984).

Sensual Reading

I
TOUCH

'L'échange de deux fantaisies et le contact de deux épidermes': Skin and Desire
NAOMI SEGAL

ALLAN SHERMAN MADE US LAUGH WITH FAMILIARITY WHEN HE CONtemplated the skin in jubilant mood in 1965, celebrating its capacity to hold us together ("it helps keep your insides in"), to give us pleasure ("nothing can match it when ya scratch it"), and to distinguish each one of us, however similarly clad in our nakedness, from everybody else ("yours fits you and mine fits me").[1] But was he really right to reassure us that skin is what we feel at home in?

In this article I want to try to explore why the skin may be a source of surprise and pleasure, a jubilation perhaps as much linguistic as sensual. It is surely no chance that discourse follows the complex lines of the body's senses with a kind of emotional tingle. The subject of touch is, I almost think by now, all there is—but it is so without being profound, penetrating (except in a way I will specify later), or deep. The discussion that follows will consist of a number of points which I have tried to collect into some kind of order but whose logic of contiguity is not so much directional as lateral. I will touch on a number of aspects of my subject. I will, of course, be superficial.

When we talk about the sense of touch, we are also talking about its two adjuncts: surface and skin. All these are modes of doubleness, an encounter that is active and passive together, whether what I touch is another body, my own body, or an object. As Sartre's Roquentin discovers one day on a beach, you may take hold of a pebble or it may let itself be taken hold of—not to know which is nausea.[2] The mode of relation of the sense of touch is lateral, extensive, traveling not (or not for long) towards but across or along. Self relates to other by means of contact—a term which is tellingly close to contagion. For after the primary relation of surface to surface by means of caress, feel, or trace, there is the secondary relation—this is as near as we will get to profundity—of an outside to an inside, container to content, being-in to coming-out. Surfaces can hold or fail to hold, be pierced or englobe, strip away or spring back. I shall try to "cover" all these aspects in the short space of this chapter.

The everyday language of the senses tends to reflect a habitual hierarchy of high to low. Touch is, along with taste and smell, one of the three "lower" senses. Grammatically, we can distinguish three main verbal forms associated with the senses which I call the active-focused, the active-unfocused, and the passive. Thus, for the "highest" sense, that of sight, we would say:

I *look at* the picture/*watch* the program (active-focused)
   French *regarder*, German *ansehen*
I *see* the moon, the moon *sees* me (active-unfocused)
   French *voir*, German *sehen*
I *look* tired (passive)
   French *avoir l'air*, German *aussehen*[3]

Similarly, for hearing: I *listen to* the music, *hear* thunder, and *sound* interested. But for the other three senses, the same verb does three different jobs, thus:

I smell a rose, I smell burning, I smell funny
I taste the soup, I taste a trace of cinnamon, it tastes bitter
I feel the velvet, I feel the sun on my face, I feel pretty

The "lower" senses are construed linguistically, then, as less readily differentiated, less accessible to the ordering processes of logic than the higher ones. The language by which we reason is infused with metaphors of seeing and hearing as equivalents of understanding; the lower senses appear to us in less finalized, more primitive but, precisely because of that, much more complex language-units which do more work, convey more variation, carry more weight.

Nietzsche defined objects as "only the boundaries of human beings."[4] Before proceeding to the question of skin and desire, I want to begin by looking at the aesthetics of surface as it appears in the work of three now largely neglected poets for whom the power of language is measured by its ability to approximate the solidity and mass of objects. As either contrast or comparison, these artists hold up to poetry the analogue of sculpture, and to themselves the models of Michelangelo, Rodin, or the Greeks. In a brilliant series of poems known as *Dinggedichte* (thing-poems), Conrad Ferdinand Meyer aspired to the condition of matter by reproducing in rhythmic forms the tracery of light and shadow thrown by a chestnut tree or the delusory solidity of rise-and-fall in a Roman fountain. In "Michelangelo und seine Statuen," he praises Michelangelo for his ability to petrify the movement of human suffering the instant before it falls, so that, in a sense, it never falls, perishes or decomposes.[5] The same coincidence of the massive and the capture of perishability in stone is celebrated by Gautier in poetry which is not only imitative of enamels and cameos, the aesthetics of the miniature (an anticipation of Lévi-Strauss's meditation on the art of the "modèle réduit"),[6] but also the power of mass:

> Tout passe. —L'art robuste
> Seul a l'éternité,
>   Le buste
> Survit à la cité.
>
> Et la médaille austère
> Que trouve un laboureur
>   Sous terre
> Révèle un empereur.
>
> Les dieux eux-mêmes meurent,
> Mais les vers souverains
>   Demeurent
> Plus forts que les airains.
>
> Sculpte, lime, ciselle ;
> Que ton rêve flottant
>   Se scelle
> Dans le bloc résistant !

[Everything passes; only robust art is eternal; the bust outlives the city. The austere medallion, discovered under ground by a workman, reveals an emperor. Even the gods die, but lines of poetry remain triumphant, stronger than bronzes. Sculpt, file, chisel: let your drifting dream be sealed in the resistant block!][7]

The logic is curious here: that poetry is both superior and equal to the qualities of stone. Elsewhere in the same collection, a woman frozen like a statue becomes the figure of the little death turned into necrophiliac fantasy. What these obsessions have in common is a fascination for surface. The desire of the other rests on her skin. When this skin is extremely pale, it produces a shower of analogies to other forms or textures of white: swandown, mother-of-pearl, snow, camelias, satin, marble, frost, ivory, the host, a candle, milk, silver, or lilies. For all that Gautier defined himself as "a man *for whom the visible world ex-*

ists,"[8] the objects of that world are never so far external that they cannot be touched. Surface in Gautier is desirable chiefly because of the promise of ambiguity suspended upon it: thus skin is impossible to tell for sure from silk, petal from cheek, pink from white; in "Contralto" a statue with its back turned to the viewer may be of either a woman or a man, and both sexes come to lust after it:

> Chimère ardente, effort suprême
> De l'art et de la volupté,
> Monstre charmant, comme je t'aime
> Avec ta multiple beauté!
>
> Bien qu'on défende ton approche,
> Sous la draperie aux plis droits
> Dont le bout à ton pied s'accroche,
> Mes yeux ont plongé bien des fois.

[Ardent chimera, supreme effort of art and sensuality, charming monster, how I love you with your multiple beauty! Though it is forbidden to come near you, under the drapery with its straight folds whose end is caught on your foot, how often have my eyes plunged!]

They haven't, though, of course, because they can't. Teasing for exactly this reason, the statue provokes because it can't be penetrated or "found out." It is, after all, in its very massiveness, nothing but an insoluble uninterpretable surface. And here I'd like to add a point about the particular risk associated with the back. For Sartre the most *en-soi* aspect of our body, one's back is what renders us the most vulnerable to the other's gaze. To be seen from behind is to be objectified, to look at a back is to objectify.

Half a century after Gautier, Rilke, himself the author of some extraordinary *Dinggedichte*, wrote two essays on Rodin. The parallel with Meyer's Michelangelo is implicit; Rodin too creates "things" which freeze gesture into solid precipitates. But here the importance of surface as the place where movement stops still is overt: "Es gibt nur eine einzige, tausendfältig bewegte und abgewandelte Oberfläche . . . Und schließlich war es diese Oberfläche, auf die seine Forschung sich wandte. Sie bestand aus unendlich viele Begegnungen des Lichtes mit dem Dinge" [There is nothing but a single, infinitely mobile and metamorphosing surface . . . and finally it was upon this surface that he concentrated his researches. It consisted of endless encounters between light and things.]⁹ Out of "die Unruhe lebendiger Flächen" [the restlessness of living surfaces] (320)—for the body consists of "lauter Schauplätzen des Lebens" [so many scenes on which life is staged] (328)—Rodin selects gesture (*Gebärde*) and around this gesture concentrates space:

> Er konnte mit einer lebendigen Fläche, wie mit einem Spiegel, die Fernen fangen und bewegen, und er konnte eine Gebärde, die ihm groß schien, formen und den Raum zwingen, daran teilzunehmen... Alle Bewegung legt sich, wird Kontur.
> [With a living surface, as if with a mirror, he could catch and move distances, and he could give form to a gesture that seemed to him great and then force space to take its part (364).... Every movement lies down, becomes contour.] (376–77)

Contour (*das Modelé*) gathers together light, air, and space on a purposeful surface which may be massive like the "Balzac," complex like the "Gates of Hell," or both at once, in erotic mode, in "The Kiss," where Rilke notes that

> man hat das Gefühl, als gingen hier von allen Berührungsflächen Wellen in die Körper hinein, Schauer von Schönheit, Ahnung und Kraft. Daher kommt es, daß man die Seligkeit des Kusses überall auf diesen Leibern zu schauen glaubt; er ist wie eine Sonne, die aufgeht, und sein Licht liegt überall.
> [it feels as though all the surfaces being touched here were sending waves into the bodies, shivers of beauty, portent and strength. That's why one seems to be able to see the bliss of that kiss everywhere on these bodies; it [the kiss] is like a sun that rises, and its light lies everywhere.] (329)

In these three poets, then, surface is where art resides, and even if the matter of the art-object is verbal rather than material, its charge is erotic, deriving from a concept of form as a kind of solidity modeled on the human body.

In Robert Mapplethorpe's "Derrick Cross" (1983), the image of a man photographed from behind as a rounded massy monolith has the power (again, something between the immediately erotic and the mediate mode of the aesthetic) of the visual ambiguities of marble and flesh, surface and mass, smooth closure against the always potentially open cleft of the backside. It is pornographic of course despite its extreme dignity because it incites us to want to break the decorum of the two-dimensional image, to go and touch, knowing as we do that this is the back of a real man whom we cannot have. If we are female and heterosexual observers, we can all the more not have him because the aesthetics of ambiguity are multiplied into desire by a complex intervention—our implicitly excluded voyeurism tacked onto the arrogance of a white man representing the body of a black man as sublime object. I will return later to this image of desire and racial difference to discuss its particular version of the relation between light and skin.

What is, I think, most remarkable about all these aesthetic readings of surface is how they avoid the philosophical norm of allowing surface its rights only in contradistinction to depth. They not only avoid the traditional relation by which surface is the inferior counterpart of depth, but also the somewhat more subtle one in which depth is its physical origin or formation. Their versions of surface as "all there is" avoid that more hazardous or even tragic reading wherein surface gets its shape by being "pushed out" (being the "expression") of something interior. Here are some examples of the latter from the notebooks of Hugo von Hofmannsthal:

> Die Tiefe muß man verstecken. Wo? An der Oberfläche.
> [The depth must be hidden. Where? On the surface]
> Es ist nichts im Innern wesentlich, das nicht zugleich im Äußern wahrgenommen wird.
> [Nothing exists in the inside which is not simultaneously perceptible on the outside]

or, in conclusion,

> Kein Stück der Oberfläche einer Figur kann geschaffen werden, außer vom innersten Kern aus.
> [No piece of the surface of a figure can be created otherwise than from the innermost kernel outwards.][10]

The fantasmatic corollary of this principle of outside/inside is an image of the surface coming away from the inner depth which has formed it and which thus continues to haunt it, pressing to "emerge." In a positive light, Proust's adolescent protagonist—who just a few pages before has evoked the impulse to describe the beauty of a field of buttercups as a substitute for eating them—represents the wish to understand what attracts him in the sight of three steeples in terms of entering or "going behind it." Suddenly, he exclaims, "leurs lignes et leurs surfaces ensoleillées, comme si elles avaient été une sorte d'écorce, se déchirèrent, un peu de ce qui était caché en elles m'apparut" [their outlines and sunlit surfaces split open like a sort of peel, and a little of what was hidden in them appeared to me]. It does not, of course; instead he writes a page of metaphors, rendering the penetration fantasy redundant to the point of reversal so that he ends up crowing with satisfaction "comme si j'avais été moi-même une poule et si je venais de pondre un œuf" [as if I were a hen that had just laid an egg].[11] In a negative light, here is Rilke's protagonist-narrator Malte Laurids Brigge, who has just marveled at how many faces people have and how they seem to recycle them, observing a woman with her face buried in her hands:

> Aber die Frau, die Frau: sie war ganz in sich hineingefallen, vornüber in ihre Hände. Es war an der Ecke rue Notre-Dame-des-Champs. Ich fing an, leise zu gehen, sowie ich sie gesehen hatte. Wenn arme Leute nachdenken, soll man sie nicht stören. Vielleicht fällt es ihnen doch ein.
>
> Die Straße war zu leer, ihre Leere langweilte sich und zog mir den Schritt unter den Füßen weg und klappte mit ihm herum, drüben und da, wie mit einem Holzschuh. Die Frau erschrak und hob sich aus sich ab, zu schnell, zu heftig, so daß das Gesicht in den zwei Händen blieb. Ich konnte es darin liegen sehen, seine hohle Form. Es kostete mich unbeschriebliche Anstrengung, bei diesen Händen zu bleiben und nicht zu schauen, was sich aus ihnen abgerissen hatte. Mir graute, ein Gesicht von innen zu sehen, aber ich fürchtete mich doch noch viel mehr von dem bloßen wunden Kopf ohne Gesicht.
>
> [But that woman, that woman: she had completely sunk into herself, right down into her hands. It was on the corner of the rue Notre-Dame-des-Champs. I began to walk softly as soon as I saw her. When poor people are thinking something over, you should not disturb them. It might still occur to them.
>
> The street was too empty, its emptiness was getting bored and tripped up my step from under my feet, kicking it around like a wooden clog. The woman took fright, and came up out of herself, too quickly, too violently, so that the face remained in the two hands. I could see it lying there, its hollow shape. It took an indescribable effort to keep my eyes on those hands and not to look to see what had been torn out of them. I shuddered to see a face from the inside, but I was more, much more afraid of that naked, raw head without a face.][12]

A contemporary artist who has reified this horror and served it up to her audience as an inversion of cosmetic narcissism is Orlan. In her video *Omniprésence IV*, she displays herself having plastic surgery done to her face. Here is how this process is described by Parveen Adams:

> Orlan's work undoes the triumph of representation. During her operation Orlan's face begins to detach itself from her head. We are shocked at the destruction of our normal narcissistic fantasy that the face "represents" something. Gradually the "face" becomes pure exteriority. It no longer projects the illusion of depth. It becomes a mask without any relation of representation. In turn this disturbs a fundamental illusion concerning the inside and the outside, that the outside provides a window onto what is represented. In one sense Orlan uses her head quite literally to demonstrate an axiom of at least one strand of feminist thought: that there is nothing behind the mask.[13]

Or as Paul Valéry observed, "The most profound thing in man is his skin."[14]

The removal of the surface—especially the surface of the head—is generally horrific. Images of scalping or flaying are the stuff of fantasy and nightmare, or of a Foucauldian world of suffering on display. As against these images, the removal of clothes should be the safe, benign, even comical version of the exposure of the inside, the offer of pleasure in the nakedness under the wraps. But our current fascination for the cross-dressed body suggests rather, I think, how far gone we are in favoring the surface over the depth, or rather, in having lost the confidence that stripping off a surface can reveal a truth. Such hero/heroines of Marjorie Garber's *Vested Interests* as Billie Tipton or the Chevalier d'Éon prove (like Gautier's unforgettable and inexhaustible Madeleine de Maupin) that you cannot find out sex by peeling off the vestments of gender.[15] In this, they are showing us the wisdom of the two children in the anecdote who are looking through a hole in the fence of a nudist camp. When one asks the other, "Which are the men and which are the ladies?" the first child replies, "You can't tell, they haven't got any clothes on."

Identity is not nudity, then, but one kind of surface, in costume no less nor more than in skin. This is aptly illustrated by the work of fine art student Joyce Harrison, in a series of photos of the finger-joints of herself and her parents, a series which also includes a family tree spun out of hair-extensions. The only black student among her classmates, she resisted her white tutors' suggestions that she might do a project on the visibility of identity. She was persuaded by an established black woman artist to try it, and when she did she also found that an attack of eczema which had troubled her since the start of her studies began to disappear.

Her close-up image of fingers, as solid on the vertical as massed tree trunks, is cross-cut by horizontal traces of white light. The image seems to me to exemplify identity as a thing-declared in contrast to the interpellation of skin as a thing-seen whether by prejudice or desire. We don't, I am sure, need to be reminded how grossly prejudice can eroticize the surface of the body of the other.

The next several examples of the expression of interrace desire were taken from three writers, all gay men, in whom the attraction of difference is expressed via the image of light on a dark surface.[16] My earliest example is from André Gide, writing in 1919:

> Il est des êtres qui s'éprennent de ce qui leur ressemble; d'autres de ce qui diffère d'eux. Je suis de ces derniers : l'étrange me sollicite, autant que me rebute le coutumier. Disons encore et plus précisément que je suis attiré par ce qui reste du soleil sur des peaux brunes.
> [Some people fall for what resembles themselves; others for what is different from them. I am one of the latter: I am drawn to what is strange, just as I am repelled by the familiar. Let us say also, and more exactly, that I am attracted by what remains of sun on brown skins.][17]

Similar images recur in James Baldwin's *Giovanni's Room* (published thirty years after the Gide text, in 1956), representing the half-admitted desire of an American for an Italian: "as he was that night, so vivid, so winning, all of the light of that gloomy tunnel trapped around his head"; or "his black hair gathering to itself the yellow glow of the wine"; or again, "Giovanni's face swings before me like an unexpected lantern on a dark, dark night."[18] And here finally is Cyril Collard in a text of 1989, using similar imagery for something more violent, exemplified in the pun of the epithet "fauve" [wild/tawny]: "Samy et ceux de sa race rayonnaient" [Samy and those of his race glowed]; "un corps simple, solaire et métissé, tendu de violences contenues" [the simple, radiant body of a half-caste boy, tense with suppressed violence]; and finally: "Il reste des taches fauves sur la mémoire en noir et blanc des corps confondus; la couleur solaire de Samy et de ses semblables que n'éteint pas l'obscurité" [Traces of that tawny colour remain on the black-and-white memory of tangled bodies: the radiant colour of Samy and his kind which the darkness cannot obscure].[19] In all these images, the effect of light seen or touched on skin becomes something not on the scale of black to white but something rather on a spectrum of cold to heat. Obviously one aspect of the image—especially in Gide or Collard—is an orientalism which associates the sun with the immediate availability of a cheap pleasure in a hot climate. But I wonder whether also this insistent image of warmth on skin might suggest a possible step forward from Fanon's castratory image of the black skin under the white mask, the black male body fetishized/feminized as the phallus exposed and destroyed, towards a recent idyllic suggestion by David Halperin that "gay desire points the way to the possibility of defetishizing difference without denying it."[20] If that were so, perhaps it would be—and I will return to this—through a nonphallic erotics of the skin.

Let me return now to the Mapplethorpe image, which is reproduced in an article by Kobena Mercer first published in 1986 and reprinted with a postscript in 1989. Commenting in 1986, Mercer makes this observation on the effect of light in the Mapplethorpe image:

> As each fragment seduces the eye into ever more intense fascination, we glimpse the dilation of a libidinal way of looking that spreads itself across the surface of black skin [. . .] There is a subtle slippage between representer and represented, as the shiny, polished sheen of black skin becomes consubstantial with the luxurious allure of the high-quality photographic print. [. . .] Here, black skin and print surface are bound together to enhance the pleasure of the white spectator as much as the profitablity of these art-world commodities exchanged among the artist and his dealers, collectors and curators.[21]

Three years later, Mercer revised this critique, seeing Mapplethorpe's transgressive and embattled gayness as a counterweight to his hegemonic whiteness. Both readings may be persuasive, and it is not my place or intention to intervene in the debate. What I want to add is something that struck me on looking closely at the reprint of the photograph on the page. The glow of this image comes not from a high-contrast black against white but from a relation among greys. The marble effect of body as sculpture here seems to control the reflection of light back to the looker in a manner that is distinct from both the sheeny effect Mercer likens to glossy photography or the kinkiness of black leather or the tracery of Joyce Harrison's image of white horizontal across a black vertical. It is perhaps for this reason that warmth, rather than light, seems the more appropriate term to describe its beauty.

In my final section I suggest how we might begin to theorize the erotics of the skin. It surely is time now to try to offer a new theory of desire, or rather a theory of love—that is, a theory that attempts to explain what Chamfort called in 1796 the "contact of two epidermises" as something which not only differs from Diderot's earlier and grosser penetrative correlative "the pleasurable rubbing of two intestines"[22] by valorizing surface over depth but also distinguishes itself from "the exchange of two fantasies"—that is, from the function of the unconscious by which, however, it will always come accompanied.

Why love, rather than desire? It seems to me probable that the familiar definition of desire as that impulse which depends on and feeds off lack can't really be superseded. For many euphemistic centuries, no doubt, this did service also as a definition of love. But as sexual and other forms of desire come to be theorized on a basis of the unconscious, what is left still unexplained is what happens to gratified desire, or how it is gratified. If desire is the motion towards, and if it can occasionally reach its goal, what happens when it spreads upon a surface? "Contact" is the key term. How do two skins touch?

It is common enough to find theories of erotic touch which emphasise relations of power. Elizabeth Grosz proposes "a model which insists on (at least) two surfaces that cannot be collapsed into one and that do not always harmoniously blend with and support each other; a model where the join, the interaction of the two surfaces is always a question of power."[23] She is right, of course, as our examination of the racialized image of sun on skin has made clear. Sartre's pessimistic representation of fleshly contact as the vegetal operation of caress as *en-soi* gives way at the end of *L'Etre et le néant* to a theory of appropriation by which I (*I* gendered masculine of course) take possession of matter by skiing or skimming across it.[24] Levinas similarly masculinizes the caress as a kind of blind exploration: "like a game with something slipping away, a game absolutely without project or plan [. . .] [which] feeds on countless hungers."[25] Alphonso Lingis connects even the gentlest physical contact with pain: "we make contact or establish community with the other in the touch that caresses his or her carnal surfaces and that is afflicted with, obsessed by, their vulnerability, susceptibility, mortality."[26] The more violent manifestations of power on skin—scarification, inscription, the scarlet letter, the penal colony—are familiar enough.

But an important development in psychoanalysis offers a different possibility. In the late 1960s/early 1970s, with articles by Esther Bick in Britain and by Didier Anzieu in France, the theory of the skin ego began to be developed. It is most fully argued in Anzieu's *Le Moi-peau*.[27] This theory takes us back to the principle I started with, drawn from linguistic and aesthetic sources—that skin/surface is always multiple and complex, synthesizing elements of active and passive, and that thus it is, in a sense, "all there is," an outside without an inside to which it must defer—viewed optimistically, it is what Allan Sherman calls "what you feel at home in [. . .] yours fits you and mine fits me!"

Like all good psychoanalytic children, Anzieu leans his theory on a number of hints by Freud, most fully developed in the later publications, *Beyond the Pleasure Principle* (1920) and *The Ego and the Id* (1923) and, especially, on an unassuming little essay of 1924 called "A note upon the mystic writing-pad." We all know those pads, still on sale at all good toyshops: they consist of a surface on which you mark lines with a pointed tool and from which, when you lift it, all trace seems to disappear—but in fact it is retained, less visibly, because the surface is in reality two surfaces of which "the upper layer is a transparent piece of celluloid; the lower layer is made of thin translucent waxed paper"; similarly, "the perceptual apparatus of our mind consists of two layers, of an external protective shield against stimuli whose task it is to diminish the strength of excitations coming in, and of a surface behind it which receives the stimuli, namely the system *Pcpt.-Cs.*"[28]

This double epiderm becomes in Anzieu's theory the *moi-peau*, or skin ego. Just as the layer on the outside controls stimulation (Freud's *Reizschutz*, Anzieu's *pare-excitation*) beneath this, as it were, and turned towards stimuli from within the subject, is "the inner layer, thinner, more flexible and sensitive, which acts as a receptor" (258). Skin is a "filmy layer with a dual face [. . .] one turned towards the outside world, the other towards the inner world: an interface, thus, which both separates and links these two worlds [. . .] the envelope of excitation and the envelope of communication and signification" (258). This double function connects sensation to thought: it is with our skin, rather than our phallus—that is, with a faculty of connection and extension rather than binary exclusivity—that we will eventually learn to think.

Anzieu finds in embryology the first cause of this double layer: every vegetable or animal skin has the dual structure of inner and outer layer, and "this ectoderm forms both the skin (including the sense-organs) and the brain" (31)—both skin and brain being alike "surface entities" (31). It is in this sense that all the other senses (lodged in the surface structures of the head) derive from and are posterior to, dependent on—if you like, "higher than"—the sense of touch.

"At birth the skin ego is a virtual structure" (125): through infancy, it is built up as a concept we will ideally take for granted. Anzieu is no better than most at rising above the routine of mother-blaming, but he has at least a new way of theorizing what happens when you pick up your crying child or tend to its grazed knee. You are restoring piecemeal or working to rebuild that fantasy of safe enclosure that is its skin ego. The mother or her substitute can do this because she is repairing an originary enclosure or envelope which is the child's infantile belief in/desire for a "shared skin" with her (62 *passim*).

And so do lovers. Lovers also create simultaneously for themselves and for each other an environment of holding and being held. Just as the young child derives confidence from being held against the strong spine of an adult or leaning its own back against the front of another body, so bodies making love increase contact by movement or rest alongside each other in sleep to recover—often through the back, precisely—that first conviction of the shared skin.

As the child develops, the other senses, in addition to awareness of such sensations as heat/cold, fullness/emptiness, grow out of the establishment of the skin ego or tactile covering and its cognates, the "envelopes of sight, sound, smell and taste" (183 *passim*), and so on. Failure to establish or conserve the skin ego may be evidenced in the sense of having a head like a sieve, or by the effort to feel or fill the skin from the inside or outside by asthma, eczema, or eating disorders, in marking oneself by masochism or protecting oneself by a "muscular armour" (126, 220). The psychoanalyst must work by gradually building or rebuilding the sense of a complete skin, recreating the maternal "bath of words" (191ff) which in childhood may have been sporadic or excessive—in the hands of a depressive or angry mother—by a regularity in time and space that is also underlaid by the absolute establishment of the "prohibition against touching" (161ff) which, Anzieu convincingly argues, universally precedes and makes possible the oedipal proscription.

Lovers transgress the law against touching and so take risks with themselves and the beloved. They both retrace the establishment of the skin ego and create a new one. Let me repeat again that I am not denying the importance of desire—nor indeed of penetration: one of the most remarkable (and almost tangentially presented) moments in this theory is the way that penetration is understood, logically enough, not as an act of breaking in or through the surface but of establishing contact between more surfaces—specifically those liminal spaces (vagina, anus, lips) which are "without a hardened layer or protective cornea acting as the shield against stimuli and with its mucous membrane exposed, so that the sensitivity and erogeneity are on the surface of the skin" (32). Similarly the moment of orgasm which, in Freud's economic/hydraulic theory, gives satisfaction because it marks the end of unsatisfaction, the restoration of an equilibrium of minimum tension, can be understood in terms of the skin ego as the moment when you fall, drop, lose, yield and are nevertheless held.

The key term I'd like to offer here is "consensuality." Anzieu uses the French *consensualité* repeatedly, meaning by it a conjunction or connection between the senses which in aesthetics would be termed synaesthesia. But (and more familiarly in English) it also signifies an exchange of mutual consents. Both kinds of consensuality together might be as good a definition of love as any other.

I want to end with a reading of Jane Campion's film *The Piano* (1991, 1993). Though I saw the film and first formulated the argument that follows before I discovered the theory of the *moi-peau*, it seems to me to begin the interpretation which that theory has helped me complete. I wanted to understand what gives that fiction its intense erotic effect—not for everyone, by any means, and not always straightforwardly along gender-divided lines—but a strangely compulsive effect which seems to be saying something about women's desire/pleasure that few other fictions have said. My reading arises out of a comparison between its triangular structure of adultery and that of *Fatal Attraction* (dir. Adrian Lyne, 1987).

Fatal Attraction is a masculine nightmare, a warning for husbands in the age of AIDS (this was the general tenor of the contemporary tabloid publicity) because it both exploits and inverts the familiar version of the adulterous triangle. An outsider threatens an established dyad; but because that outsider is a woman she threatens it uncannily. In this traditionally penetrative fantasy of sexual irruption, the subject of forced entry is female and familial: she enters more insistently because she is an already containing unit, herself both penetrated by and penetrative of the man's psychological space.

In *The Piano*, it is also a question of the entry into a person's protected space and of colonization. Desire is triangulated and cooptative but differently so. The key differences are temporal and spatial, using the inevitability, the motion-towards of desire in a way that replaces sadism with curiosity, and showing how bodies can reach each other in a mode that somehow resembles the playing of a piano.

The adulterous triangle in this film consists of a woman and two men, the most common pattern in traditional representations of adultery which, with their oedipal freight, tend to show an already assigned woman sought by a younger man. But here the married woman stands at the apex of the triangle, consistently focalized, alongside neither of the men. And, somewhat like Lyne's Alex Forrest and very much like Hawthorne's Hester Prynne, she starts out doubled by an illegitimate daughter whose existence declares her sexuality and represents one mode of access between her and the world. It is the multiplicity and substitutability of these modes of access that I want to examine.

Ada's muteness is not explained and is presented in the first frames as a state that she both has chosen and is powerless to reverse.[29] "Not a handicap but a strategy," a multiplication and dissemination of the possible resources of communication,[30] her silence marks out very clearly the way in which an originating choice (or "will," as the characters describe it) both frees up and restricts the actions that follow. This film, like the other, multiplies and fetishizes the channels between subject and object; but it reverses the triangulation which sees the "third" element as invasive, and presents it instead as a putting out, a means towards the other. Where the daughter of Beth, the wife in *Fatal Attraction*, was a possession that could be stolen from her, Ada's daughter is an extension of herself that is broken from her. It is not surprising that when Beth is hurt it is by a shattering of the whole body, and when Ada is hurt it is by the cutting off of one of her fingers, the spoiling of a complete set, what her mutilator calls "clipping her wings."

There are many objects and modes of mediation, some more

subtle than others. Bonnets resemble scallop-shells "designed to concentrate acoustic information,"[31] crinolines become tents, skirts leading-reins, shirts dusters, the wooden slats of a packing-case or a rough-hewn cottage let sound out or voyeurism in. The main fetish-object is, of course, the piano: both desired thing and part of self, it is bulky, inert, biddable, and sensual; its cumbersomeness and beauty make it the possession no one can hold with certainty, like their own body.[32] It ends the film imagined undead beneath the sea and still, even after Ada's graphic birth out of the amniotic bubble, keeping one version of her body suspended umbilically above it. In the opening moments of the film, there is a shaft of red, a color only rarely seen,[33] and through it (like the light seen through fingers, behind which a child might hide its face, thinking that makes it invisible) a piping voice identifies itself as Ada's "mind's voice" and announces that she stopped speaking when she was six. This, we will discover, is just after or just before she began to play the piano. Thus the instrument allows the child's preservation as voice inside her body and its voluntary-involuntary expression, a model of psychoanalytical *Aufhebung*.

We are tempted perhaps to think it is her daughter Flora's voice. Unlike the Maoris, whose difference is marked fairly carefully in superiority and mimicry,[34] her doubling of her mother is both functional and reciprocal. It is a double Venus that is brought forth and landed on the beach, and the adequation and exploitation of the child as substitute for speech is shown when she pronounces Ada's aggressive message to the sailor and only escapes his fist by hiding in her mother's skirts. She has the rights of monogamous enjoyment of her mother: like Ellen, the daughter in *Fatal Attraction* she is there in the bed when the husband visits at the end of the day and it is her he offers to kiss rather than the woman.

The child and the piano are alternative communicators of the woman's physical desire. For Stewart, both Ada and her piano are his to buy and sell; Baines at once recognizes its mediatory function. He first takes her to it, standing as audience to the complete unit of mother/child/instrument on the beach; then he uses it to bring her to him, listening silently as she reappropriates it by playing. From this point, the child as mediator becomes redundant to the newly formed unit of woman, piano, and man. It is of course essential that Baines cannot read, so that the instrument is at first the only means between them. Gradually, through the simultaneously comic, threatening, and reassuring eroticism of Baines's clumsy "bargain," the woman's body reenters the communicative circuit, replacing both piano and child.

I will return to the development of dyadic communication in a moment. First, there is more to say about the human mediators. Flora, cast off as she becomes the object rather than the interpreter of her mother's will and coopted by the patriarchal symbolic society of the Scottish colonizers, makes an expected move from the mother/daughter cell into the fostering oedipal. Continuing to wear her angel costume—the Hebrew for "angel" translates as "messenger"—she will act as transmitter of judgment and carrier of keys. But before the story is over, she will undergo a second transfer, from Ada's bed to Baines's, and she will end up turning healthy cartwheels in another triangular family, the least traditional of all.

Stewart plays his assigned role as disruptor of adulterous love, but he too is also used as something peculiarly connective. In the interlude of her imprisonment, Ada plays only in her sleep, and when she makes an unexpected move towards her husband, seems to "play" on his body in a similarly somnambulist way. What makes this moment so affecting is that it remains in excess of what it proposes. Ada's erotic approach is not simply the redirection of a sexual appetite that Baines has aroused and Flora cannot satisfy. Two scenes represent her night visits: in the first, the screenplay describes her motive as "a separate curiosity of her own"; in the second, she is "moved by his helplessness, but distanced, as if it has nothing to do with her."[35] With a detachment hanging somewhere between compassion and cruelty, Ada touches but will not let herself be touched. But what unmans and maddens the husband most is how she touches him: with the back of her hand upon the back of his body. This special mode of caress is reserved elsewhere only for the sea, the child, and the piano.

In many languages other than English, the word used for the keys of a piano is associated with the faculty of touch (French *touches*, Italian *tasti*, German *Tasten*) and connected with a verb of blind or quasi-blind feeling, groping (*toucher/tâtonner, tastare, tasten*). In describing Ada's silence as strategy rather than disability, Campion is both right and wrong: she has extended the reach of her senses, transferring voice into an extra modality of touch. Stewart is unmanned by this; Baines understands and reciprocates. It is this which makes the sexuality of this film unusual.

George Baines's mediation between cultures is etched on his

brow. The tattoo does not simply make him a cross between Tarzan and Mellors; it is also the sign of his bilingualism, the ability, like Ada's, to transfer himself and his desire from one mode to another. She cannot speak, he cannot read; she plays, he listens; he touches, she touches. Like Stewart, Baines talks stiltedly—here, Harvey Keitel's struggle with the accent was useful—and, like him also, he struggles to hear Ada speaking, but whereas the former intuits her wishes "in his head," Baines helps her to move her voice out onto the surface of her skin.

Colonization comes from and operates by the structures of capitalism: grading, marking, and counting out. Analogous to piano keys and fingers, numbered territorial stakes measure out the landscape and buttons are supposed to pay for it. These are Stewart's coinage. Baines and Ada begin with black and white keys, black overclothes and white underclothes; but at a certain moment, the bargaining stops and with it the grading of access which is undoubtedly one mode of the erotic, creating an appetite in both the heroine and the audience. Baines is after all, like the husband, a colonial exploiter, but less absolutely, not so much an owner as a mediator and interpreter. Implicated nonetheless, he buys the piano and expects to buy Ada; but let us not forget that Ada is as hard a bargainer as he is and it is he who stops the negotiations first.

Erotic violence is not always chaotically invasive: Sade, quite the reverse, creates an atmosphere of graded cruelty by his obsessive enumeration, space within space, sectioning off of days, cells, or tortures. It is no chance that Stewart cuts off just one finger: he can then grade the threat on into the future, "another and another and another." Thus the gentle striptease of the unerect Baines is also potentially coercive, but he stops when he has reached her skin. What follows is the transformation of the temporal erotic onto a multiplied surface which is the whole extent of the person (inside and out, we may understand) now accessible without destruction.

In *The Piano*, then, adulterous triangularity is reinterpreted: not as the other who invades or irrupts into an enclosed thing that can be punctured or shattered, but instead as the condition of the complex movements of desire through its own involuntarinesses into diverse forms which meet other forms at the tips of the fingers. Both these cinematic fictions are post-AIDS: *Fatal Attraction* is indeed about the perils of penetration, of man by woman and woman by man, of hallowed spaces by their own fracturability and violence, and of frames by the seduction of a false imaginary. *The Piano* is about the extensability of desire upon a surface that is its own mediation.

NOTES

Unless otherwise stated, all translations from French and German are my own, and reference is given to the original text.

"The exchange of two fantasies and the contact of two epidermises," Sébastien-Roch Nicolas Chamfort, *Maximes et pensées* (Neuchâtel: Paul Attinger, [1796], 1946), 89.

1. Allan Sherman, "Skin," from the LP *The Best of Allan Sherman*, Valiant Records, 1965.

2. Jean-Paul Sartre, *La Nausée* (Paris: Gallimard, 1938), 10, 13.

3. It is interesting to note that German uses differentiating prefixes while French and English have distinct verbs for the three modes of sight; also that the French verb *sentir* does duty for both the senses of smell and touch, as well as the emotion of feeling, which as in English and German (*fühlen*) carries the burden of our sentimental as well as our sensorial life.

4. From no. 48 in Friedrich Nietzsche, "Morgenröthe," *Werke*, sec. 5, vol. 1 (Berlin and New York: Walter de Gruyter, [1887], 1971), 49.

5. Conrad Ferdinand Meyer, "Schwarzschattende Kastanie," "Der römische Brunnen," "Michelangelo und seine Statuen", in *Werke in 2. Bänden, Erster Band: Gedichte* (Berlin and Weimar: Aufbau-Verlag, 1970), 7, 34, 65.

6. Claude Lévi-Strauss, *La Pensée sauvage* (Paris: Plon, 1962), 33–37.

7. Théophile Gautier, "L'art," in *Émaux et camées* (Lille and Geneva: Droz, [1857], 1947), 131–32.

8. Quoted by Edmond and Jules Goncourt in the entry for 1 May 1857 in their *Journal: Mémoires de la vie littéraire 1851–1863*, vol. 1 (Paris: Fasquelle et Flammarion, 1956), 343, their italics. The poems referred to in this and the next paragraph are "Le poème de la femme," "Coquetterie posthume," "Symphonie en blanc majeur," "A une Robe rose," "Étude de mains," "La Rose-thé."

9. Rainer Maria Rilke, *Gesammelte Werke*, vol. 4 (Leipzig: Insel, 1930), 383, 309. Further references will be given in the text.

10. Hugo von Hofmannsthal, *Gesammelte Werk: Aufzeichnungen* (Frankfurt: Fischer, 1959), 47, 40, 70.

11. Marcel Proust, *A la recherche du temps perdu*, vol. 1 (Paris: Gallimard, 1954), 182.

12. Rainer Maria Rilke, *Die Aufzeichnungen des Malte Laurids Brigge* (Eschwege: Suhrkamp, [1910], 1975), 10.

13. Parveen Adams, *The Emptiness of the Image* (New York and London: Routledge, 1996), 145.

14. Paul Valéry, "L'idée fixe," in *Œuvres complètes* (Paris: Gallimard, 1960), 215.

15. Marjorie Garber, *Vested Interests* (New York: Routledge, 1992).

16. For a fuller exploration of how gay desire is made descriptive in modern French writing, see Christopher Robinson, *Scandal in the Ink* (London: Cassell, 1995), chap. 9.

17. André Gide, *Si le grain ne meurt* [1926], in *Journal 1938–1949; Souvenirs* (Paris: Gallimard, 1954), 565.

18. James Baldwin, *Giovanni's Room* (Harmondsworth: Penguin [1956], 1990), 45, 61, 157.
19. Cyril Collard, *Les Nuits fauves* (Paris: Flammarion, 1989), 35, 39, 98.
20. David Halperin, review of Leo Bersani, *Homos*, in *London Review of Books*, 23 May 1996, 25.
21. Kobena Mercer, *Welcome to the Jungle* (New York and London: Routledge, 1994), 183–84.
22. Denis Diderot, *Supplément au voyage de Bougainville* [1772], in *Œuvres* (Paris: Gallimard, 1951), 998.
23. Elizabeth Grosz, *Volatile Bodies* (Bloomington and Indianapolis: Indiana University Press, 1994), 189.
24. Jean-Paul Sartre, *L'Être et le néant* (Paris: Gallimard, 1948), 466, 672–73.
25. Emmanuel Levinas, *Le Temps et l'autre* (Paris: Presses universitaires de France, 1983), 82–83. I am grateful to Seán Hand for this translation.
26. Alphonso Lingis, *Foreign Bodies* (New York and London: Routledge, 1994), 185.
27. Didier Anzieu, *Le Moi-peau* (Paris: Dunod, [1985], 1995). References to Anzieu will be given in the text.
28. Sigmund Freud, "A note upon the mystic writing-pad" [Notiz über den Wunderblock] in *The Standard Edition of the Complete Psychological Works of Sigmund Freud*, vol. 19, ed. and trans. James Strachey (London: Hogarth and the Institute of Psycho-analysis, 1961), 229, 230.
29. Kate Pullinger, who wrote the book of the film (abandoned by Jane Campion after a couple of chapters), explains that "Ada is mute because at six, when she contradicted the adults, she was ordered not to speak again that day and she decided to stay silent for ever" (Marianne Brace, *The Guardian*, (18 April 1994): 11). Whatever the originating event—and why should it not be the smallest of traumas?—the result is necessarily something other than its occasion.
30. See Campion's interview with Ian Pryor, *Onfilm* 10, (9 October 1993): 25; also Valerie Hazel, "Disjointed articulations: The Politics of Voice and Jane Campion's *The Piano*," paper presented at the Centre for Women's Studies, Monash University in March 1994.
31. Adam Mars-Jones, "Poetry in Motion," in *The Independent*, (29 October 1993): 26.
32. Campion, who cites one of her motives as the wish "to explore the relationship between fetishism and love" (Katherine Dieckmann, *Interview* 27 (1 January 1992): 82), stresses the characteristics of the piano as inert object, and a number of critics note the analogy with the ship of *Fitzcarraldo*. But it is interesting to remember that her original title referred not to the object but to *The Piano Lesson*, which has been followed exactly in the French version, while the Italian pluralizes it into *Lezioni di Piano*.
33. For example, here, in the patterned curtain behind which Baines waits naked, in Flora's Red Riding Hood cloak and in the blood which splashes on her white apron.
34. Campion has claimed that the original interest in making a film set early in New Zealand colonial history arose from her fascination with the "European cross-dressing" of Maoris in the mid nineteenth century (see Geoff Andrew, "Grand entrance," *Time Out* [20–27 October 1993]: 24). More generally, she contrasts her "strange heritage as a pakeha New Zealander" with the Maori

sense of history (Campion, *The Piano* screenplay [London: Bloomsbury, 1993], 135). She has since been accused of Orientalism and her portrayal of the Maoris in the film as too simplistically based on a noble savage/repressed Britishers contrast. See for example the debate between Richard Cummings and Stella Bruzzi in the letter pages of *Sight & Sound* (February 1994): 72, and (March 1994): 64.

35. *The Piano* screenplay, 90, 93.

WORKS CITED

Adams, Parveen. *The Emptiness of the Image*. New York and London: Routledge, 1996.

Andrew, Geoff. "Grand entrance," *Time Out* (20–27 October 1993): 24.

Anzieu, Didier. *Le Moi-peau*. Paris: Dunod [1985], 1995.

Baldwin, James. *Giovani's Room*. Harmondsworth: Penguin [1956], 1990.

Brace, Marianne. *The Guardian* (18 April 1994).

Campion, Jane. *The Piano* screenplay. London: Bloomsbury, 1993.

Chamfort, Sébastien-Roch Nicolas. *Maximes et pensées*. Neuchâtel: Paul Attinger [1796], 1946.

Collard, Cyril. *Les Nuits fauves*. Paris: Flammarion, 1989.

Diderot, Denis. *Œuvres*. Paris: Gallimard, 1951.

Dieckmann, Katherine. *Interview* 27 (1 January 1992): 82.

Freud, Sigmund. *The Standard Edition of the Complete Psychological Works of Sigmund Freud*, vol. 19. Edited and translated by James Strachey. London: Hogarth and the Institute of Psycho-analysis, 1961.

Garber, Marjorie. *Vested Interests*. New York: Routledge, 1992.

Gautier, Théophile. *Émaux et camées*. Lille and Geneva: Droz [1857], 1947.

Gide, André. *Journal 1938–1949; Souvenirs*. Paris: Gallimard, 1954.

Goncourt, Edmond et Jules de. *Journal: Mémoires de la vie littéraire 1851–1863*. Paris: Fasquelle and Flammarion, 1956.

Grosz, Elizabeth. *Volatile Bodies*. Bloomington and Indianapolis: Indiana University Press, 1994.

Halperin, David. Review of Leo Bersani, *Homos*, in *London Review of Books*, 23 May 1996.

Hazel, Valerie. "Disjointed Articulations: The Politics of Voice and Jane Campion's *The Piano*," Paper delivered to the Centre for Women's Studies, Monash University in March 1994.

Hofmannsthal, Hugo von. *Gesammelte Werk: Aufzeichnungen*. Frankfurt: Fischer, 1959.

Lévi-Strauss, Claude. *La Pensée sauvage*. Paris: Plon, 1962.

Levinas, Emmanuel. *Le Temps et l'autre*. Paris: Presses universitaires de France, 1983.

Lingis, Alphonso. *Foreign Bodies*. New York and London: Routledge, 1994.

Mars-Jones, Adam. "Poetry in Motion." *The Independent*, 29 October 1993.

Mercer, Kobena. *Welcome to the Jungle*. New York and London: Routledge, 1994.

Meyer, Conrad Ferdinand. *Werke in 2. Bänden, Erster Band: Gedichte*. Berlin and Weimar: Aufbau-Verlag, 1970.
Nietzsche, Friedrich. *Werke*, sect. 5, vol. 1, "Morgenröthe" (Berlin and New York: Walter de Gruyter: [1887], 1971.
Proust, Marcel. *A la recherche du temps perdu* , vol. 1. Paris: Gallimard, 1954.
Pryor, Ian. Interview with Jane Campion, *Onfilm* 10 (9 October 1993).
Rilke, Rainer Maria. *Die Aufzeichnungen des Malte Laurids Brigge*. Eschwege: Suhrkamp [1910], 1975.
Rilke, Rainer Maria. *Gesammelte Werke*, vol. 4. Leipzig: Insel, 1930.
Robinson, Christopher. *Scandal in the Ink*. London: Cassell, 1995.
Sartre, Jean-Paul. *L'Être et le néant*. Paris: Gallimard, 1948.
Sartre, Jean-Paul. *La Nausée*. Paris: Gallimard, 1938.
Sherman, Allan. "Skin," from the LP *The Best of Allan Sherman*. Valiant Records, 1965.
Valéry, Paul. *Œuvres complètes*. Paris: Gallimard, 1960.

The Touch of the Other on the Threshold of Sex; or The Skin between Levinas and Irigaray
DAVE BOOTHROYD

INTRODUCTION

THIS TEXT ADDRESSES BOTH THE MATTER AND SENSE OF TOUCH AND its figuring in the chiastic threshold between the phenomenon and discourse, taking as its focus the "dialogue" on touch which takes place between Emmanuel Levinas and Luce Irigaray (as evidenced in Irigaray's writings). It is directed at that zone of discursive encounter between their bodies of thought concerning the nature of the contact between *the same* and *the other*. It holds that the "contact" of touching is not only thematically approached by Irigaray in her philosophical reflections on Levinas but also intertextually instantiated therewithin. Addressing the theme of touch in Irigaray's reading of Levinas raises the question of what she embraces of his thinking on the relation to alterity, and of what she comes to regard as its limits with respect to her own attempts to articulate an "ethics of sexual difference." In her reading of Levinas's account of Eros, his phenomenology of the caress, and the figuring of touch in relation to these, Irigaray identifies and describes the nature of his failure to recognize the significance of sexual difference to the "origin" of the ethical. It is in the context of their respective accounts of the touch and touching of the other that this essay will explore the connection between touch and the sexing ethical sensibility.

From a critical point of view, the importance of Levinas's thinking for Irigaray has often been commented upon.[1] What might be described as her most "intimate" engagement with Levinas, takes place, principally, in the essay "The Fecundity of the Caress," which forms the final chapter in *An Ethics of Sexual Difference*.[2] Later I shall turn to her other direct, and significantly, "interrogative" approach to Levinas, undertaken in the later essay "Questions to Emmanuel Levinas: On the Divinity of Love."[3]

The first essay is a commentary on the "Phenomenology of Eros" chapter of Levinas's *Totality and Infinity*.[4] In it she considers the significance of touch within Eros for the articulation of an "ethical" relation to alterity; a relation in which neither the one nor the other is subjected, across (their) difference, to a subalternization. It attempts to describe how ethical discourse is held to emerge out of the threshold of contact between one and the other, and how the experience and thought of each is immanently related to the specificity of their sexuate (*sexué*) incarnation.

The style of the discursive phenomenology Irigaray adopts in her engagement with Levinas could perhaps be described as "materialist immanentism"; it is a thinking which emerges out of the contact zone between two sexuate (*sexué*) bodies of thought. Its critical tactic is to articulate the contactual possibilities of a "flesh" whose becoming-word (in being thematized) reverts at every instant into the very sensuality out of which it emerges. She speaks in terms of the *morphology* of bodily contact between sexed bodies and directs her attention to the unthematized sensuality of touching the other.[5] The "bodymorph" is a notion which expresses the unthematized facticity of the sexed body, which is only ever visible, or representable, when clothed in discourse. In so far as "touching" can be attributed to such a "body," it is a touching in which the distinction between word and thing, or language and experience, has not yet been made. It will be my contention here that this is also to be understood in terms of the textual encounter which is "reading"; and that it is helpful to think of Irigaray's reading of Levinas as a kind of readerly embrace, an encounter in which the irreducibility of sexual difference comes to the fore. This essay will retrace the movement of this "embrace." Irigaray's sense of the necessity of a passage through Levinas's thinking on alterity, and her specific critical appropriation of it, led her to formulate what could be described as a "sexed response." I will attempt to show that the difference between them becomes the scene of an intertextual instantiation, or staging, of the "touch of the other" as literary performance.

For Levinas, the phenomenological experience of the "threshold" of erotic contact, in general, is discerned, as such, *in the withdrawal* from the one-on-one, fleshy encounter between two lovers, from what Levinas regards as the "voluptuosity" of touching skins, in which the "I" is prone to lose itself in the indulgent carnal embrace. But in this insistent characterization of the withdrawal as the failure of transcendence, Irigaray identifies a certain sex-blindness, or, to be more precise, a certain sex-numbness: Levinas's account misses the irreducible "morphology" of the sexual difference between male and female, with the result that it neither accounts for the difference of the touching sexes (which refers, synecdochally, also to the female sex organs),[6] nor addresses the important matter of how touching differs in the cases of male/female, male/male, and female/female contacts. Consequently, he misses the significance of the "fact" that women are (*within* their sex) "constantly touching themselves," as Irigaray says, *from the inside*—a notion she variously expresses, often in the discursive formulations centered around the trope of "the lips" (*les lèvres*). Briefly, this "(l)abi(a)lity" of woman gives rise to a sex-specific philosophy of exteriority (being); on which basis Irigaray proposes, in turn, that the ethics of sexual difference cannot be separated from the ethics of Eros. Eros figures, therefore, not only in what is ordinarily understood by prediscursive sexual interaction between individuals, but also at the level of relations between the sexes in society in general. But, to discuss this synecdochal repetition of themes—of what happens between touching bodies and what happens in society at large—in terms of either structure and logic, or in the inadequate phenomenological terminology of "levels," would be misleading here. Irigaray's "discursive phenomenology" seeks to avoid getting caught up in the philosophical problem of "transcendentality" by bracketing the problem of *how* sensation becomes language. And there is throughout her work a certain calculated philosophical disregard for *how* the touch across sexual difference ontogenetically figures and figures in societal relations.

To get a grip on how the ethical might be said to have its origin in the touch "in between" or "across" sexual difference, in the separation, or interruption, of the touching of touching skins, we need now to slip between Levinas and Irigaray in order to get a sense of friction arising from their contact. Both phenomenological and discursive-narrative styles of theorizing touch could be said to share this nonphilosophical "origin" of the interstitial "bodily encounter." Irigaray's major undertaking here is to claim that such body-to-body contact (*corps-à-corps*), and the thinking which ensues from it, is from the first, or prediscursively, a scene of contact framed by sexual difference.

THE THRESHOLD OF TOUCH: ASYMMETRY AND RECIPROCITY

Irigaray's indebtedness to Levinas in "The Fecundity of the Caress" is not at issue here. The focus of attention is rather on her relation to Levinas expressed in the form of her reflections concerning the ethical significance of sensual contact of touch with other bodies. Her critique of Levinas is Levinasian to the extent to which, in this amorous intertextual encounter, it seeks to retain for itself, on the basis of a reanalysis of sensibility, an ethical understanding of the tactility of contact. She is, nonetheless, at pains to identify the ethical limits of Eros, as Levinas figures these in terms of its role in "fecundity" (which takes the birth of the *male* child as the perpetuation of the father and of patriarchy), and in relation to his making this the source of the fundamental experience of "myself as other." Against this preoccupation of the masculine philosopher with himself—as she later comes to express this in "Questions"—Irigaray presents her account of maternity as a noninstrumental model for the body-to-body relation to the child in birthing, and as the model of the *feminine* relation to the other. This figure of "birthing" is not, however, restricted to the phenomenon of sexual reproduction. As Cathryn Vasseleu has recently written in her discussion of Irigaray in relation to Levinas: "Erotic pleasure is an imaginary beginning, a birth after and before the present which will never have taken place."[7] Concomitantly with this, Irigaray presents an account of fecundity *between lovers* in Eros, which does not depend, as it does for Levinas, on its "offspring" for its ethical significance. She attempts, as Tina Chanter has astutely shown, to develop Levinas's ethical thinking by "sexing" the caress;[8] by thinking the movement of difference "reverting to sameness" without the reversion, at the same time, to structural forms of subalternization of the beloved (*l'aimée*) and the lover (*l'amant*), and of women in their relations to men.[9]

As already noted, the suggestion here is that Irigaray's texts performatively exemplify a touching textual encounter in what they might be said to stage in their reading of Levinas. Hers is through and through a "sensual reading" in that it is written from within, and exemplifies discursively the form of an amorous, erotic embrace. It is from within the "erotico-exegetical" contact she initiates between them that she refuses the meaning of the feminine attributed to (erotic and other forms of) contact by Levinas, in his account of Eros. She sets out to recover the ethical significance of Eros by means of her own discursive phenomenology of touch within the caress, which she understands in terms of absolute passivity. This leads her to insist on an account of touch which acknowledges that from the first, touching itself is sex specific (*sexué*). Hence, it is in relation to the sensual proximity of touching, rather than in the light of conceptual reason, that the ethics of eros may be articulated.[10]

In this respect, Irigaray directs us back to the original birth of sexual difference in the separation of one from the other, recalling the philosophically underexamined relation to the mother, birthing, and the womb. It is a part of her discursive strategy of privileging sexual difference as the "precondition" of separate singular existence in general: Eros requires and gives rise to the separation of two from the oneness of the lovers engaged, as if fused together, in the erotic caress.

Along with Levinas, at least to a certain degree, Irigaray directs us to "the sensual pleasure of birth into a world where the look itself remains tactile" and from there seeks to examine how "sensual pleasure can reopen and *reverse*" the "construction of world" (*Ethics*, 185). From a philosophical point of view, this calls for a "return," of some sort, from the given situation of mastery (of which patriarchy is the generic form), and it marks Irigaray's location in relation to the tradition of philosophical "returns" (repetitions and turnings) running through Hegel, Nietzsche, Merleau-Ponty, Heidegger, and Derrida. *She* "returns" in a gesture of *undoing* directed at the mastery of the masculinist constructionism of the subject which has been responsible for the political subalternization of woman; a subalternization which implies, moreover, the denial of woman's "natural" relation to her element.[11]

Irigaray has of course written at length and throughout her oeuvre about the need for feminism to think in terms of a "sexed culture," but the crux of her engagement with Levinas is not so much focused on the highly complex level of symbolic exchange as on the most simple contact of touching skins; of the lubrication of touching bodies and sensual contact with the other across epidermal membranes; with what happens "in between" two skins. She directs us, to adopt a Levinasian idiom, to the "signifyingness" of such contact prior to its (discursive) signification, or prior to the (philosophical) decision of its meaning. And it is this chiasmus of the phenomenological and the discursive which Irigaray brings to the thinking of sexuate incarnation.

> On the horizon of a story is found what was in the beginning: this naive or native sense of touch, in which the subject does not yet exist. Submerged in *pathos* or *aeisthesis*: astonishment, wonder and sometimes terror before that which surrounds it. (*Ethics*, 185)

These opening sentences of "The Fecundity of the Caress" recall Levinas's "phenomenological" thesis of the hypostasis of the "substantive," singular existent which takes up its position in anonymous existence (*il y a*) in the form of a relationship of enjoyment and nourishment: as an indulgence in pure, undifferentiated sensibility. Unreflected and unrepresentable—and in this sense prephenomenological—the sense *par excellence* of this aeisthesis is touch: touch is the "source of all the senses" (*Ethics*, 192). Levinas's account of the encounter with the other in Eros, as much as the encounter with the other in the ethical relation, which he calls the "face to face," requires that the existent has accomplished this autochthonous movement of existence as the precondition, or substantive basis, for entry into the relation to the other.[12] This is a moment, says Irigaray, in which Levinas's phenomenology remarks a form of "Eros prior to any Eros defined and framed as such. The sensual pleasure of birth into a world where the look itself remains tactile" and "still carnal" (*Ethics*, 185).

In such unreflected Eros, the relation to the other permits no distinction between environment and (what reflection later comes to regard as) the other person. In this pure sensuality, which is neither "consciousness of . . ." nor representation, but rather enjoyment (*jouissance*),[13] self and other are not yet born: *only on reflection* can we *think*, along with Irigaray, of "the touch of the caress" as being a *co*-existence and "untouched by mastery" of one over the other. There is an Edenic innocence in the blind gropings of erotically intertwined bodies; unfinished, unframed, undefined "flesh," in which the distinction between sensual touch and what can be thought by means of the metaphorical displacement of "touch" has not yet taken place. As Vasseleu says, "Tactility is generic sensibility which constitutes the opposition of interiority and exteriority."[14] In this the alterity of the other is neither known nor encountered *as such*: importantly for Levinas, it is therefore a figure of the nonethical.

It is from within this threshold (*seuil*) of the touching between two lovers—rather than between the lover (*l'amant*) and the beloved (*l'aimeé*)—that Irigaray refers us to the communal reciprocity (a reciprocity without negation) of the Eros she seeks to "ethicize." Where Levinas finds "profanation" and failure of ethical contact,[15] Irigaray will attempt to demonstrate—by means of her "literary touch"—that sexual difference is the sensible, material condition for the ethical. She is aiming to demonstrate that Eros is ethical; that the ethical is conterminous with the "experience," or interstitial contact, of sexual difference; that the questions of sexual difference and ethics cross over one another; moreover, that all of these metaphorically displaced contiguities are never entirely removed from the "actual" discontiguities of two caressing bodies (and the literary engagement of two *corpora*): "Touch [. . .] remains palpable flesh on this side of *and beyond the visible*" (*Ethics*, 192: my emphasis).

Sameness and Difference

It is not surprising, on reflection, that Irigaray's explicit engagement with Levinas focuses on the relatively short section of *Totality and Infinity* entitled "The Phenomenology of Eros," for it is the "outcome" of the erotic encounter in Levinas which is decisive for the meaning of sex, or the sexuate being (of each one). For Levinas, to use a metaphor of elevation and directionality, Eros is to be regarded as a halfway stage between the unicity, or separateness, of the existent (accomplished as nourishment and enjoyment in relation to the elemental, or undecided being) and the ethical relation to another person, through which the "I" is oriented toward the absolutely other "beyond the face." In Levinas's account, the opening of the ethically decisive "difference" is dependent on the separation of the same and the other who face one another. Eros for Levinas could therefore be said to have a critically decisive function: it bridges the gap between solipsistic elemental life (*vivre de* . . .) and the "straightforwardness" of the face in the face-to-face, or ethical, relation.[16] It is not surprising either, then, that Irigaray seeks to expose and reject this account of Eros, which implicates the feminine as the instrumental link or bridge to the beyond, namely to *his own* transcendence (*Ethics*, 202). In Levinas, Eros has the function (though it itself does not know it) of fecundation: it is instrumental to, and results in, the birth of the child. The child, born of the erotic encounter, is Levinas's "trope" of infinitude coming to pass in the human context, despite that fact Eros, by nature, neither knows this nor aims at knowledge at all.

The feminist response to Levinas has understandably focused on this preoccupation with the offspring of Eros *qua* the *son*, and on the instrumental role of woman in Levinas's schema.[17] However, as an alternative to engaging with this reception and this problematic, I seek here to follow that aspect of Irigaray's response, which undertakes to return to the primordial scene of Eros from within the intimacy of the two who do not yet know they are *not one*, and to see how touch can be made the basis for a reinscription of sex (difference) *within* Eros. This move is intended, on her part, to refute Levinas's "profanation thesis" and to replace it with a model of the "reversal" of Eros in the service of an ethics of sexual difference. In other words, it ultimately seeks and calls for the reciprocal acknowledgment of sexual difference as the origin of the ethical.

It is in a comparison of Levinas's and Irigaray's thinking of the "sameness," or rather the "sexed-ipseity" of the "I" or the "one," respectively, that the importance of the liminality implicit in the touch of the other in Eros is to be traced. Irigaray proposes an account of erotic contact which relocates it in the elemental, an idea to which I shall turn shortly. For Levinas, emphatically, "elements and things remain outside respect and disrespect." Existence and the position the existent holds with respect to existence in general are, for Levinas, essential to the condition of separation and openness to the other. But, "in themselves" they are a "profanity": being at home (*chez soi*) in the elemental is a kind of nonethical form of life; it is an indulgence. The ethical comes to me *from* the other, not from within my elemental existence. The relation to the elemental is, nonetheless, held by Levinas to be decisive for the "upsurge" of the existent into being such that it can turn toward the other.[18] Against this background metaphysics of elemental life, Eros is seen as a kind of unthinking groping in the dark, from which the existent is never startled or awakened into reflection; the feeler and the felt, the touching and the touched, are neither separated nor separable as such—they are, to use a significantly visual metaphor, unreflected: "only the face in its morality is exterior" to such (an) existence.[19] My touching the other's skin is a touching or sensibility that does not distinguish between the thingly surface touched and the other as "ethical subject."

Touching on Merleau-Ponty

The ethical limitation of Eros, on Levinas's account, results from its confusion between need and desire. This distinction is one that is central to his entire account of the relationship between sensibility and transcendence. In Eros, the ethical desire for the other, as it moves towards its object, is confused: it is life wholly at the level of appetite—it is not, in this respect, different from hunger. It exists as an "irresponsible animality"[20]—which Irigaray will claim Levinas ultimately identifies with the feminine (see "Questions," 113). It moves toward the other but does not, in this movement, distinguish the other from exteriority in general. It is rather in the nature of its *withdrawal* from Eros that it can come to know the significance of its yearning for satiation through contact, and also how this differs from—and is inferior to—the ethical obligation which comes to it from beyond the erotically confusing threshold of need/desire, which marks the limit or boundary of its sameness. In Eros, the ambivalence of the touching/being touched—its nondistinction or nondifference—refers this touching "couple" back to its own sameness—the touched one being *nothing other* than the instrumental accomplishment of its own sameness.

Irigaray takes this aspect of Levinas's remarks on touch and the elementality of the sense of touch into her reading of Merleau-Ponty in the essay "The Invisible of the Flesh" (*Ethics*, 151–84), in which she examines his famous "The Intertwining—The Chiasm."[21] This is the chapter which precedes "The Fecundity of the Caress" in *An Ethics of Sexual Difference*, and it focuses, in particular, on the passages concerning auto-affection, or touching-oneself. It is by way of this reading of Merleau-Ponty's essay that I shall now attempt to clarify what it is that she finds lacking in Levinas's account of the caress.

In her engagement with Merleau-Ponty Irigaray develops an account of how touch is the "primary" sense and makes this primacy central to her analysis of how the traditional prioritizing of vision works in the service of patriarchy and "mastery." Her reading is broadly in accord with the Merleau-Pontean phenomenological gesture of a return to prediscursive experience, but she finds that his analysis of this "experience" in terms of the intertwining of sensibility/intelligibility, or passivity/activity ("it is as though our vision were formed in the heart of the visible"),[22] rethinks vision *by analogy* with touch. Consequently, it "returns the privilege to the *seer's* look" (*Ethics*, 152). It thus misses the most important distinction of touch, namely, that touch is a sensibility "more passive than any passivity of and within my own touch" (*Ethics*, 170), "more passive than any voluntary passivity" (*Ethics*, 195), touch is a sensibility to *the touch of the other person*. It is the touch of the other which awakens me from my slumberous bathing in the visible. I am not touched *by* the visible: I am touched only by the other. Merleau-Ponty's famous discussion of the toucher and the touched is undertaken in terms of the "subject" of touch which "experiences" itself, as such, in the phenomenon of auto-affection. In her own return to prediscursive experience, Irigaray shows that this account of touching, which is expressed in terms of the relationship between, or rather dissolution of, the interior/exterior divide, takes their intertwining as the interstitial origin of the subject. This is a subject whose existence is (to use the term favored by Levinas) accomplished in the form of a self-reflexive movement. But whereas Merleau-Ponty stresses the unity of the subject's body as both "sensible mass" and "the mass of the sensible,"[23] Irigaray emphasizes the "*solipsistic* character of this touch(ing) between the world and subject; of this touch(ing) of the visible and the seer in the subject itself" (*Ethics*, 157: my emphasis). For Levinas, "solipsism" characterizes the elemental life of the existent in separation from being in general, and he argues that the ethical comes from elsewhere, namely, beyond this material basis upon which its singularity depends. Without leaving the level of the elemental, Irigaray seeks to reject this solipsism of the toucher/touched distinction played out, as it were, internally, *within the same* and to address instead the "question of the other as touched and touching" (*Ethics*, 157).

Although Merleau-Ponty attempts to think the material union of the visible and vision, of the seer and the seen—indeed, this move is indispensable to the rethinking of touch in Irigaray's own text—he nonetheless remains committed to a model of the subject's hypostasis which leaves it closed in upon itself in the act, or rather movement, of auto-affection. And, whereas Levinas seeks to breach this circuit of sameness by directing us toward a "metaphenomenology," or "ethicophenomenology," of sameness as *response* to that alterity which approaches (me) from beyond, "accusatively" and as "obligation,"[24] Irigaray's tactic is to direct her reader back to the sameness which is "not one," both in and of itself—namely the female sex (*sexe*). She thus develops a critique of the Merleau-Pontean account of the becoming-one of sameness *qua* "the subject as flesh," on the basis of thinking "female flesh" as the materiality of woman's sexuate being. Her readings of Merleau-Ponty and Levinas find them both to be culpable of missing the role of sexual difference in the ontogenesis of the singular existent, and that their similarity on this matter is held to be evident, above all, in their accounts of touch. They are both held to associate touching with a loss of self or with the threat of such a loss. What Levinas specifically adds to this scenario, according to Irigaray, is a theory of the divine which comes from beyond the body to body (*corps-à-corps*) of the erotic encounter; an encounter which is, moreover, a profanation of the divine due to its being mistaken for it. Consequently, the fecundity which is accomplished by the birth of the child, on the Levinasian model, is what comes to save Eros from being what it otherwise would be, namely, a form of sacrilege. Against this channeling of Eros into procreation, Irigaray refers Eros to a fecundity prior to any procreation, to that which is to be rediscovered in (the) touching (of) the other.

The crux of Irigaray's critique of both Levinas's and Merleau-Ponty's accounts of the "life" of the substantive existent, "living from" or "intertwined" in being, is that contact as the touch *between women* is different from that between men—or, more precisely, where men are involved (with one another or with women). Of course, this is not to remark a collapse back into some genre of philosophically unexamined, psychological theorizing, or into a soma-aesthesiology of sexual preference. Far from it. Irigaray is here developing a radical discursive-phenomenology of the female sex and its relation to itself, as "the sex which is not one." Unlike the model's self-same, solipsistic existence which she finds in Merleau-Ponty and Levinas, in which "sexedness" is "lost" in consuming passions of one sort or another, Irigaray claims the existence of an internal relation of self-sameness: one which occurs from within the female sex, so to speak, in its "nature." This condition is something expressed in an array of tropes in Irigaray, but directly discussed, for example, in terms of mother/daughter relations, the (female) bodily bifurcation of birthing, and refigured, notably, in the form of the unique (and yet simultaneously doubling) "phenomenon" of woman's giving birth to herself, or rather, to *her own sex*.

In Irigaray's texts, these refigurings of the relation to the self are "read off" the form of the female body, or rather, the female bodymorph. The bodymorph can be thought of as a sort of discursive, *langue*-like substrate supporting the particular, *parole*-like discourse of female difference. It is not accessible to phenomenology in the classical sense, nor is it constructed out of "pellicles" of lived experience (as Merleau-Ponty suggests of the body in his discussion of color in "The Intertwining"). It is above all else, a model or figure of the female body's sexed specificity prior to its reflection, *qua* sexed, in thought. It is "sexedness" at the level of the purely sensible: discernible only in the touching between one and another, between two who come into contact in the sensibility of touching, in "the caress," and who have *not yet withdrawn* into the "oneness" of their identities.

The bodymorph for Irigaray is the surface which supports the specificity of sexuate tactility: it is the substantive surface of touch. It serves as the "medium"—a medium which is prior to what it mediates, namely language and sense—of the sensual, material inscription of sexual difference. The body for Irigaray, as for Merleau-Ponty, is not a seen thing distinct from the seeing, but the seen/seer (non-)distinction is, on her account, always marked by sexed specificity prior to its identification as a sexed-thing. Her discourse aims to recover sexual difference from the oblivion in which it is lost in the thinking that thinks individual existence on the basis of its relation to the world (something which is re-marked always on the ground of an act of negation, of one sort or another).[25]

The account of touch as sexed with which Irigaray leads us back to a reexamination of the touching of the other (within the caress), and into her engagement with Levinas, is preceded, in her reading of Merleau-Ponty, by a comparison of the touching hands with what she describes as a touch "more intimate than that of the one hand taking hold of the other" (*Ethics*, 161), namely that of the "two lips" (*les lèvres*). The "lips" figure the touching of mucous membranes; that "most intimate interior of the flesh [. . .] threshold of the passage between the inside and the outside" (*Ethics*, 179). It is this other threshold of contact, of the tactile itself, that Irigaray insists upon.

The touching lips are a figurative displacement of the female sex (*sexe*),[26] and an alternative cultural decoder/reencoder to, for example, the tropes of masculinist *phallocentrisms*; they figure also in her alternative account of auto-affection. Auto-affection is wholly affective and "fecund," without any lack, or need for any kind of movement: "A phenomenon that remains in the interior, does not appear in the light of day, speaks of itself only in gestures, remains always on the edge of speech, gathering the edges, *without sealing them*" (*Ethics*, 161). Difference within sameness, oneness within twoness: this (trans)figures the female sex as that which in its nature differs within itself. Touch is not, however, simply a figure for making visible the tangible. Nor is this discourse of Irigaray's simply a representation of some indirectly addressed, essential nature of the female sex (as some of her critics have supposed). The implicit thesis is that language and sensibility are only distinguished by reflection, and its corollary is that only "female language" can accomplish the sexual reinscription of the female body unreflected in the light of masculinist reason. Such an undertaking "extends," moreover, to the sexing of culture at large, sculpting it anew neither on the basis of an underlying, amorphous sensuality of erotic frenzy (a masculine erotics), nor by means of the heavy hand of theory (the masculine instrument of touch, mastery and self-gratification), but by means of a touching-forming contact with the other, one which is based on an erotics of the caress as feminine touch. In Irigaray's schema, it is the figure of the lips which articulates this touching which does not have recourse to the visible: it identifies a touching within the touching of the same sex and an auto-erotics of feminine "sameness."

Irigaray *corps-à-corps* Levinas

The requirement for an encounter which is ethical "at the point of contact" is immanent to the "erotic exegesis" of Levinas which Irigaray's reading undertakes: it is exegetical in the sense of being "readerly" in so far as it constitutes also the intertextual moment or instantiation of the ethical contact. Neither "text" nor "flesh" is given precedence in this encounter; nor are the intertextuality and intermateriality of touch to be distinguished. In any case, it should not be supposed that what our language names "the phenomenon"—the familiar everyday skin against skin of touching others—is any less in need of a "reading" than whatever is referred to as "the text."

To counter the relegation of the undecidable toucher/touched of Eros to the subethical, Irigaray's text rejoins with the Levinasian text in a kind of textual-erotic embrace which returns to the erotic moment in a phenomenological gesture aimed at the rediscovery of the intimacy of which it speaks. This intimacy is variously referred to as "the intimacy of that first house of the flesh [. . .] intimacy of the mucous" and as "porosity [. . .] the most profound intimacy [. . .] [which] crosses itself like a threshold"

(*Ethics*, 189–91). The fluidity of intertextual crossings is characteristic of Irigaray's highly original "erotico-exegetical" or "amorous" readings (these are her own terms), such that in a performative, staged *withdrawal*—corresponding also to the moment of "philosophical" reflection in her text—the signifyingness of her sex is revealed, and revealed otherwise than in terms of its being an instrumental bridging of the earthly and the divine (as Levinas would have it). It is at this point, in effect, that she stages her breaking with, or withdrawal from, her intimate intertextual "embrace" with Levinas. In the following passage, which I suggest can also be read as an homage to Levinas's part in all this, or at least to Levinas as reinscribed in the folds of her text, she reevaluates "fecundity" in terms of reciprocal "birthing" of the kind described above:

> Prior to any procreation, the lovers bestow on each other—life. Love fecundates both of them in turn, through the genesis of their immortality. They are reborn, each for the other, in the assumption and absolution of a definitive conception, each one welcomes the birth of the other, this task beginning where neither he nor she has met—the original infidelity. Attentive to that weakness which neither one could have wanted, they love each other as the bodies that they are. (*Ethics*, 190)

Reciprocity rather than asymmetry; reciprocity without a resultant equality—the birth of sexual difference out of Eros is performed here in the form of an exegetically sexed response. Where Levinas thinks the separation of the subject in relation to anonymous being, Irigaray seeks to relocate this decisive moment within the *severance* of the erotic embrace: separation amounts to the "condition" of being in sexed-contact. Their sexed *corpora* encounter one another on the territory of elemental Eros. The encounter with the other in nakedness, skin against skin, is a nudity "before the fall," before any possibility of profanity and immodesty in exposure to alterity: it is before *any* law is given; before the law of the phallus is instituted. It is a feminine sensibility, then, expressed in terms of touch and touching, which gives access to this (feminine) "truth." Rather than the feminine being a bridge to transcendence, it names and relocates the scene of the "original separation" within the female body, or more precisely, the female sex—metaphorically and meta-morpho-logically expressed by means of the trope of the female sex: the lips (*lèvres*).

If "The Fecundity of the Caress" can be seen as an expression of the intimacy of Irigaray's embrace of Levinas, in which it is in the breaking-off from this "sensual reading" of Levinas that the sexuate "identity" of two can be thematized, then it is to her second, "post-erotic" reading of Levinas that we can look in order to get a sense of, so to speak, how it was for her.

This text is notably entitled "*Questions* to Emmanuel Levinas: On the Divinity of Love"; in it Irigaray interrogates Levinas and claims to expose the unquestioned patriarchal basis of his "theological philosophy." In this respect, she suggests, he does not hold true to his own phenomenological insights, in particular with regard to "the caress," which, she says, in representing to him the threat of profanation, indicates also that "the function of the other sex as an alterity irreducible to myself eludes [him]" ("Questions," 110). She contends that this represents a repetition of the traditional rejection of sensuality in the form of the sensual contact between bodies and ultimately leads to the ethical failure of his account of the caress. This account, she says,

> does not touch the other [. . .]: To caress for Levinas consists, therefore, not in approaching the other in its most vital dimension, the touch, but in the reduction of that vital dimension of the other's body to the elaboration of a future for himself. ("Questions," 110)

His ethics, therefore, does not reach the other in her/his actuality—a future event—it aims at the future as "ungraspable," that philosophical (non-)object of the male philosopher's desire *par excellence*. The feminine other is reduced in all this philosophy to "an immediate object of desire" and she is "left without her own specific face" ("Questions," 113–15).

In returning to the theme of touch (starting from the "experience" of touch) within the caress of Levinas, Irigaray's two texts, "The Fucundity of the Caress" and "Questions," taken together, restage that moment of "sexed separation," showing it to be independent and "later" than the auto-erotic movement of the feminine, or self-touching. Irigaray's feminine figure of "labiality" is independent of and prior to women's entry into relations with men. The argument attempts to restore to sexual difference its revolutionary potential: the thesis of the *non*-substitutability of female for male, their irreducible difference, is a call for nothing less than an alter-ation of every cultural form and of every hitherto "unsexed" cultural structure, form, entity, belief, truth, and so on. She suggests, for instance, that we consider the consequence of substituting a male God with a female God and the "upheaval in the symbolic order" that this would necessitate.[27] No matter how extensive (masculinist) cultural totalitarianism may be, no matter the extent of its figurative hold on the imagination, it can nonetheless be perpetually disrupted by the simple touch of the other. This "positive," even optimistic, conclusion is tenable because the ethics of contact is exposed, repeatedly, in "the loss of boundaries which takes place for both lovers when they cross the boundary of the skin into the mucous membranes" ("Questions," 111). No matter what changes the future technologies of procreation may bring, or how varied the cultures of parenting may be, such crossings of the skin, whatever they might come to mean, are unlikely to go out of style.

NOTES

1. E.g. Tina Chanter, *Ethics of Eros* (London: Routledge, 1995); Margaret Whitford, *Philosophy in the Feminine* (London: Routledge, 1991); Kate Ince, "Questions to Luce Irigaray," in *Hypatia* 11: 2 (1996): 122–40.

2. Luce Irigaray, "The Fecundity of the Caress" in *An Ethics of Sexual Difference*, trans. Carolyn Burke and Gillian Gill (Ithaca: Cornell University Press, 1993), 185–217. References to this and other essays in this volume will be given in the text with the abbreviation *Ethics*.

3. Luce Irigaray, "Questions to Emmanuel Levinas," in *The Irigaray Reader*, ed. Margaret Whitford (Oxford: Blackwell, 1991), 178–89. Further references will be given in the text with the abbreviation "Questions."

4. Emmanuel Levinas, *Totality and Infinity*, trans. Alphonso Lingis (Pittsburgh, Penn.: Duquesne University Press, 1969), 256–66.

5. Cf. Judith Butler, *Bodies that Matter* (London: Routledge, 1993); Jane Gallop, *Thinking through the Body* (New York: Columbia University Press, 1990); Dave Boothroyd, "Labial Feminism: Body against Body with Luce Irigaray," in *Parallax* 3 (1996), 361–86.

6. Cf. Gallop, *Thinking through the Body*.

7. Cathryn Vasseleu, *Textures of Light: Vision and Touch in Irigaray, Levinas, and Merleau-Ponty* (London: Routledge, 1998), 113.

8. Chanter, *Ethics of Eros*, 221.

9. Irigaray uses the masculine and feminine variants of these terms to reflect the different relations of lovers to the "objects" of their love: "In "The Fecundity of the Caress," I used the term "woman lover" (*l'amante*) and not only, as Levinas does, the word "beloved" (*aimée*). I wanted to signify that the woman can be a subject in love (*un sujet amoureux*) and is not reducible to a more or less immediate object of desire" ("Questions," 115).

10. Cf. Vasseleu, *Textures of Light*.

11. For a discussion of the political implications of Irigaray's feminism and the "feminist political," see my "Sexual Politics and Sexual Difference," chap. 12 of Terrell Carver and Veronique Mottier (eds.), *Politics of Sexuality* (London: Routledge, 1998).

12. Cf. Levinas, *Existence and Existents*, trans. Alphonso Lingis (The Hague: Martinus Nijhoff, 1978).
13. Cf. Levinas, *Totality and Infinity*, 136–37.
14. Cf. Vasseleu, *Textures of Light*, 115.
15. Levinas, *Totality and Infinity*, 257.
16. *Totality and Infinity*, 262.
17. For example, see Chanter, *Ethics of Eros*, especially 198–207.
18. Cf. Levinas, *Existence and Existents*.
19. Levinas, *Totality and Infinity*, 262.
20. Levinas, *Totality and Infinity*, 263.
21. Maurice Merleau-Ponty, *The Visible and the Invisible*, trans. Alphonso Lingis (Evanston, Ill.: Northwestern University Press, 1964).
22. *The Visible and the Invisible*, 130–31, cited by Irigaray in *Ethics*, 152.
23. *The Visible and the Invisible*, 136, cited by Irigaray in *Ethics*, 166.
24. These are terms which are prevalent in Levinas's later work, *Otherwise than Being; or Beyond Essence*, trans. Alphonso Lingis (The Hague: Martinus Nijhoff, 1981).
25. Cf. Irigaray, *I Love to You*, trans. Alison Martin (London: Routledge, 1996), especially 1–17. Irigaray expresses her philosophical commitment to thinking the negative, but she understands this to be primarily in relation to sexual difference rather than to exteriority: "The negative in sexual difference means an acceptance of the limits of my gender and recognition of the irreducibility of the other. It cannot be overcome, but it gives a positive access—neither instinctual nor drive related—to the other" (13).
26. Gallop, *Thinking through the Body*, 97.
27. The substitution of a female for a male God is here clearly not merely a matter of theology, but of all onto-theologies and whatever remains of them in their deconstructions.

Works Cited

Boothroyd, Dave. "Labial Feminism: Body against Body with Luce Irigaray." *Parallax* 3 (1996): 361–86.

———. "Sexual Politics and Sexual Difference," chap. 12. *Politics of Sexuality*. Edited by Terrell Carver and Veronique Mottier. London: Routledge, 1998.

Butler, Judith. *Bodies that Matter*. London: Routledge, 1993.

Chanter, Tina. *Ethics of Eros*. London: Routledge, 1995.

Gallop, Jane. *Thinking through the Body*. New York: Columbia University Press, 1990.

Ince, Kate. "Questions to Luce Irigaray" in *Hypatia* 11: 2 (1996): 122–40.

Irigaray, Luce. "The Fecundity of the Caress." *An Ethics of Sexual Difference*. Translated by Carolyn Burke and Gillian Gill. Ithaca: Cornell University Press, 1993.

———. *I Love to You*. Translated by Alison Martin. London: Routledge, 1996.

———. "Questions to Emmanuel Levinas." *The Irigaray Reader*. Edited by Margaret Whitford. Oxford: Blackwell, 1991.

Levinas, Emmanuel. *Totality and Infinity*. Translated by Alphonso Lingis. Pittsburgh, Penn.: Duquesne University Press, 1969.

———. *Existence and Existents*. Translated by Alphonso Lingis. The Hague: Martinus Nijhoff, 1978.

———. *Otherwise than Being, or Beyond Essence*. Translated by Alphonso Lingis. The Hague: Martinus Nijhoff, 1981.

Merleau-Ponty, Maurice. *The Visible and the Invisible*. Translated by Alphonso Lingis. Evanston, Ill.: Northwestern University Press, 1964.

Vasseleu, Cathryn. *Textures of Light: Vision and Touch in Irigaray, Levinas, and Merleau-Ponty*. London: Routledge, 1998.

Whitford, Margaret. *Philosophy in the Feminine*. London: Routledge, 1991.

Long Distance Love: On Remote Sensing in Shakespeare's Sonnet 109
IAN MACLACHLAN

> O, never say that I was false of heart,
> Though absence seemed my flame to qualify.
> As easy might I from my self depart
> As from my soul, which in thy breast doth lie.
> That is my home of love; if I have ranged,
> Like him that travels I return again,
> Just to the time, not with the time exchanged,
> So that my self bring water for my stain.
> Never believe, though in my nature reigned
> All frailties that besiege all kinds of blood,
> That it could so preposterously be stained
> To leave for nothing all thy sum of good;
>   For nothing this wide universe I call
>   Save thou, my rose; in it thou art my all.

SOMEONE IS CALLING, CALLING WITH THE REASSURANCE OF A LONGdistance love. Wherever he has been, he has always been as close as this—right here with you; couldn't you sense it? So near, and yet so far. If, that is, he has indeed been away—it's far from clear. Perhaps he's just seemed a little absent; perhaps he hasn't quite been feeling himself. In any case, although he *may* have been away, he has never been out of touch. He's getting in touch to say he's always been in touch. Can we keep in touch from a distance? And when we touch, what is it that always comes between us? What happens when we touch each other?

Let's put the question in French; the French, after all, are supposed to be good at this sort of thing. What happens when *on se touche*? As Derrida points out in his essay on Jean-Luc Nancy, "Le Toucher," the reflexive form in French can signal either an action performed on oneself—to touch oneself—or a reciprocal action, although we shall come to question this reciprocity—to touch each other.¹ Beginning already to unbalance the apparent symmetry of the reciprocal sense of this reflexive form, Derrida follows Nancy in proposing the solecistic construction *se toucher toi*, translated by Peggy Kamuf as "to self-touch you."² The *se toucher toi*—self-touching-you—suggests, first of all, that the two senses of the reflexive form must inhabit one another. Like any reflexive form, the notion of "touching oneself" installs a division in the self as subject and object, such that the self is already relayed through alterity. And, in a preliminary gloss that we shall later come to complicate, in touching you I must also feel myself touching you: I must self-touch you.

We may also say, and this already begins to complicate our account of the ambivalent "self-touching-you," that there can be no touching without loss of contact. Something always intervenes to disrupt the apparent immediacy of touch, whether it be a case of touching oneself or touching the other; touching presupposes interruption, lest touch simply vanish into consubstantiality. The resistance of skin as I feel myself touch you is testimony to this interruption, but this is not to deny the contact of touch. And if the distance of an interruption inhabits the contact of touch, then a possibility of touch may also inhabit the interruption of distance, for example the distance of writing: "Whether we wish it or not, bodies are touching each other on this page, or else, this page is itself that touching [*attouchement*] (of my hand writing, of your hands holding the book). This touch [*toucher*] is infinitely diverted, deferred [*différé*]—machines, transport, photocopies, eyes, still other hands have intervened—but there remains the minute, tenuous, stubborn speck, the infinitesimal dust of a contact which is everywhere interrupted and everywhere pursued."³ The infinite diversion and deferral of this touching is only underscored by my citation of these lines on this page, here. But what then of *staying* in touch with you? If touch always involves interruption, perhaps the only means of staying in touch would be to touch without touching, to elude the limit of the other's touch; one would have to get under someone's skin, to touch their heart, the intangible seat of feeling.

So our addresser, in asserting the constancy of his feelings, his touching fidelity, will want to touch his lover's heart. "Our addresser": let's call him "Shakespeare," although everything we shall go on to say about the addressee of this poem will also hold for the addresser, and will prevent us from identifying the source of this utterance with a particular individual living in Stratford and London from 1564 to 1616. Shakespeare's poem should go to the heart, perhaps in the sense that Derrida describes in "Che cos'è la poesia?": "I call a poem that very thing that teaches the heart, invents the heart, *that which*, finally, the word *heart* seems to mean and which, in my language, I cannot easily discern from the word itself."[4] However, going to the heart is no simple matter, especially when, as Shakespeare declares in the opening lines of the poem, he has never been anywhere else but in his lover's heart. How very touching. Unless, of course, he's just being tactful. Tact or touch? A heart false or true? How could one tell proximity without distance, presence without absence? We simply cannot tell; it's a necessary condition for making this call to the heart that one can never be sure of the sincerity of the call, which in no way inhibits the capacity of the poem to touch the heart—quite the opposite, as we shall see. Let's take him at his word, then. We haven't much choice, and in any case, the giving and taking of words, not to mention their give and take, turns out to be precisely what we're concerned with here.

Wherever he has been, he has always been in touch with his lover—more than in touch: intangibly, impossibly close. The one in the other, his soul in the other's breast: lovingly enfolded, a chiasmus of self and other, of spirit and flesh. It is in the other's heart that he is at home—his "home of love"—home, of course, being where the heart is. To leave that home, in the heart of the other, would be like leaving himself. Let's note in passing that, by dint of the sort of good fortune that may always befall a text such as to confound conclusive discrimination between chance and design, the typography of the Quarto text underscores this division in "my self." But what would departing from oneself mean, if that "self" *begins* in departure, *is* only itself outside of itself in a movement which is never self-contained?

Let us say that the self ceaselessly constitutes itself in the promise to return home, in the heart of the other. Neither self-contained nor simply enclosed in the other, the self—the subject of the poem, Shakespeare, let's say—is compelled to perform a two-step in relation to the other, or rather a *pas de deux*, in which we should discern a double *pas*—a step and *not* a step[5]—as well as a "not-two," for in this relation of self to other, one plus one is always more or less than two. It is this necessity of the *pas de deux* which compels the shuttling movement of departure and return announced hypothetically to describe the relation to the "home of love," in the heart of the other: "if I have ranged, / Like him that travels I return again." It is also in the nature of this shuttling two-step that the circle of departure and return remains incomplete: neither departure nor return can ever be said to be accomplished. Wherever Shakespeare goes, he never loses touch with the other, can never get the other out of his system, whence perhaps the hypothetical "if I have ranged." But even "now" when he is "here" in his "home of love," he is not quite back where he started, outside of himself. (If by now there is some confusion as to which departure we are talking about—from self or from other—then it may be said that this confusion arises precisely from the irresolvably chiastic relations at issue here.) Return is never complete, if only because the movement of return transfigures both the point from which one departed and the one returning, as we may even read in the shift of pronoun that separates "I" from "I" in Shakespeare's poem: "Like *him* that travels . . ."[6]

But the promise to return remains, a promise to self-touch-you implicit in the apostrophizing call of this poem. The apostrophe already announces the unachievability of the return it promises, installing a distance in the proclaimed immediacy of the relation to the other. Furthermore, the form that this apostrophe takes—"O, never say . . ."—indicates that the ineluctable interruption in the relation to the other is concomitant with an interruption in the self-relation of the subject. The call to the other is *already* a response, the apostrophe of the poem re-marking an always prior relation to the other, an absolutely anterior engagement with or promise to the other which is endlessly held out, since it can never be fulfilled once and for all. Let us note here what Derrida says about this prior engagement or affirmation in the essay "Ulysses Gramophone: Hear Say Yes in Joyce." He begins with an allusion to Molly Bloom's reversal of the line from Goethe's *Faust*, "Ich bin der Geist, der stets verneint": "Before the *Ich* in *Ich bin* affirms or negates, it poses itself or pre-poses itself: not as *ego*, as the conscious or unconscious self, as masculine or feminine subject, spirit or flesh, but as a pre-performative force which, for example, in the form of the 'I' [*je*] marks that 'I' as addressing itself to the other, however undetermined he or she is: 'Yes-I,' or 'Yes-I-say-to-the-other,' even if *I* says *no* and even if *I* addresses itself without speaking."[7] The promise to the other re-marked by apostrophe can only be made on the condition that its fulfillment can never be assured. By virtue of the dissymmetrical relation in which the other always precedes and exceeds the subject, a promise to the other must always be cast into the unknown, for if its destination were known in advance, the promise would never even be issued, but would instead remain stalled in the circulation of the same, in a short-circuit of *ego* and *alter ego*.

The "O" which calls home—a call made from the heart to the heart of the other, the "home of love," an "O" which promises the circle of return, reappropriation, homecoming—in the distance opened by the call and without which the call could not take place, finds the circle broken in an interruption which alone makes the call possible. This is the catastrophe of apostrophe as the very condition of apostrophe, the divisibility of the letter as the condition of the letter's dispatch, the circle of issue and receipt broken by the necessary crossing, or chiasmus, of destiny and chance: a game of noughts and crosses, absence and presence.

No precaution can entirely eliminate the chance of this indirection. Even the adoption of a secret code, or pet name, could not vouchsafe a message to a unique destinee, in as much as such a code or name would still have to be subject to a minimal requirement of decipherability. This is clearly the case at the moment when Shakespeare's poem might be said to be marking its destination, in the address to "thou, my rose." In a sequential reading of the Sonnets as they are ordered in the Quarto, this particular form of address, echoing after an interval the same address used frequently in the early sonnets, may be seen as reasserting the constancy of Shakespeare's feelings towards the same addressee, notwithstanding the absence—literal or figurative—recorded in line 2 of this sonnet and more fully treated in Sonnets 100–104, for instance. More precisely, as Shakespearean scholars tell us, it's possible that this "rose" marks the identity of Shakespeare's "sweet boy" as the Earl of Southampton, Henry Wriothesley, a name which in Shakespeare's time could be pronounced "rose-ly." But we would also have to note, among other things, that the address to "my rose" participates at the same time in a tradition of courtly love poetry.[8] In so far as we may decipher a proper name in this address, therefore, it only provides a particularly salient example of what we may call, after Derrida, the impropriety or commonality of the proper name, which can only succeed in naming to the extent that it compromises its claim to unique designation.[9]

Even a declaration of love, then, can only reach the other, touch the heart of the other, on the condition of possibly going astray, of being received by some other. We may also suggest, with Nancy, that love *is* that declaration, the promise of "I love you," a promise which, he stipulates, is not a performative:

> But "I love you" (which is the unique utterance of love and which is, at bottom, its name: love's name is not "love," which would be a substance or a faculty, but it is this sentence, the "I love you," just as one says "the cogito")—the "I love you" is something else. It is a promise. The promise, by constitution, is an utterance that draws itself back before the law that it lets appear. The promise neither describes nor prescribes nor performs. It does nothing and thus is always vain. But it lets a law appear, the law of the given word: that this must be.[10]

We might qualify this by saying that the promise of love is a performative in abeyance or, in a formulation to which I shall return shortly with the help of Derrida, that it is a promise of synchrony which is only possible on the basis of an anachrony that inhabits the promise, the anachrony that opens the future—of the passage from me to you , and of the uncertain fulfillment of the promise. It is in the uncertainty of that future that the promise may always touch some other. In other words, the promise of love can only be made with the risk of a certain *two-timing*. It so happens that Shakespeare's poem invites the question: what time is love?

At first sight, the poem would seem to have us believe that love is timeless, eternal: "Just to the time, not with the time exchanged." The line appears to reassert the writer's constancy, his touching fidelity, which dissolves the passage of time and completes the circle of departure and return in a single moment. But I want to argue that the logic of reading this poem compels us to a different understanding of love's timelessness, and for that matter, of the so-called timelessness of this love poem, which would only be timeless in the sense that its time always remains to be accomplished: a timelessness, therefore, which is historical through and through. This same line which appears to annul the passage of time requires itself to be read in two times, and demands that we read "time" twice, differently: time as punctual moment and time as interval or delay. And these two times must be read as inhabiting one another if one is to be able to read them at all. The chance of encountering the other, the chance of a declaration of love reaching the other, can only be sustained in this anachronous opening to reading, to the other. The promise of synchrony must be held open by anachrony.

Some passages from Derrida's "Aphorism Countertime" may help us here. I should just remark briefly that "aphorism" functions here in a manner analogous to what we have said about promises and declarations: in order to function here, now, it must be open to the time of the other: "I love because the other is the other, because its time will never be mine. The living duration, the very presence of its love remains infinitely distant from mine, distant from itself in that which stretches it toward mine and even in what one might want to describe as amorous euphoria, ecstatic communion, mystical intuition. I can love the other only in the passion of this aphorism. [. . .] Conversely, no contretemps, no aphorism without the promise of a now in common, without the pledge, the vow of synchrony, the desired sharing of a living present. In order that the sharing may be desired, must it not first be given, glimpsed, apprehended?"[11] Or to say it again, differently: I can only love because, from the outset, my time is never quite my own. I can only touch you because I never quite feel myself. I am already outside of myself: from the beginning, impure, corrupted, "stained." "My nature" is already unnatural, "preposterously" so, "preposterous"—a word of recent coinage in "Shakespeare's time," meaning "unnatural," "reversed," what should be "after" coming "before."

It is only on the condition of this anachronous promise of synchrony that I can "save thou," that I can hold you, and only you, apart from all that is not you. To "save thou" in this way, to hold you apart from all the destinations which my address may touch, to keep you safe from that indirection, I have to "save thou." But, in that same gesture, I have to run the risk that I may "save thou," that I may exclude you from that very address, which will have to take its chances to have that unique chance of "saving thou." Perhaps, recalling Nancy's elaboration of the promise of love cited earlier, love just *is* that risky address. Perhaps, Shakespeare's poem just *is* love, but above all not in the sense that it enacts what it appears to utter, nor indeed in the sense of a verbal icon which would embody what it appears to describe, for that would be precisely to forestall and thus to doom the promise of love: whence the necessity of a "perhaps." If the poem does hold out the promise of love, then it would be on the condition that it never quite accomplish itself as enactment or embodiment.

It is only on this same condition of the promise that I can touch "thou, my rose"; you—the other who precedes and secretly inhabits me, the other who is prior to self-identity and to the determinations of ontology, who survives the opposition of being and nothingness, "nothing" and "this wide universe." You who open and hold open the narcissistic relation, whom I love beyond myself—within beyond "my self." Let's get back in touch with Derrida one more time:

> When I speak to you, I touch you, and you touch me when I hear you, from however distant it comes to me, and even if it is by telephone or by letter. But of course, in order for me to be touched in this way by you, I have to be able to touch *myself*. In the "self-touching-you," the "self" is as indispensable as you. A being incapable of touching itself could not bend itself to that which absolutely unfolds it, to the totally other who, as totally other / like all others [*comme tout autre*], inhabits my heart as a stranger. It is necessary to love *oneself / each other* [*Il faut s'aimer*], says every "I love you," and without this (impossible) auto-affection, without the reflected experience of impossible auto-affection, without the ordeal of the possibility of this impossibility, there would be no love.[12]

It is only through these impossible crossings—of destiny and chance, of my time and your time, of me and you—that the circle of love may be held open. From me to you, sealed with a kiss, **X**

NOTES

1. Jacques Derrida, "Le Toucher" [Touch / to touch him], trans. Peggy Kamuf, in *Paragraph* 16:2 (1993): 122–57. It will be clear that my discussion is indebted to the work of Derrida in a more thoroughgoing manner than is attested in these notes. I implicitly rely, for example, on the related notions of iterability and destinerrance: for an account of iterability, see "Signature Event Context," in Derrida's *Limited Inc*, trans. Samuel Weber and Jeffrey Mehlman (Evanston, Ill.: Northwestern University Press, 1988), 1–23; destinerrance is especially prominent in the essays collected in Derrida's *The Post Card: From Socrates to Freud and Beyond*, trans. Alan Bass (Chicago: Chicago University Press, 1987).

2. Nancy introduces this formulation in his *Corpus* (Paris: Métailié, 1992), 36. I give Peggy Kamuf's translation of this passage, cited by Derrida in "Le Toucher" (137): "*To self-touch you* (and not 'oneself')—or again, identically, *to self-touch skin* (and not 'oneself'): such is the thinking that the body always forces to go further, always too far. In truth, it is thought itself that forces itself in this way, that dislocates itself: for all the weight, all the gravity of thought—which is itself a *weighing*—in the end goes toward nothing else than to *consenting the body*. (Exasperated consent.)"

3. Nancy, *Corpus*, 47. The necessity of interruption is repeated a few pages later: "Two bodies cannot simultaneously occupy the same place. Thus, not you and I at the same time at the place where I am writing, at the place where you

are reading, where I speak, where you listen. No contact without a gap" (41: my translations for this and the previous passage from *Corpus*).

4. "Che cos'è la poesia?" trans. Peggy Kamuf, in *A Derrida Reader: Between the Blinds*, ed. Peggy Kamuf (London and New York: Harvester Wheatsheaf, 1991), 222–37; this passage on 231. On the "invention of the heart," let us also note Nancy's remarks, in the section of his essay "Shattered Love" entitled "The Heart: Broken": "Actually, the heart is not broken, in the sense that it does not exist before the break [*brisure*]. But it is the break itself that makes the heart. The heart is not an organ, and neither is it a faculty. It is: that *I* is broken and traversed by the other in its innermost presence and at the outermost limits of its life. The beating of the heart—rhythm of the partition of being, syncope of the sharing of singularity—cuts across presence, life, consciousness. That is why thinking—which is nothing other than the *weighing* or testing of the limits, the ends, of presence, of life, of consciousness—thinking itself is love" ("Shattered Love" trans. Lisa Garbus and Simona Sawhney, in Nancy, *The Inoperative Community*, ed. Peter Connor (Minneapolis and London: University of Minnesota Press, 1991), 82–109; this passage on 99: translation modified. The French text of "L'amour en éclats" is in Nancy's *Une Pensée finie* (Paris: Galilée, 1990), 225–68.) I leave these lines without commentary for the moment, in the hope that the latter part of my discussion will at least echo them.

5. Derrida develops the notion of the *pas* as "step" and "not (a step)" in a number of essays, most notably in his text on Blanchot, from whom he inherits the term, entitled "Pas," collected in *Parages* (Paris: Galilée, 1986), 19–116.

6. But I mean to suggest that there is something at issue here quite other than such a limited transfiguration. To cite Nancy again, from "Shattered Love": "*I* do not return from [love] [Je *n'en reviens pas*—idiomatically, "I can't get over it"], and consequently, something of *I* has definitively got lost or split apart in its act of loving. That is undoubtedly why *I* return (if the image of return is even appropriate here), but *I* return broken: I come back to myself, or I come about [*j'adviens*], broken. The 'return' does not annul the break [*brisure*]; it neither repairs it nor sublates it, for the return in fact takes place only across the break itself, keeping it open. Love re-presents *I* to itself broken (and this is not a representation). It presents this to it: he, this subject, was touched, sliced into, in his subjectivity, and he *is* from then on, for the time of love, opened by this slice, broken or cracked, however slightly. He *is* so, which is to say that the break or the wound is not an accident, and neither is it a property that the subject could relate to himself. For the break is a break in what is proper to him [*sa propriété*] as subject; it is, essentially, an interruption of the process of relating oneself to oneself outside of oneself. From then on, *I* is *constituted broken*" (96: translation modified).

7. "Ulysses Gramophone: Hear Say Yes in Joyce," trans. Tina Kendall and Shari Benstock, in Jacques Derrida, *Acts of Literature*, ed. Derek Attridge (New York and London: Routledge, 1992), 256–309; this passage on 298.

8. On these points, see for example the editorial comment on line 2 of Sonnet 1 in John Kerrigan's edition of *The Sonnets and A Lover's Complaint* (Harmondsworth: Penguin, 1986), 170.

9. On the question of the proper name, see for example Derrida's *Signéponge/Signsponge*, trans. Richard Rand (New York: Columbia University Press, 1984).

10. Nancy, "Shattered Love," 100.

11. "Aphorism Countertime," trans. Nicholas Royle, in *Acts of Literature*, 414–33; this passage on 420–21.

12. Derrida, "Le toucher," 140.

Works Cited

Derrida, Jacques. *Signéponge / Signsponge*. Translated by Richard Rand. New York: Columbia University Press, 1984.

———. *Parages*. Paris: Galilée, 1986.

———. *The Post Card: From Socrates to Freud and Beyond*. Translated by Alan Bass. Chicago: Chicago University Press, 1987.

———. *Limited Inc*. Translated by Samuel Weber and Jeffrey Mehlman. Evanston, Ill.: Northwestern University Press, 1988.

———. "Che cos'è la poesia?" Translated by Peggy Kamuf, in *A Derrida Reader: Between the Blinds*. Edited by Peggy Kamuf. London and New York: Harvester Wheatsheaf, 1991, 222–37.

———. "Ulysses Gramophone: Hear Say Yes in Joyce." Translated by Tina Kendall and Shari Benstock. *Acts of Literature*. Edited by Derek Attridge. New York and London: Routledge, 1992, 256–309.

———. "Aphorism Countertime." Translated by Nicholas Royle. *Acts of Literature*, 414–33.

———. "Le Toucher" (Touch / to touch him). Translated by Peggy Kamuf. *Paragraph* 16:2 (1993): 122–57.

Nancy, Jean-Luc. *Une Pensée finie*. Paris: Galilée, 1990.

———. "Shattered Love." Translated by Lisa Garbus and Simona Sawhney. *The Inoperative Community*. Edited by Peter Connor. Minneapolis and London: Minnesota University Press, 1991, 82–109.

———. *Corpus*. Paris: Métailié, 1992.

Shakespeare, William. *The Sonnets and A Lover's Complaint*. Edited by John Kerrigan. Harmondsworth: Penguin, 1986.

II
EARS

*Tintern*abulation: Poetry Ringing in the Ears
SCOTT BREWSTER

IN HIS FOREWORD TO GEOFFREY HARTMAN'S *THE UNREMARKABLE Wordsworth*, Donald G. Marshall makes a potentially remarkable claim. He states that Hartman possesses an uncanny ear for sounds in poetry: "Hartman's gift is the power to hear echoes and to write a criticism as echo-chamber. This is not quite what is called 'intertextuality,' for what is at stake is not the disseminated play of signifiers, but having 'ears to hear.' "[1] Although he acknowledges that Hartman does not "become one" with the poet he is reading, Marshall contends that "any separation of the critic from the poet being read will interrupt and still the reverberations which animate the reading."[2] This ideal nonseparation of critic and poet, permitting poetry's echoes to ring out clearly, implies an intimate connection at a distance. Poetry's good vibrations bring the act of reading into being, its lines tingling with potential meaning. Literary analysis, and poetry, are inescapably woven into the structure of telecommunications: the phenomenon of touching, thinking, or feeling across distance touches upon the idea of the telegraph, the telephone, and telepathy, although Wordsworth's writing does not coincide historically with such technological and conceptual developments.

Marshall suggests a curious sort of intentionalism, proposing that reading is a matter of waiting for a collect call from the writer via a flawless literary telephone exchange. Yet questions remain: who or what might "call" in poetry, and what is the nature of this call? To alter the metaphorical mode of conveyance, Marshall exhibits a faith in a system of registered post by presuming that a poem, like a telephone call or letter, always reaches its addressee. At the same time, he suggests that a text's structure of address—its reverberations—"animate" or constitute its reading process. In a telecommunication network, signals may go astray or fail to reach their intended destination, since the possibility of what Jacques Derrida terms "destinerrance" accompanies every transmission.[3] Tracing this logic of misdirection through Derrida's work on poetry, Timothy Clark points out that "the movement of poetic communication, or rather experience, cannot be mapped onto a familiar tripartite division of sender, a relay and a receiver"; the poem brings "what it relates into being by force of its own event."[4] This posits an addressee who does not exist in advance of a text: thus the poetic event is less an authoritative dispatch than an act of chance or interruption that constitutes the reader. Keeping its ear open, the echo-chamber of criticism elicits and receives calls from poetry that are uncanny and incalculable. Returning to the ear (as echoes do), we might be able to reconfigure Marshall's remarks and propose poetry, echoing Nicholas Royle, as a strange and uncertain type of telephony.[5]

This essay listens into certain acts of calling in the poetry of Wordsworth, Coleridge, and Keats. It eavesdrops on "Lines Composed a Few Miles above Tintern Abbey" and "The Solitary Reaper," "Frost at Midnight" and "Ode to a Nightingale," poems attentive to music from a distance and which also hear themselves speak. In doing so, it sets up a dialogue with the critical assumptions underlying Marshall's comments. Resonant with tolling bells, echoes, and noises off, these poems locate the subject in an ecstatic, haunted sensorium. Each text longs to hear and to issue pure sound, to let itself reverberate with "dizzy raptures" and yet to speak authoritatively. Entranced by the call of the other to become a medium or communication channel, the text simultaneously privileges and radically dissolves the power of voice as the index of the subject's punctual integrity. The sweet, strange sounds of an otherness that is at once irreducibly remote and intimate, belated and immediate, traverse the poems' temporal and spatial relations, and they ring with uncanny (h)earsay. The notion of invisible communication, of reading at a distance in a fashion that disorders space and time, can be understood not only in thematic terms but also as structurally necessary in these texts. The problem of trying to get in touch with the poets behind these intensely meditative poems (which are nonetheless addressed to someone) is that the reverberation of poetry is precisely that which interrupts or disorders critical analysis.

As Derrida notes in *The Ear of the Other*, "[t]he ear is uncanny . . . an organ for perceiving difference."[6] Observing that the ear "can make or let happen . . . [it] is the most tendered and open organ" (33), he elaborates a notion of otobiography, whereby the *autos* of autobiographical discourse (associated with the speaking subject) becomes transformed into *otos*, the structure of the ear. In a discussion of Nietzsche's *Ecce Homo* and *On the Future of Our Educational Institutions*, Derrida discerns otobiography as a matter of committing one's name and one's writing to the future, (perhaps impossibly) anticipating its reception in advance. As he points out, the testamentary survival and comprehension of Nietzsche's work depend upon the reader countersigning these texts in the writer's own name:

> it is the ear of the other that signs. The ear of the other says me to me and constitutes the autos of my autobiography. When, much later, the other will have perceived with a keen-enough ear what I will have addressed or destined to him or her, then my signature will have taken place. (51)

Derrida contends that every text answers to and articulates this testamentary structure. As in autobiography, whose "signature is entrusted to the other, one who comes along so late and is so unknown," a text is "signed only much later by the other" (51). Thus identity, and textuality in general, are always mediated through and by otherness, the self's articulation consigned to the keen, but undesignated, ears of posterity.

As Derrida insists we hear, the oscillation between hearing and speaking characterizes for Nietzsche the relationship between state, teacher, and student:

> You must pay heed to the fact that the *omphalos* that Nietzsche compels you to envision resembles both an ear and a mouth. It has the invaginated folds and the involuted orificiality of both. Its centre preserves itself at the bottom of an invisible, restless cavity that is sensitive to all waves which, whether or not they come from the outside, whether they are emitted or received, are always transmitted by this trajectory of obscure circumvolutions. (36)

Nietzsche envisages the university system as an "umbilical cord." Linked to the paternal body of the state, the student is induced into the role of teleprinter, with the teacher (who merely simulates the mother) dictating "the very thing that passes through your ears and travels the length of the cord all the way down to your stenography" (35–36). This stenography is both dictation and utterance: what your ears transcribe is what the master deciphers of a text that precedes him, and from which he is suspended by a similar umbilical cord.

This umbilical dependence of paternal genealogy simultaneously appropriates maternal power and acknowledges that autobiographical discourse inherits itself from two parents, a mother and a father. The ears of the writer, and the hearing of posterity, must be attuned to this double signing. As Derrida observes, in *Ecce Homo* Nietzsche effectively declares that "I am two, my father and my mother" (53). Of necessity, the *autos* proclaims "I am the (masculine) dead the living (feminine) and I am destined to them" (21). The educational establishment requires equally keen ears to discern this destiny. The academy must nurture, and let itself be nurtured by, the national mother tongue, a domain "in which the pupil must learn to act correctly" (22). Although similar to the double signing at work in autobiography, Nietzsche's testamentary structure of learning more explicitly treasures and effaces the "living feminine." Derrida comments that woman "never appears at any point along the umbilical cord, either to study or to teach." The mother is both a faceless extra and a constitutive echo in the system:

> She gives rise to all the figures by losing herself in the background of the scene like an anonymous persona. Everything comes back to her, beginning with life; everything addresses and destines itself to her. She survives on the condition of remaining at bottom. (38)

Plugged complicitly into the academy, a "criticism as echo-chamber" must avoid becoming an empty shell for the mother tongue purified of the figure of the maternal. To recall this figure who lives silently on, we must come back to her through the ripples of her echo. To hear this figure ring through poetry, we must have keen ears.

To sound out the otopoetics—the reception of an other's signature and acts of countersigning—that Derrida traces, we might start by paging Wordsworth's tintinnabulatory poem, which responds to an earlier call pealing across the West Country. "Frost at Midnight,"[7] one of Coleridge's "Conversation" poems dated February 1798, takes a few months to elicit a return call: "Tintern Abbey"[8] is dated July 1798. In the opening line of "Tintern," sound is both secondary and generative. The "sweet inland murmur" resounding in the inner ear re-presents, as if for the first time, a "wild secluded scene." Sound has a calming, benign effect on the inner eye: the eye can be "made quiet by the power / Of harmony" (48–49). This harmonious power mutes or filters out "the din / Of towns and cities" (26–27), curing the tinnitus of "the fretful stir / Unprofitable, the fever of the world" (53–54). Nature can also entrance and overwhelm hearing: the speaker is passionately haunted by "The sounding cataract" (77). Here overpowering sound evokes the veiling of the eye: Hartman argues that the "inner voice" of Wordsworth's poetry points both to visionary sight and the fear of a terrible blindness.[9]

Predominantly, however, hearing makes one see, in a prophetic and educational sense:

> For I have learned
> To look on nature, not as in the hour
> Of thoughtless youth, but hearing oftentimes
> The still sad music of humanity,
> Not harsh nor grating, though of ample power
> To chasten and subdue.
>
> (89–94)

The poet learns to look by listening, an obedient student of this "music" that nature passes down the years. The poet declares himself a lover

> of all the mighty world
> Of eye and ear, both what they half-create,
> And what perceive; well pleased to recognise
> In Nature and the language of the sense
> The anchor of my purest thoughts, the nurse,
> The guide, the guardian of my heart, and soul
> Of all my moral being.
>
> (108–12)

The ear produces and perceives, constructing and learning from the language of sense. Nature nurtures and instructs, a moral guardianship replicated by the poet, who receives and imparts this mother tongue to a "dear sister." Harold Bloom reads "Tintern Abbey" through his map of misprision as a "Scene of Instruction,"[10] a text countersigning its poetic precursor and countersigned by its successors. According to Bloom, the poem functions within poetic tradition as an echo-chamber: "I suspect that 'Tintern Abbey' is the modern poem proper, and that most good poems written in English since 'Tintern Abbey' inescapably repeat, rewrite, or revise it."[11] The poem's testamentary structure consigns itself to another through repetition and generation, revision and singularity. The spectrum of soothing and haunting sounds echoes the text's movement between retrospection and projection. The murmuring Wye not only reawakens the "aching joys" of "my boyish days" (74), it animates "pleasing thoughts / That in this moment there is life and food / For future years" (64–66). The poem's echo-chamber sets the ear ringing with "recognitions dim and faint" (60) and resonates with "unremembered pleasure" (32).

The visionary possibilities of hearing are given clearest articulation in the closing lines, when the subject contemplates being out of earshot of the addressee yet still projects a scene in which its voice is preserved:

> and in after years,
> When these wild ecstasies shall be matured
> Into a sober pleasure, when thy mind
> Shall be a mansion for all lovely forms,
> Thy memory be as a dwelling-place
> For all sweet sound and harmonies, oh! then,
> If solitude, or fear, or pain, or grief,
> Should be thy portion, with what healing thoughts
> Of tender joy wilt thou remember me,
> And these my exhortations! Nor, perchance,
> If I should be where I no more can hear
> Thy voice, nor catch from thy wild eyes these gleams
> Of past existence, wilt thou then forget
> That on the banks of this delightful stream
> We stood together, and that I, so long
> A worshipper of Nature, hither came
> Unwearied in that service—rather say
> With warmer love, oh!, with far deeper zeal
> Of holier love. Nor wilt thou then forget,
> That after many wanderings, many years
> Of absence, these steep woods and lofty cliffs,
> And this green pastoral landscape, were to me
> More dear, both for themselves, and for thy sake.
> (138–60)

Similarly to the poem's opening, the ear is conceived as both passive and active, derivative and constitutive. The poem searches for a posthumous line through to the future, a connection that depends upon an ear that listens and an ear that signs, on hooking up with a "dear sister" who can receive *and* produce its memorable message: "Nor wilt thou then forget." It anticipates the "sweet sounds" it commits to the memory banks of the future.

The beloved sister, putative beneficiary of the text's "will," is expected to hold the line, lending a keen ear (like the reader) to the harmonies bestowed by this poetry. In the testamentary structure of this poetic meditation, the sister is destined to become the ear of the other that signs.[12]

Like the nurturing mother tongue of Nature, this female inheritance differs markedly from the patrilineal descent that perpetuates the educational system as envisaged by Nietzsche. Anonymous, silent but guaranteeing life, the feminine is inseparable from the figure of the reader, invoked and erased by the text's self-narration. By calling to its descendants, this poetry of the future attempts to live on, to sign or reproduce itself, to determine or guarantee its reception in the ear. This signing depends upon the ear of its absent other, the feminine that will outlive the masculine voice, who will have ears to listen "If I should be where I no more can hear" (148). The sensual, progenitive reading of the ear, eternally entrusts one's name to the maternal, the living feminine survivor.

The ear's relation to death, posterity, instruction, gender, and prophetic vision echoes through Coleridge's "Frost at Midnight." The strangely apposite thing about this poem about strangeness is that it conducts a conversation with precisely no one. The inmates of the cottage are at rest, leaving the speaker to address a sleeping "Babe" that cannot hear. All save the speaker are enjoying some shut-eye, or rather shut-ear. For all the emphasis on calm, the frost's windless ministry and the reiteration of "quiet" in the closing line, the text's solitude and silence is perturbing: "Tis calm indeed! so calm, that it disturbs / And vexes meditation with its strange / And extreme silentness" (8–10). The slumbering infant's gentle breathings remain audible in the text's "deep calm," and possess the power to fill up "the interspersèd vacancies / And momentary pauses of the thought" (45–47). The "stranger" that "flutters" on the grate (a piece of soot) makes itself heard at the very center of domestic or family space. The anthropomorphic stranger's unsettling of the silence is both close and remote, and the disturbance brought about by this "sole unquiet thing" (16) constitutes noise from nowhere: the motion of the ghostly familiar, which according to Coleridge's note portends the arrival of an absent friend, issues from and arrives at no specified location.

In this disquieting midnight, "the numberless goings-on of life" are "Inaudible as dreams" (12–13). The speaker's recounted daydreams are highly audible, however: they resound with memories of

> the old church-tower,
> Whose bells, the poor man's only music, rang
> From morning to evening, all the hot fair-day,
> So sweetly, that they stirred and haunted me
> With a wild pleasure, falling on mine ear
> Most like articulate sounds of things to come!
>
> (28–33)

The wild pleasures produced by these sweet sounds are uncannily "Presageful"(25), fondly remembered yet still heard. They mimic the sensual rapture anticipated for the infant:

> so shalt thou see and hear
> The lovely shapes and sounds intelligible
> Of that eternal language, which thy God
> Utters, who from eternity doth teach
> Himself in all, and all things in himself.
> Great Universal Teacher! he shall mold
> Thy spirit, and by giving make it ask.
>
> (58–64)

Calling on the eye, ear, and mouth, learning involves "giving" in a double sense. The Universal Teacher imparts "eternal language"; the pupil's ear gives to (receives) this teaching, but also gives (donates) to the ear a response and gives that language life. The text's paternal network recalls Nietzsche's "umbilical cord of the university." In the poem, the speaker's vision anticipates and performs this process of induction, the teacher whispers right into the ear-duct, in fact. This projects the child as receiver of eternal wisdom, a situation that demands the infant respond to an invocation at the utmost distance. Yet what should the infant need to "ask" if the message is merely relayed as if by teleprinter? The text proposes an ear which dictates and generates a voice: in this scene of instruction, one does not just receive the other's voice or signature, one must also produce it. Deriving in Coleridge's poem from a Universal Teacher who "doth teach / Himself in all," learning transmits itself through a combination of inherited tradition and autodidactism. Thus neither teacher, speaker, nor infant are transformed into "a diaphanous mouthpiece of eternal pedagogy" (*Ear of the Other*, 4). Eternal language speaks itself through master and student, father and son, speaker and listener, a patrilineal cord whose ear depends upon the "invaginated folds" and "involuted orificiality" of a feminine biotechnology. The immanence of this mother tongue is countersigned, its line of credit extended, by a living feminine that overhears.

"Frost at Midnight" chimes with such an umbilical structure. As Richard A. Rand remarks, the text opens and closes with the effects of signature,[13] underlining the complex sense of lineage at work in the poem. Induced to "see and hear" by the Universal Teacher, the speaker transcribes the wild and haunting pleasures of the past and bestows them on the infant. The abstruse schoolday musings are consigned to a futurity: the poem's subject hears these articulate sounds spontaneously, yet in remembering countersigns its childhood self, rendering it posthumous. The entrancing church bells, ostensibly recalling the idle fancies of youth, sound the listener's death knell, the impress of its "silent icicles" (73) resonating through the poem. The bells haunt the self, tolling out its own "strange / And extreme silentness." The text meditates on the message it can bequeath to the future; in sweet seasons to come, who will have ears to hear "the eave-drops fall" in "trances of the blast" (70–71)? Where, in fact, does the poem's uncanny, silent communication network end? Only the text's spectral presence, the "secret ministry of frost" (72), enjoys an acoustics beyond static and interference: it possesses the power to "freeze" the sound of falling eave-drops. Stirred by the text's "shapes and sounds intelligible," it is the reader who eave(s)drops on the poem's traffic, lodged like a listening device that records and rewrites what it overhears. To return to Derrida's aural topography, this positions the reader as a restless ear sensitive to all waves. The reader is a ghostly listener; in registering the poem's posthumous endurance, we simultaneously hear our own death and live on, transmitting our own posterity, in the present of its utterance. In its restlessness, "Frost at Midnight" has less confidence than "Tintern Abbey" that someone will tune into its frequency when its speaker is no longer around to "hear."

Keats's "Ode to a Nightingale"[14] concludes by echoing down another valley, ringing once more with invisible communication, attributable in this case only to a disembodied voice divorced from any stable, originating source or location. The poem exemplifies Shelley's notion of the poet as a nightingale "who sits in darkness and sings to cheer its own solitude with sweet sounds."[15] As in "Tintern Abbey" and "Frost at Midnight," hearing in Keats's ode is equated with prophetic or entrancing inner sight: the "viewless wings of poesy" (33) suggests a visionary blindness, yet the poem wavers between synaesthetic delight and a painful, intoxicating excess. The ode is subject to a form of sensory deprivation, afflicted by a ringing in the ears and an indistinct field of vision. Unseen, pure breath or airy spirit, the nightingale is in the act of departure. Even as its song inspires with rapture, it fades away. The enchanting but deathly sound of this intangible creature is buried, its voice issuing from the "embalmèd darkness" (43) that the speaker imagines as an ideal resting place. A phantasmal "Dryad" or "Darkling," the nightingale's plaintive anthem drifts out of the text until it is "buried deep / In the next valley glades" (77–78). As in "Frost at Midnight," ringing bells drown out phantasies of immortality or self-identicality. The word "forlorn," "utterly lost" in its archaic sense,[16] implies that poetry has revoked its claims to assume an ecstatic, transcendent voice: it is irreducible to a "self-same song," and sounds a "forlorn" warning bell "To toll me back from thee to my sole self" (72). Silence beckons the poem back to its own solitude, suggesting Maurice Blanchot's sense of a poetic language that does not speak:

> The defining characteristic of ordinary language is that listening comprises part of its very nature. But at this point of literature's space, language is not to be heard. Hence the risk of the poetic function. The poet is he who hears a language which makes nothing heard.[17]

A graphic silence is also discernible by leafing through the text's "verdurous glooms," as if by turning the pages of a directory for a missing entry. Although Eleanor Cook[18] has traced the ways in which the motif of a heavenly bird has been deployed in poetry, one intertextual echo not generally made to be heard by critics in relation to Keats's nightingale is that of Philomel. Her silence "So rudely forced,"[19] Philomel is an analogue of tongueless desire, her fate a fable of primal silence and violence. Mute and invisible, the figure of Philomel is nonetheless voiced, resonating with uncanny insistence. This insistence may be attributed to what Jean-François Lyotard describes as "the effect on language of the force exerted by the figural," a force which "hinders hearing but makes us see." The figure of Philomel may thus function as "a tongue lost in a hallucinatory scenography, the first violence."[20] The myth of Philomel commits a haunting signature to the future, one that the nightingale's song validates or countersigns.

Violent echoes that gather around a mysterious female figure ring across yet another "vale profound" in Wordsworth's "The Solitary Reaper."[21] The "Highland lass" overwhelms the valley with plaintive songs of "old, unhappy, far-off things / And battles long ago" (19–20). Sweeter than the nightingale or the cuckoo, the young woman's "melancholy strain" is an enchanting but foreign tongue. Her enigmatic song commends a legacy for the poet to countersign:

> Whate'er the theme, the maiden sang
> As if her song could have no ending;
> I saw her singing at her work,
> And o'er her sickle bending;
> I listened till I had my fill,
> And as I mounted up the hill,
> The music in my heart I bore
> Long after it was heard no more.
>
> (25–32)

Bent over her sickle, this "maiden" harvests her inheritance. She resembles a Mother Time that severs the paternal umbilicus, her voice commemorating the ruins of masculinity that lie scattered over ancient battlefields. The poem has no ear for the father, its song resounding through a solitary female voice. As representatives of the living feminine, singer, poet, and reader connect with and cut the patronymic cord. Although "everything addresses and destines itself to her" this young woman, unlike Nietzsche's feminine, does not lose herself in the background of the scene. In her, this enduring music originates, survives, and returns. O'er-brimming vessels, maternal carriers, our ringing ears bear the song into the future. Registering in the hollow of the ear, heard but also disturbing and transforming the utterance of the text, these nightingales constitute (like the sister in "Tintern Abbey" and both speaker and child in Coleridge) the ear of the other that signs.

The nightingale's enigmatic transmissions, and the difficulty of dictating a message from "beyond," perform the telephonic reading experience instituted by "Ode to a Nightingale" and "The Solitary Reaper." Each poem sends forth a barely audible call from no place, its echoes frustrating the ear and veiling the eye, yet nevertheless provoking a response from an addressee who has picked up the receiver. Their leavings of voice, and their conversations with "Tintern Abbey" and "Frost at Midnight," perhaps illustrate Roland Barthes's reflections on telephonic communication:

> on the telephone the other is always in a situation of departure; the other departs twice over, by voice and by silence: whose turn is it to speak? We fall silent in unison: crowding of two voids. I'm *going to leave you*, the voice on the telephone says with each second.[22]

Haunted by the void of separation and silence, their lines full yet consigned to an uncertain destination and recipient, these poems depart like Barthes's telephone conversations. To risk nonarrival or misdirection, to reverberate posthumously: such lost connections echo the fate of writing. This seems a likely cue to ring off: now it is the turn of another to call.

NOTES

1. Donald A. Marshall, foreword to Geoffrey H. Hartman, *The Unremarkable Wordsworth* (London: Methuen, 1987), ix.
2. Marshall, *The Unremarkable Wordsworth*, ix.
3. On the logic of the epistolary and telecommunication, see Derrida's *The Post Card: From Socrates to Freud and Beyond*, trans. Alan Bass (Chicago: University of Chicago Press, 1987) and "Telepathy," trans. Nicholas Royle, *Oxford Literary Review* 10 (1988): 3–41.
4. Timothy Clark, "By Heart: A Reading of Derrida's 'Che Cos'è la poesia' through Keats and Celan," *Oxford Literary Review* 15: 1–2 (1993): 67.
5. Nicholas Royle, *Telepathy and Literature: Essays on the Reading Mind* (Oxford: Basil Blackwell, 1991), especially 162–79.
6. Jacques Derrida, *The Ear of the Other*, trans. Peggy Kamuf and Avital Ronnell, ed. Christie V. McDonald (Lincoln and London: University of Nebraska Press, 1988), 33, 51. Further references will be given in the text.
7. Samuel Taylor Coleridge, *Select Poetry and Prose*, ed. Stephen Potter (London: Nonesuch, 1971), 79–81. Subsequent quotations from this work are cited parenthetically in the text.
8. William Wordsworth, *Selected Poems*, ed. D. W. Davies (London: J. M. Dent, 1994), 114–18. Subsequent quotations from this work are cited parenthetically in the text.
9. Hartman, *The Unremarkable Wordsworth*, 22.
10. Harold Bloom, "The Scene of Instruction: 'Tintern Abbey,'" in *William Wordsworth: Modem Critical Views*, ed. Harold Bloom (New York: Chelsea House, 1985), 123.
11. Bloom, "Scene of Instruction," 118.
12. See also John Barrell's discussion of Dorothy's "use" in "Tintern Abbey," in *Poetry, Language, and Politics* (Manchester: Manchester University Press,1988), 141–67.

13. Richard A. Rand, "Geraldine," in *Untying the Text: A Post-structuralist Reader*, ed. Robert Young (London: Routledge, 1981), 312.
14. John Keats, *The Complete Poems*, ed. John Barnard (Harmondsworth: Penguin, 1986), 346–48. Subsequent quotations from this work are cited parenthetically in the text.
15. Percy Bysshe Shelley, "A Defence of Poetry," in *Poetry and Prose*, ed. S. Reiman and J. Powers (New York: Norton, 1977), 486.
16. Barnard, in Keats, *The Complete Poems*, 657n.
17. Maurice Blanchot, *The Space of Literature*, trans. Ann Smock (Lincoln and London: University of Nebraska Press, 1989), 51–52.
18. Eleanor Cook, "Birds in Paradise: Uses of Allusion in Milton, Keats, Whitman, Stevens and Ammons," *Studies in Romanticism* 26: 3 (1987): 421–33.
19. T. S. Eliot, "The Waste Land," in *Collected Poems 1909–1962* (London: Faber, 1985), 66.
20. Jean-François Lyotard, "The Dream-work Does Not Think," trans. Mary Lydon, *Oxford Literary Review* 6: 1 (1983): 32.
21. Wordsworth, *Selected Poems*, 301. Subsequent quotations from this work are cited parenthetically in the text.
22. Roland Barthes, *A Lover's Discourse: Fragments*, trans. Richard Howard (London: Jonathan Cape, 1979), 114–15.

WORKS CITED

Barrell, John. *Poetry, Language and Politics*. Manchester: Manchester University Press, 1988.

Barthes, Roland. *A Lover's Discourse: Fragments*. Translated by Richard Howard London: Jonathan Cape, 1979.

Blanchot, Maurice. *The Space of Literature*. Translated by Ann Smock. Lincoln and London: University of Nebraska Press, 1989.

Bloom, Harold. "The Scene of Instruction: 'Tintern Abbey.'" *William Wordsworth: Modern Critical Views*. Edited by Harold Bloom. New York: Chelsea House, 1985, 113–35.

Clark, Timothy. "By Heart: A Reading of Derrida's 'Che Cos'è la poesia' through Keats and Celan." *Oxford Literary Review* 15, nos. 1–2 (1993): 43–78.

Coleridge, Samuel Taylor. *Select Poetry and Prose*. Edited by Stephen Potter. London: Nonesuch, 1971.

Cook, Eleanor. "Birds in Paradise: Uses of Allusion in Milton, Keats, Whitman, Stevens, and Ammons." *Studies in Romanticism* 26, no. 3 (1987): 421–33.

Derrida, Jacques. *The Post Card: From Socrates to Freud and Beyond*. Translated by Alan Bass. Chicago: University of Chicago Press, 1987.

Derrida, Jacques. "Telepathy." Translated by Nicholas Royle, *Oxford Literary Review* 10 (1988): 3–41.

Derrida, Jacques. *The Ear of the Other*. Translated by Peggy Kamuf and Avital Ronnell. Edited by Christie V. McDonald. Lincoln and London: University of Nebraska Press, 1988.

Eliot, T. S. *Collected Poems 1909–1962*. London: Faber, 1974.

Hartman, Geoffrey. *The Unremarkable Wordsworth*. London: Methuen, 1987.

Keats, John. *The Complete Poems*. Edited by John Barnard. Harmondsworth: Penguin, 1984.

Lyotard, Jean-François. "The Dream-work Does Not Think." Translated by Mary Lydon. *Oxford Literary Review* 6, no. 1 (1983): 3–34.

Rand, Richard A. "Geraldine." *Untying the Text: a Post-Structuralist Reader*. Edited by Robert Young. London: Routledge, 1981.

Royle, Nicholas. *Telepathy and Literature: Essays on the Reading Mind*. Oxford: Blackwell, 1990.

Shelley, Percy Bysshe. "A Defence of Poetry." *Poetry and Prose*. Edited by S. Reiman and J. Powers. New York: Norton, 1977.

Wordsworth, William. *Selected Poems*. Edited by D. W. Davies. London: J. M. Dent, 1994.

Bodies of Resonance
RACHEL JONES

> I do not see the history of the West as homogeneous. There have been singularities within it. Openings come from the writings of some familiar philosophers, such as Nietzsche, Diderot, Kierkegaard, Bergson or Foucault. But we need also to look in some unfamiliar places: in texts by past women writers who register that they must count as abnormal, peculiar or singular in terms of the dominant models of the self—and then go on to make imaginative or theoretical adjustments. (Christine Battersby, *The Phenomenal Woman: Feminist Metaphysics and the Patterns of Identity*)

IN THE ABOVE PASSAGE, THE FEMINIST PHILOSOPHER CHRISTINE Battersby stresses the importance of locating subversive "openings" within the history of the Western subject if woman is not to be continually positioned as the "other" of a masculinized self. Battersby also emphasizes that women writers who themselves "register" the singularity of their identity in relation to the dominant norms of selfhood can work with the "radical transformative potential" offered by the very difference/s they embody.[1] In what follows, I will suggest that the much-neglected work of the German expressionist writers Paula Ludwig and Claire Goll constitutes one of the "unfamiliar places" we might look to find such openings in the history of the West. More specifically, I will focus on the ways in which these two writers use images of music subversively to explore the constitution of selves and of texts.

Through images of sound, resonance, and touch, Ludwig and Goll radically rework the subject's relation to materiality as well as to difference, thus transforming the space-time of the self. In the first section of this chapter, I will site this transformative work in relation to the feminist philosophy of Luce Irigaray. Subsequent sections will then examine particular texts by Ludwig and Goll in detail. In the case of Ludwig, I will argue that her poetry disrupts and reworks a specifically Kantian model of the modern subject, whereas I will suggest that Goll's work subverts an oppositional model of identity whose genealogy stretches back through Western metaphysics to Plato. I will begin, however, with a brief biographical introduction to Ludwig and Goll, which will aim to make them a little less unfamiliar.

Paula Ludwig (b. 1900, Altenstadt, Austria; d. 1974, Darmstadt) and Claire Goll (b. 1891, Nürnberg; d. 1977, Paris) are two of the many women who participated in and contributed to the literary, artistic, and cultural activities of German expressionism. However, like many of the women whose part in this diverse and explosive movement has been virtually forgotten, Paula Ludwig's richly poetic voice has been silenced in the history of European modernism. There exists a collected edition of her writings, which includes a short biographical essay,[2] but apart from a few short articles and despite winning the George Trakl prize in 1962, her work has received little critical attention, in either English or German. In this paper, I will explore poems from her collection *Die selige Spur*, published in 1920.[3]

Claire Goll, on the other hand, has a somewhat notorious place in literary history as the self-appointed muse and guardian of the work of her more famous husband, the expressionist and surrealist Yvan Goll. Perhaps best known for her scandalous and often hilarious autobiography (*Ich Verzeihe Keinem*), comparatively little attention has been paid to her as a poet and writer of fiction except as the coauthor of several texts with Yvan.[4] Recently, much of her work has been republished, and there has been a resurgence of interest in her writing. This is primarily reflected in two studies: the 1994 conference and subsequent book, *Yvan Goll—Claire Goll: Texts and Contexts*, which includes an insightful essay by Margaret Littler using Irigaray to analyze the gendering of Claire Goll's relation to literary modernism; and a booklength study of Goll's early work by Verena Mahlow, published in 1996.[5] These studies notwithstanding, however, there has been little research focusing on the particular early texts which I will examine here, namely, some poems from her collection *Mitwelt* (1918), and a short story, *Der Gläserne Garten* (1919).[6]

Ludwig's life became interwoven with that of Claire Goll in the 1930s, when Paula Ludwig became the lover of Claire's husband, Yvan. The painful relationship of these two female authors in later years, a relationship constructed around a dominant male figure, has overshadowed the ways in which they are linked more productively through their early writings, where their voices resonate with shared subversions. In the specific texts to be analyzed here, both Goll and Ludwig use music to dislocate the notion of a stable, autonomous, and self-contained subject. Read with the French philosopher Luce Irigaray, such dislocations are clearly gendered: they displace identity constructed via boundaries that exclude difference, including sexual difference, only to re/contain it as the other of the same.

In her book *Speculum of the Other Woman*, Irigaray weaves her way through the history of Western philosophy, showing how the seemingly genderless, universal category of the human subject both depends on and erases difference exactly because it privileges the sameness of all subjects.[7] The subject depends on marking himself off from that which is other and on making the other a reflection, albeit inverted, of himself, to reaffirm his view of himself and his world. Irigaray offers a compelling account of the ways in which woman has functioned as the other and the object against which Western metaphysics has constituted its (male) subject; thus, to borrow a chapter title from *Speculum*, "Any Theory of the 'Subject' Has Always Been Appropriated By the 'Masculine.' "[8] The normative maleness of the subject is consistently affirmed via his constitutive opposition to the figure of woman, while this opposition simultaneously excludes sexual difference from the realm of proper selfhood and perpetuates the myth that the human subject is a neutral and universal ideal. Woman cannot be added into the category of the subject because the specificity of embodied sexual difference can be seen only as interfering with the purity of the "self-as-same."

Irigaray's subversive mimicking of the patriarchal genealogy of the subject brings into view the ways in which woman's potential for disruption has been contained by an endlessly convoluted variety of moves, each of which has redefined her differences in the subject's terms. Woman is lack or excess, monstrous materiality or maternal corporeality, *jouissance* or threat, but always that "otherness" against which the boundaries of a masculinized subject are secured. When man gets bored by the limits of an identity he has set up just a little too securely, the feminine can also represent a space where the bounds of his ego can be transcended and his identity reworked. Always an object and never a subject, woman is a resource for extending both man's knowledge and his subjectivity.

Irigaray asks what would happen if woman refused to be positioned by a male gaze as the other and object of the subject; she asks what would happen if this object started to speak.[9] She suggests that between subject and object, self and other, there may be spaces for another self, one that refuses and exceeds the masculine logic of an oppositionally constituted self-as-same. However, I would agree with Christine Battersby that Irigaray's own analysis tends to homogenize the history of Western philosophy, such that it "remains the expression of a seamless masculine imaginary."[10] Thus Irigaray makes it difficult to see the spaces within different philosophical systems as well as within the imagination of the West more generally where woman's excessive "otherness" could become productively disruptive. In what follows, I will argue that both Ludwig and Goll produce such disruptions, exploring modes of spatial and temporal organization that are radically different from those which generate the oppositional subject-object relations that secure the identity of the autonomous, masculinized self. I will suggest that in this way, these authors can be read as generating "imaginative adjustments" with rich implications for the theorizing of the self and its relation to the matter of the senses. In particular, both writers use images of music to explore alternative modes of subjectivity, opening spaces for difference and for potentially female selves.

In his introduction to the first edition of *Die selige Spur*, Hermann Kasack describes Ludwig as the "naive nature of woman" through which the "simple voice of the people" speaks:

> Although it seems obvious [. . .], that here the naive nature of woman [. . .] is revealed, yet it still might be worth adding as an aside [. . .]: the poetess Paula Ludwig had no knowledge of any exemplary literature. [. . .] in her is risen again the simple voice of the people, which speaks untouched by foreign things, united only by the word.[11]

This gendered account of literary genius privileges Ludwig precisely because she lacks any active artistic capacity. Her supposed lack of training contributes to making her the archetypal woman writer for Kasack: she is a passive vehicle for "the people's" unmediated simplicity and will not interfere with their voice through any literary inventiveness of her own. Kasack finally reduces her to a channel for the "Blood of eternity: *Vox humana*."[12]

In this way, Kasack constructs Ludwig's female nature as unformed and unknowing receptive matter, through which an eternal genealogy of humanity can be propagated. She is the instrument through which the pure voice of the "human" spirit can resound without (her) interference. However, her mute passivity as the material through which this voice is transmitted excludes her from being properly part of its active, vocal, and incorporeal identity. As Irigaray has shown, this structure whereby female matter acts as the necessary (and necessarily excluded) ground of a "universal" humanity has underpinned Western metaphysics from Plato on—Kasack is certainly not alone. However, as I will show, Ludwig's texts themselves work to destabilize both the construction of receptive matter as inertly passive, and the notion of a single and unified "human" voice.[13] In one of her most powerful poems, Ludwig uses a musical image to disrupt the specific construction of the modern, Enlightenment subject:

> Die Ferne steht, eine blaue Harfe,
> in die deine schlafenden Sinne greifen.
> Mond verweilt zwischen den Saiten,
> den tönenden Wimpern deiner Augen.
>
> Grau ist die Stadt und Regen
> hängt über den Häusern.
> Keine Spur zeugt von der Nähe der Sonne,
> und keine Hand hebt mir ihr Leuchten.
>
> Aber die Ferne steht, eine blaue Harfe.
> Durch den blaßen Tag tönt es mich an
> und füllt meine Seele.

[The distance stands, a blue harp, / played by your sleeping senses. / Moon lingers between the strings, / the resonating lashes of your eyes. // Grey is the town and rain / hangs over the houses. / No trace shows the nearness of the sun, / and no hand lifts its light towards me. // But the distance stands, a blue harp. / Through the pale day sounds reach me / and fill my soul.][14]

In the first stanza of this poem, the other who is addressed is positioned as both playing the strings of the harp, the figure of distance, and as being the harp: her eyelashes are the resonating strings. The image of the strings of the harp contributes to the tension produced in the very first line: its blueness confirms a notion of distance evoking the wide spaces of the horizon, the sky or even the sea. However, this "wide blue yonder" is curiously static—"es steht," "it stands"—and the harp itself suggests a spatiality divided between the lines of the strings: the blue distance seems here to be already divided up as if by a grid. When the strings later become the eyelashes of the sleeping self addressed by the poet, they form a kind of grid through which this slumbering one sees, a frame for dreaming eyes. This framed gaze held *within* the strings/lashes is thus differentiated from the sleeping senses which play the strings as if from *outside* or above.

These images of a divided and organized subjectivity recall a particular version of the modern Enlightenment subject. The notion of a framework organizing spatiality together with a self that is structurally split between the framed gaze and the unknowing senses invokes not so much the Cartesian attempt at self-presence in the *cogito*, as the Kantian model of the transcendental subject. Hence in what follows, I will show how the specificity of Ludwig's disruptive images, particularly that of the resonating strings or lashes, can most productively be read within the context of Kant's philosophy of the subject.

For Kant, human subjects can never know either themselves or objects unconditionally; man has no immediate access to "things in themselves" or to the ideal noumenal realm beyond the conditions of human perception. However, the senses do provide us with access to the phenomenal world, the world of appearances, through a manifold of sensory intuition. To make sense of this world at all, it is necessary to posit a stable subject who exists though time. This subject functions as a permanent *structural* reference point to which all perceptions can be related. At the same time, however, as this subject is never simply "given" as such, to position ourselves as permanent subjects we must also construct *objects* of perception. The imagination schematizes (or maps) the manifold of sensory intuition in ways that allow for the configuration of an external world of objects that remain stable enough both in space, and across time, for an enduring subject to be posited against them as a single perceiving consciousness. The Kantian subject only comes into being as a persistent self by being positioned as the correlative of an external objective reality, that is, against that which is "not-self." Subject and object are thus interdependent, oppositionally related and constructed simultaneously though a complex spatio-temporal grid.

Hence, even our sense-impressions are never simply immediate but are conditioned by the pure *forms* of space and time. That which appears as external to us appears via outer sense as existing in space, but because all appearances are determinations of the consciousness or inner state of the perceiver, they all appear in time, which conditions the relation of representations in a perceiving subject. As our sense-impressions thus already appear in space and time, the imagination can construct schemata that act as templates through which we recognize particular arrangements of space in time as unified objects. This space-time grid and the subject and objects constructed through it are transcendental: they are the necessary conditions of reality as it exists for man because they structure his experience of the phenomenal world.

Ludwig's image plays out this complex structure in a subversive way. For Kant, the forms of space and time and the imagination's templates form the invisible conditions of sensory perception. In the poem, though both space and the gaze of the subject are framed, far from remaining invisible, this frame has been projected into space where it is played *by* the senses. Although there are tensions in Kant's account of space, considered as the aesthetic form of intuition, space is "given" as an infinity which, despite lending itself to being divided up into bounded parts or units, cannot be represented as the sum of its parts.[15] As Kant reminds us in the *Critique of Judgement* in his analysis of the sublime, the infinity invoked by the imagination's encounter with vast objects can never be represented as a whole, in its totality.[16] For Kant, then, the distant horizon represents an infinity of as yet unimagined and hence unobjectified spaces which draw the mind on in endless search of the new. In Ludwig's poem, by contrast, the distance which should open into an alluring infinity is already presented as if framed by a grid. Nonetheless, Ludwig's poem is far from presenting an image of the external sensory world as wholly organized and objectified through a framework determined in advance. Whereas for Kant, sensory/sensible matter is incapable of ordering itself and requires organization via an a priori space-time frame, as we shall see, in Ludwig's poem, the material world of the senses is active in ways that allow it to participate in the shaping of the spatio-temporal meshes of reality.

Hence in Ludwig's poem, the frame of the strings—which becomes the lashes framing the gaze—does not in fact organize sensory perception by dividing external space into contained and containable unities. Far from being invisibly *determined* by such an organizing grid, the senses here *play* the strings, making the framing lashes resonate. Ludwig cannot be read here as simply reasserting the primacy of an immediate sensory encounter with nature. In this image, perception is still mediated. The senses interact with the spaces between the frame—with the world of objective nature represented by the moon—only *through* the frame. Nonetheless, *how* the strings frame space, the specific forms this framework generates, depends on how the senses play them, on how the strings vibrate, at what frequencies and for how long. Moreover, if they are to resonate at all, the strings must be able to move: the spaces around the strings must be fluid enough to let them vibrate and receptive enough for vibrations to be transferred into them as sound.

This musical frame depends not only upon its own elasticity but also on the flexibility and reciprocity of the spaces between the strings. It does not simply impose spatial forms upon an inert materiality, nor do its meshes contain within fixed boundaries the sensory spaces where sound resonates. Rather, the shaping of the spaces of the objective world *through* the frequencies of the strings is simultaneously the shaping *of* the strings into specific vibrations. The patterning of the strings cannot be identified completely separately from the pattern of the spaces between, for each is generated by shared resonances which flow through one to the other. Thus neither the frame, nor the world constructed through it, is stable, fixed, or contained. For Ludwig, the objects of the sensible world are not constituted as units of space enclosed within firm boundaries. Thus in turn, without permanently bounded objects, no subject can here be positioned as a stable and enduring focal point.

As the senses play the strings in their sleep, they do not knowingly determine how the strings move: the exact form this frame takes is not given in advance. Rather, the strings form a sensitive surface of mediation. Their vibrations are generated by an ongoing process of interrelation between the senses, which "play" the strings, and the sensible world caught within the strings, whose fluid movements shape the sound these strings produce. The strings constitute relations through resonance, and these resonances become their own temporary form/s. They are a site across which vibrations are transferred which leave neither the spaces between the strings nor the strings themselves intact or untouched. Finally, as the strings are also the resonating lashes shaping perception, the perceiving subject itself is here imaged and imagined as such a resonating surface constituted between the play of the senses and a fluid objective spatiality. This subject is neither permanent nor a bounded unity, but is not therefore formless. Its shape is spread across a set of vibrating strings and is constituted in the manifold fluxing relations between them, temporary patterns of harmony or dissonance.

Ludwig thus radicalizes Kant's transcendental insight that human perception is conditioned by undermining the idea that these conditions are universally determined a priori. In Ludwig's image, how you see is generated immanently along with what you see. Her image can be read as constructing a sensible transcendental, not because the senses simply determine what one sees, but because the grid determining perception is embedded in and generated by patterns of relation shaped between the sensing self and the sensible world. For Ludwig, the self is not projected via this transcendental frame as a permanent formal unity, as it is for Kant. Rather, the self has become a mediating surface whose form is generated through the perception it, in turn, conditions. This self emerges as a particular site with and within the sensible world, as a particular set of related harmonics.

To turn briefly to the other two stanzas of the poem, Ludwig sharply contrasts this dream logic with a grey and dreary reality, where no hand raises its light for the poet—"keine Hand hebt mir ihr Leuchten." Yet in the final stanza, the poet's soul is filled with the touch not of a hand but of vibrations of sound which reach through her day from the distance, the blue harp. More usual conceptions of spiritual life are here subverted: the soul as it is usually conceptualized—immaterial, amorphous—is not so much suited to being a container as to being contained by the body. At the same time, the movement of sound through the dreary city emphasizes those qualities of music employed in the first verse: music relies exactly not on containment but on the possibilities of transference through matter as resonance. Being filled with sound is not so much a matter of becoming a container as becoming permeated with sound, vibrating through and through. In this poem, the soul itself seems to become another kind of resonating, manifold surface, transformed by tonalities which are themselves transformed by the nature of the material through which they move. For if the soul becomes vibrantly materialized in sound, frequencies and vibrations have become the site of an animate identity. The harp seems to hold open another possibility of being, another kind of life. Exactly because this other world is built on the model of sound and not sight, the poet is not entirely excluded from this other mode of existing: it can permeate her everyday world.

In other poems, Ludwig uses images of sound or music similarly to disrupt the distinctions between the soul or self as immaterial but active, and the body or matter as inert passivity. In one poem she writes of a lost love for whom a bell tolls:

> Und ich weiß
> wenn ihr Ton anrührt meine Stirne,
> werde ich traurig sein.
> [And I know / when its tone touches my forehead, / I will be sad.][17]

In this image Ludwig specifically emphasizes that sound is also a touch. Its vibrations do not respect supposed distinctions between inner and outer: it can pass through and across bodies. Music here communicates emotion not by moving an inner soul but via the forehead. This touch suffices to affect the self, which is once again shaped by a surface receptive to vibrations, a sensitive skin. Such receptivity is not passivity: though the sound transforms the self, it is also transformed as it touches the forehead from the resonances of a bell into those of emotion. Oppositional distinctions between inner and outer, between what belongs to the self and what to external spatiality are here not so much blurred as displaced. It is not that the sound of the bell cannot be distinguished from the affective vibrations into which it is transformed, but that nonetheless, the sound moves between the surface of the self and the space around it, inhabiting both and inhabiting each *differently*.

In both of the poems discussed, the self is not constructed via relations which exclude otherness in the manner of the Kantian subject, whose identity is secured against an external materiality contained within the forms of a bounded objectivity. However, *because* the self in Ludwig's poems is not constructed by means of such oppositional exclusion, it does not run the risk of losing its identity and dissolving into indeterminacy or chaos via contact with otherness or materiality. The self is shaped across a sensual surface which is not a barrier but a site of mediation, transference, and permeability; what becomes part of oneself can simultaneously belong to another space, shaped differently in each according to the specific material conditions allowing for such transference. Hence the "knowledge" of the one who knows that the touch of a particular sound will cause her sadness is not the product of a purely conceptual act of consciousness. Rather, this is an embodied knowledge of the way skin and sound will interact, of the way different materialities respond to and transform each other, a knowledge that could only be born of memories carried in the living skin itself.

Finally, the self in Ludwig's poems is the embodied site of a multiplicity of possible connections which are not determined by a given "natural" order: in the images discussed in detail here, sound is associated not with the ears, but with eyelashes and forehead. Thus connections are generated according to the needs of communication or transference, both between the poetic self and otherness within the poems, and between the poem on the page and the reader. The images in "Die Ferne steht" cannot be mentally mapped onto the familiar structures of the modern subject, and neither can they be read as composing a unified image-scape, for the self addressed by the poet both plays the harp and is the strings thereby set in motion. Both the images and the self they figure are complex, metamorphosing, and multiple. Moreover, Ludwig's synaesthetic images of resonating lashes and forehead reclaim those parts of the body most associated with an identity constructed via the gaze or the intellect and reinscribe them into a mode of embodied, sensual selfhood based on sound.

Claire Goll's early work invokes similar qualities of sound and music to reimagine the self. In several of her poems, she uses the verb *rauschen*, which suggests a symbiosis of sound and movement, or a movement characterized by sound rather than by what can be seen, a murmuring wind, for example, or rushing waters. This relation between sound and spatiality is invoked in her 1918 poem "Gebet," for example, which culminates in an intense, mystical encounter with the divine:

> Und wieder in der dunklen Bucht deines Abends
> Knie ich am tiefen Abgrund deiner Stille hin,
> Wenn die rauschenden Sonnen und Sterne
> In der schwarzen Kuppel der Nacht
> Wie unaufhörliche Glocken schwingen.

[And in the dark bay of your evening again / I kneel down at the deep abyss of your stillness, / When the rushing suns and stars / in the black cupola of the night / swing like incessant bells.][18]

The poetic subject here kneels at the edge of a deep abyss which is mirrored by the black cupola of the night. The spatial orientation of this subject is destabilized because the limitlessness associated with both spaces means that no clear boundary can be drawn between them: night and abyss are merging depths of darkness. The dark void beneath the poet recalls the infinity of nature which becomes "an abyss" for the imagination in the Kantian sublime.[19] For Kant, however, such an encounter ultimately reaffirms the subject's capacity to strive towards totality and the supersensible, and thus enables him to transcend nature and resecure the boundaries of his identity against the sensible, material world.[20] For Ludwig's poetic subject, by contrast, the encounter with the abyss does not allow a transcendence of nature and the sensible, but instead simultaneously opens into the darkness of an animate materiality where suns and stars rush and swing like unceasing bells. Material nature is here no longer an inert realm which passively lends itself to ordering by a subject who can thereby orient himself securely against its objectified forms. Instead, the relation between sound and motion, emphasized by the comparison of the rushing stars to incessantly resounding bells, is used to invoke a dynamic and unstable materiality which would disorient any Kantian subject.[21]

In Goll's short story *Der Gläserne Garten*, images of music are employed to explore the ways in which a female self might be differently constituted, that is, without depending on a founding opposition to an objectified other. Specific musical imagery plays a key role in this text, a richly poetic account of the relationship between two women, Ylone and Venera. Though the temporality of the story is complex, at the beginning the women are together but inhabit their shared space uncertainly. Ylone then undergoes a rite of passage by becoming involved with a man, Claudio. In this section Goll provides a devastating account of the reduction of woman in a heterosexual economy to the specularized object of male desire, an account that startlingly prefigures Irigaray's critique in *Speculum*. Ylone works through the impossibility of living with Claudio as a subject in her own right in a letter to him, and returns to Venera. Throughout the text, Goll builds on a complex series of images such that by the end, the two women occupy a different if precarious world, one where they are selves together.

The focus of this story is not so much erotic love as the growth of a relationship which enables the two women to discover a form of identity. As such it is reminiscent of Plato's account of love in the *Phaedrus*, particularly as it was reworked in the Neoplatonism of the German Romantics. In loving the beauty of the beloved, Plato's lover is in fact loving a reflection of the beauty of the eternal Forms. As long as his love is properly disciplined—that is, is not physical or sensual but is focused purely on the beauty of his beloved—this beauty serves as a medium through which the lover is able to recall the "absolute beauty" of the Forms.[22] For the romantics, Plato's specular economy of desire not only swiftens the soul's recollection of the ideal realm, but most importantly, in the vision of his beloved, the lover ultimately accesses his own true form and thus comes to know himself. The relation of the lover to the beloved (and vice versa) is always the reflective relation of one to himself: "So now the beloved is in love, but with what he cannot tell. [. . .] [H]e is like a man who has caught an eye-infection from another and cannot account for it; he does not realise that he is seeing himself in his lover as in a glass."[23] Goll's text uses music to disrupt this model of oppositional and specular self-relation and to develop an alternative model of fluid interrelation between selves who retain their differences.

When Ylone leaves Venera to become Claudio's lover, she almost loses herself in an uncontrollable mimicry, passively modeling and remodeling herself on what he needs:

Du warst künstlich bis zur Entwertung. Du warst kaum mehr Du vor Angst. [. . .] Besinnungslos steigerst du dich, deine Gesten, deine Worte, formtest um und schufst neu. Stürztest aus einem Lächeln, das geliehen war, in die Pose einer Fremden, hattest hundert Gesichte in der Minute, entblößtest alle Menschen, die in dir waren, warst naive Verständnislosigkeit und greisenhaftes Erkennen.
[You were so artificial that you devalued yourself. You were almost too frightened to be you any more. [. . .] Insensibly you worked yourself up, your gestures, your words, reshaping and creating anew. Falling out of a borrowed smile into a stranger's pose, having a hundred faces per minute, laying bare all the people inside you, naively blank and knowing beyond your years.][24]

Her actions testify to her knowledge that to become the object of Claudio's gaze, she must become a pure and passive reflection of his endlessly projected desires. In a kind of hysterical mime of the specular role of the Platonic beloved, she mindlessly heightens and exaggerates her appearance, metamorphosing through gestures and poses which do not belong to her. Mimicking all the others he might like to see, she is alienated from her excessive appearances. The complexity of her potential identities is reduced to a succession of objectified poses. Ylone herself accuses Claudio of only being able to love her when she is reduced to this one-dimensional form, and as having no ear for a certain irreducible multiplicity whose nuances cannot be captured within his reductive gaze:

> Du hast einen Menschen an mir geliebt, und da waren so viele andre in mir [. . .] aber du überhörtest ihre hundert Nuancen, und ich mußte dich in der hundersten über die anderen neunundneunzig hinwegtäuschen, weil deine Liebe nur die eine ertrug."
> [You loved one person in me, and there were so many others in me . . . but you ignored their hundred nuances, and by means of the hundredth I had to deceive you about the other ninety-nine, because your love could only support the one.] (223)

Furthermore, after Ylone has left Claudio, Venera swears revenge on him for having reduced not just Ylone but both women to a single object specularized by his gaze: "Ich hatte ja nicht nur seine Blindheit zu rächen, nein, vor allem, daß er dich genommen und uns beide gemeint hatte" [I had to take revenge not just for his blindness, no, above all, that he had taken you and meant us both] (225). Claudio can only see one at a time. Thus in relation to Claudio, who lacks an ear for difference/s, Ylone's love "umspannt dich . . . von Kopf zu Füßen *wie eine Oktave*" [My love encompasses you . . . from head to toe *like an octave*] (224). Her love is reduced to an encompassing unity, to the musical relation which emphasizes sameness and the power of the tonic, such that though two notes are played they sound as one, each reinforcing itself in the other. For Claudio, as for Plato's lover, the other is only a reflection of himself.

Ylone's inherent multiplicity makes it clear that Claudio's failing in seeing the two women as one is not that of failing properly to distinguish two individual unities. Rather he fails to see that the women do not fit into any model based on self-contained individuality: Ylone's self is inherently manifold, it contains otherness *within*. Goll uses another musical image, that of the fermate, the pause, to suggest this self based on a relationality which does not reduce the other to a mere version—or inversion—of the same.

Drained by her experiences with Claudio, Ylone returns to Venera, where "Dein Blick wurde fester, hielt auf mir aus wie eine Fermate, sah mich und dich in mir und wußte" [Your gaze became steadier, dwelt on me like a fermate, saw me and you in me and knew] (222). In a moment of suspended self-recognition, Ylone's gaze rests on Venera like a musical pause, and she sees both herself and Venera *in* Venera. The pause is the holding of a note, notes, or rest beyond their notational worth. The *Brockhaus-Wahrig Deutsches Wörterbuch* defines the *Fermate* as a "lengthening or pause sign over a note or rest whose worth is thus extended for an undetermined time."[25] The fermate is thus an undetermined expansion of time which nonetheless will come to have its own determinate shape. The pause cannot be strictly separated from the initial playing of the notes whose sound is suspended but for which time does not simply stop: sound resonates, time deepens as tonalities are allowed to expand beyond a regular beat. Within the suspension of the fermate, sound moves not in a linear progression but in a vibration across its own dimensions. These dimensions give shape not only to the time of the pause itself but resonate across and through the music: the suspended notes emphasize certain harmonies but also take on certain resonances according to how they connect to the piece as a whole. The fermate is not closed within the bounds of an irretrievable and absolute unity: instead, its sound shapes and is shaped by a continuum of change from and into which it seeps.

Thus as Ylone's eyes rest as in a pause, she does not only see herself in Venera but also sees Venera. Venera's doubleness as both reflecting surface and reflected object indicates that she is not simply a screen onto which Ylone projects her own image to see only *herself* more clearly. There is no single site of Venera's identity onto which Ylone can be completely mapped. Rather, Ylone sees herself in another together with this other: self and other coexist without merging into one. In this moment of self-knowledge, the self does not specularize herself in the other like the Platonic lover. In Venera, Ylone finds a space structured not by boundaries which close off the other and reduce it to a flat surface of reflection. Rather, Venera opens a space structured by the shape of her relation with Ylone, a space where the two women do not define themselves through an oppositional specularity but where "einer [wird] im anderen so stark werden, daß man nebeneinander stehen kann" [one (will) become so strong in the other that each can stand side by side] (224).

Thus neither Ylone nor Venera is clearly distinguishable as subject or object of the gaze. Neither one nor the other singly determines what can be seen of them: what can be seen is the shared space of their relationality. Ylone's singular, different identity, which exceeds this shared space insofar as she remains the viewer and not just the object of the gaze, nonetheless is only recovered through this spatiality in which both women are gathered together. Venera is thus more like the concave eye of the fermate, gathering together a space between herself and Ylone where each can be more clearly seen as their relation is suspended and given space to re/sound. Like the space between one moment of music and the next, Venera provides a resting place where resonances are temporarily stilled and so perceived more clearly, their depths explored before they move on in a multiplicity of possible resonances where they will sound differently because certain harmonies, certain relations have been emphasized, drawn out, thickened. Containment dissolves into a manifold of multiplicity-producing difference. This growing of identity through the other neither reflects nor produces a self-contained subject.

Thus towards the end of the text Venera describes herself as a mirror which has preserved the complexity of Ylone's identity, which did not become bound up in Claudio's world. However, though she allows Ylone to look into her to discover herself, Venera is once again a subversive mirror:

> Du konntest dich in mir wie in einem Spiegel sehen, der dein Bild von früher unverändert zurückwarf. Aber ich verhängte diesen Spiegel sorgfältig, um dich nicht zu erschrecken [. . .]. So ließ ich dich stückweise und in Zwischenräumen einsehen in mich, damit du dich langsam wieder aufbauen konntest wie ein Mosaik, aus dem ein Sturm einige Steinchen gebrochen hat.
> [You could see yourself in me as in a mirror that reflected your earlier image unchanged. But I hung this mirror carefully so as not to shock you [. . .]. In this way, I let you see into me bit by bit and in interstices/gaps, so that you could slowly piece yourself together again, like a mosaic, from which a storm has broken some small tiles]. (229–30)[26]

Ylone's lost self is not preserved whole in a single original form, but has to be built up again piece by piece, through multiple partial configurations generated in interstices, spaces between, through which patterns of interrelation can emerge both between different aspects of her complex, manifold self, and between herself and Venera. No single one of these relations contains her essence. Such an identity, composed through interrelations, finds an echo in Irigaray's essay "When Our Lips Speak Together": "between our lips, yours and mine, several voices, several ways of speaking resound endlessly, back and forth. One is never separable from the other."[27] Similarly, then, together with and in Venera, Ylone becomes herself. Identity is here no longer based on the oppositional exclusion of the "other," either via Platonic specularization, or via Kantian objectification. Nonetheless, Ylone does not dissolve into indeterminate ambiguity because otherness and difference/s have been brought within the self. Rather, she is like a mosaic, whose pattern is shaped by the interstices determining the relations of each piece to those around it; Ylone's self is shaped *with* otherness in productive and reciprocal relations.

Towards the end of the text, Venera finally describes how music flows from Ylone's hands and her voice breaks forth like a song: "Da floß ein leiser Wind aus den Fächern deiner Händen: Musik.... Und einmal brach deine Stimme zwischen den Tasten auf wie ein Lied" [Then a light wind flowed from the hollows of your hands: music.... And once your voice broke forth between the [piano] keys like a song] (230). The word *Tasten*, the keys between which Ylone's voice resounds, also suggests the touch by which these keys are played: as a verb it suggests feeling one's way towards something. The image can be read as a musical translation of the mosaic-mirroring, where pattern and order emerge through the interstices, for Ylone's is a syncopated voice which emerges between the keys, between the touches through which music flows from her hands. Sounding between, her voice and fingers together feel their way towards a new music. Ylone's voice takes shape as one note touches on another: her song is composed within—and between—other patterns of sound which stream from her fingers and hands. Ylone's music, like that of Ludwig's harp, is not restricted by the deadening construction of matter as inert or inanimate. Her song emerges between touches as a sound embedded in a resonating materiality; its sound voices an embodied as well as a relational identity.

Ylone's voice in this final section recalls another voice invoked at the beginning of the text, when Ylone and Venera were as yet unseparated by Claudio and alone together, lost in an intense, boundless love. A voice from a distance disturbs Venera, calling up shadows and making her turn back towards another moment in the past when she and Ylone were together. This memory recalls her to the present and to the necessity of losing Ylone, who is about to leave to live with Claudio. As Goll specifically describes this distant voice as singing from Gluck's opera *Orphee*, it at first seems to position Venera as Orpheus, who according to the myth turns back to look at Eurydice as he leads her out of Hades and by doing so loses her forever.

Goll's reference to Gluck's text is knowing: written for a castrato, the role was rewritten in the nineteenth century for alto voice, and thus became a role for women.[28] The notion of a woman singing to another woman immediately disrupts the heterosexual logic of opposition underpinning the myth, where a passive Eurydice is left in the darkness which Orpheus transcends in life and in his artful laments, whose absent object she becomes. Venera's voice cannot be so simply separated from that of her lover, for as we have seen, like the two lips in the Irigaray essay cited above, they are "neither one nor two" and refuse clear demarcation into subject and object of desire.[29] Hence, it is not in fact Venera, but Claudio whom Ylone later positions as Orpheus. She has always struggled to follow him—"ich habe mich bemüht, dir nachzuwerden" [(I struggled to follow you [lit: become like you])—and yet he "kamst niemals dahin, wo ich mir selbst am dunkelsten war." (never came to those places where I was darkest to myself] (223). Venera, however, does go with Ylone into the dark spaces, into the pauses, gaps, and interstices, the fermate, in which Ylone's self, far from being lost, finally takes on its own living form. Far from condemning her to darkness, Venera enables the voice of Eurydice as Ylone finally to be heard.

Goll's invocation of specific musical structures not only subverts the Platonic account of love, but also disrupts Plato's exposition of the proper production of meaning. Plato writes in the *Phaedrus* that the written word is lifeless and "sterile" matter which cannot legitimately give birth to truth, knowledge, or beauty. Such things can only be properly brought to life via the spoken word passed from one living soul to another, miming the immediacy of the Forms.[30] In Goll's text, though Ylone finds her true form in a voice borne on the air, Goll's synaesthetic image of this music as emanating from hands and in relation to touch works in a similar way to Ludwig's attachment of music to the eyelashes or forehead. It disrupts any simple reading of Ylone's song as the pure breath of a disembodied soul. Thus, though like Ludwig, Goll explores music's ability to pass between one and another, as I suggested above, she also emphasizes that the self borne on music is born of an *embodied* relationality. Moreover, in invoking Gluck's opera, Goll emphasizes that music also lives through specific texts and scores, through inky materiality, and hence through a *body of work* as a site where a self takes shape. In Goll's subversive reworkings of Orpheus, dead ink becomes resonating shadows that transform to produce their own offspring: through the dark interstices of the fermate emerges Eurydice, the female self condemned to a lifeless objectification by philosophers such as Plato and Kant.

Thus for Goll as for Ludwig, music's airborne physicality produces the self through the resonances of an animate materiality, and reinscribes textuality as a body of manifold resonance. By re/figuring the sensuous encounter with music, these writers imaginatively transform both self and text which are allowed to take flight, not towards the static Forms of the Platonic soul nor the self-contained unity of the Kantian subject, but as resonating bodies of becomings. Both Goll and Ludwig explore modes of identity where the self is not permanently secured via an oppositional relation to an excluded "other," in the manner of Kant's objectified matter or the specularized beloved of (Neo-)platonism. Instead, the perceiving subject is like the vibrating strings in Ludwig's poem, shaped via the interaction of senses and sensible matter, a resonating site whose patterns of resonance cannot be separated from the patterning of the spaces between. This self-as-resonance emerges with and through the shaping of an otherness with which it remains in productive interrelation, holding open the possibility of further transformations. Similarly, Goll's female selves take shape in the dark space of the fermate, a shared interstice where the particular identity of each is generated through relations of harmony and dissonance, sameness and difference that bind identity together with difference.

Thus, for both the authors examined here, the figure of music becomes vital to the refiguring of selves shaped together with otherness such that differences remain incorporated within manifold, material identities. This refiguring begins to answer Irigaray's question about what might happen if the "object" and "other" refused to submit passively to the gaze of a male subject and instead began to speak. Both Ludwig and Goll find ways of articulating the space-time of subjects who emerge through an animate materiality and who can thus retain the specificity of sexual difference and female embodiment. For both writers, such selves are most richly embodied by the fluid materiality of music, which refuses a topography of visible boundaries and instead creates space and time through patterns of timbre, tempo, vibration, and harmonic relations.

It is precisely a model of selfhood produced by taking sound, rather than sight, as the norm which is explored by Battersby, in her recent work on feminist metaphysics. Drawing on the writings of Deleuze and in particular Kierkegaard, Battersby uses music, together with a perceptual model based on sound, to rethink identity. In place of the self whose identity is secured by an oppositional relation to an objectified "other," Battersby offers a model of a "scored" subject where identity is shaped by embodied patterns of repetition, echo, and rhythm which emerge out of flow.[31] Her analysis pays particular attention to (nonlinear) memory and temporal depth in ways that would productively extend and enrich the alternative models of selfhood based on music and sound which I have explored in texts by Ludwig and Goll. Indeed, as I hope to have shown, the writings of Ludwig and Goll are "singularities," imaginative openings within the history of the West whose potential for feminist philosophy is stressed by Battersby herself. The model of self-as-resonance which unfolds through their texts contributes to the collaborative project of rethinking a female identity where "[n]either fully autonomous nor completely determined, the self is produced relationally: in the resonances between self and other; in a 'present' that is a generative caesura between future and past."[32]

Notes

1. Christine Battersby, *The Phenomenal Woman: Feminist Metaphysics and the Patterns of Identity* (Cambridge: Polity Press, 1998), 56.
2. Paula Ludwig, *Gedichte*, ed. Christiane Peter and Kristian Wachinger (Munich: Langewiesche-Brandt, 1986).
3. Paula Ludwig, "Die selige Spur," in *Die neue Reihe* 22 (Munich: Roland Verlag Albert Mundt, 1920); reprinted in Paula Ludwig, *Gedichte* (9–29; 301–303).
4. Claire Goll, *Ich verzeihe keinem* (Bern and Munich: Sherz Verlag, 1976).
5. Eric Robertson and Robert Vilain, eds., *Yvan Goll—Claire Goll: Texts and Contexts*, IFAVL 23 (Amsterdam: Rodopi, 1997); see especially the essay in this volume by Margaret Littler, "Madness, Misogyny, and the Feminine in Aesthetic Modernism: Unica Zürn and Claire Goll" (153–73). Verena Mahlow, *"Die Liebe, die uns immer zur Hemmung wurde . . .": Weibliche Identitätsproblematik zwischen Expressionismus und Neuer Sachlichkeit am Beispiel der Prosa Claire Golls*, Studien zur Deutschen und Europäischen Literatur des 19. und 20. Jahrhunderts, vol. 31 (Frankfurt am Main: Peter Lang, 1996).
6. Claire Studer, *Mitwelt* in *Der rote Hahn* 20 (Berlin, Wilmersdorf: Verlag Die Aktion, 1918); Claire Goll, *Der Gläserne Garten. Zwei Novellen* (Munich: Roland Verlag Albert Mundt, 1919); reprinted in Claire Goll, *Der Gläserne Garten: Prosa 1917–39*, ed. Barbara Glauert-Hesse (Berlin: Argon, 1989), 215–30. Studer was Claire's name from her first marriage; her maiden name was Aischmann.
7. Luce Irigaray, *Speculum of the Other Woman*, trans. Gillian C. Gill (New York: Cornell University Press, 1985).
8. Irigaray, *Speculum*, 133.
9. Irigaray, *Speculum*, 135.
10. Battersby, *The Phenomenal Woman*, 56.
11. Hermann Kasack, "Vorwort," in *Die selige Spur*, 8. As no published English translations are available of either Ludwig's or Goll's texts, all transla-

tions provided here are my own. I would like to thank Adrian Armstrong, Christine Battersby and Georgina Paul for their generous assistance and advice as regards these translations; any clumsy phrasing which remains is of course wholly my responsibility.

12. Ibid.

13. Kasack's sentimental vision is fundamentally misplaced on a more empirical level too: although *Die selige Spur* was published when Ludwig was only twenty, by this time she was a single mother supporting herself by working in artists' studios in Munich and was also part of the artistic circle surrounding Stefan George, which included her most famous female contemporary, Else Lasker-Schüler. To position her as the naive innocent is to overlook both the complexity of her life and the early and substantial links she made with contemporary artists and writers.

14. Ludwig, *Die selige Spur*, 11.

15. See Immanuel Kant, *Critique of Pure Reason*, trans. Norman Kemp Smith (London: Macmillan, 1929), 69 [A25; B39–40]. Note that although Kant here positions space as an infinity "given" in a priori intuition, he also suggests that space is the pure *form* of intuition (that is, not "given"): *Critique of Pure Reason*, 170–71 [B160–61n]. These very tensions indicate the importance for Kant of accounting for space in ways that make it possible to posit a persistent subject (the transcendental "I"). References to the *Critique of Pure Reason* give the pagination for Kemp Smith's translation, followed in square brackets by the pagination of the *Akademie* text of the first and second editions, referred to as A and B respectively (*Kants Gesammelte Schriften*, 29 vols. (Berlin: Preussische Akademie des Wissenschaften, 1900–85), vols. 3 and 4).

16. See Immanuel Kant, *Critique of Judgement*, trans. Werner S. Pluhar (Indianapolis, Ind.: Hackett, 1987), sec. 26, 107–14 [5: 251–57]. The numbers in square brackets again indicate the location in *Kants Gesammelte Schriften*.

17. Ludwig, *Die selige Spur*, 17.

18. Studer, *Mitwelt*, 15.

19. See Kant, *Critique of Judgement*, sec. 27, 115 [5: 258].

20. For a rigorous analysis of Kant's account of the sublime with particular reference to its gendering, see Christine Battersby, "Stages on Kant's Way: Aesthetics, Morality, and the Gendered Sublime," in *Feminism and Tradition in Aesthetics*, ed. Peggy Zeglin Brand and Carolyn Korsmeyer (University Park: Pennsylvania State University Press, 1995), 88–114.

21. Goll uses the verb *rauschen* in a similar way in at least one other early poem, "Gedicht," where it invokes a lost state of animate materiality: "Nichts rauscht mehr von dir, / Sonne, / Wind, / Stern" [No more rush of you, / Sun, / Wind, / Star] The poem is taken from her 1922 collection, *Lyrische Films* (Basel, Leipzig: Rhein, 1922), 33.

22. Plato, *Phaedrus*, ed. Walter Hamilton (Harmondsworth: Penguin, 1973), 62 [254].

23. Plato, *Phaedrus*, 64 [255].

24. Goll, *Der Gläserne Garten*, 221. Further references will be given in the text.

25. *Brockhaus-Wahrig Deutsches Wörterbuch*, 6 vols. (Wiesbaden: Brockhaus; Stuttgart: Deutsche Verlags-Anstalt, 1980–84), vol. 2 (1981), 711; my translation.

26. The word *Zwischenräume* denotes both gaps in space and intervals in time.

27. Luce Irigaray, "When Our Lips Speak Together," in *This Sex which Is Not One*, trans. Catherine Porter (New York: Cornell University Press, 1985), 205–18 (209).

28. For a detailed discussion of the intense debate that has raged about Orpheus's sex since Berlioz transcribed the part for contralto in 1859, see Wendy Bashant, "Singing in Greek Drag: Gluck, Berlioz, George Eliot," in *En Travesti: Women, Gender, Subversion, Opera*, ed. Corinne Blackmer and Patricia Smith (New York: Columbia University Press, 1995), 216–41.

29. Irigaray, "When Our Lips Speak Together," 207.

30. See Plato, *Phaedrus*, 95–101 [275–78].

31. See chap. 9, "Scoring the Subject of Feminist Theory: Kierkegaard and Deleuze", in Battersby, *The Phenomenal Woman*, 176–97.

32. Battersby, *The Phenomenal Woman*, 184.

Works Cited

Bashant, Wendy. "Singing in Greek Drag: Gluck, Berlioz, George Eliot." In *En Travesti: Women, Gender Subversion, Opera*. Edited by Corinne Blackmer and Patricia Smith. New York: Columbia University Press, 1995.

Battersby, Christine. "Stages on Kant's Way: Aesthetics, Morality, and the Gendered Sublime." In *Feminism and Tradition in Aesthetics*. Edited by Peggy Zeglin Brand and Carolyn Korsmeyer. University Park: Pennsylvania State University Press, 1995.

———. *The Phenomenal Woman: Feminist Metaphysics and the Patterns of Identity*. Cambridge: Polity Press, 1998.

Brockhaus-Wahrig Deutsches Wörterbuch. 6 vols. Wiesbaden: Brockhaus; Stuttgart: Deutsche Verlags-Anstalt, 1980–84.

Goll, Claire. *Lyrische Films*. Basel, Leipzig: Rhein, 1922.

———. *Ich verzeihe keinem*. Bern and München: Scherz Verlag, 1976.

———. *Der gläserne Garten: Prosa 1917–1939*. Edited by Barbara Glauert-Hesse. Berlin: Argon, 1989.

Irigaray, Luce. *Speculum of the Other Woman*. Translated by Gillian C. Gill. New York: Cornell University Press, 1985.

———. "When Our Lips Speak Together." In *This Sex Which Is Not One*. Translated by Catherine Porter. New York: Cornell University Press, 1985.

Kant, Immanuel. *Critique of Pure Reason*. Translated by Norman Kemp Smith. London: Macmillan, 1929.

———. *Critique of Judgement*. Translated by Werner S. Pluhar. Indianapolis, Ind.: Hackett, 1987.

Littler, Margaret. "Madness, Misogyny, and the Feminine in Aesthetic Modernism: Unica Zürn and Claire Goll." In *Yvan Goll—Claire Goll: Texts and Contexts*. Edited by Eric Robertson and Robert Vilain. IFAVL 23. Amsterdam: Rodopi, 1997.

Ludwig, Paula. *Die selige Spur*. Die neue Reihe, no. 22. Munich: Roland Verlag Albert Mundt, 1920.

———. *Gedichte*. Edited by and afterword by Christiane Peter and Kristian Wachinger. Munich: Langewiesche-Brandt, 1986.

Mahlow, Verena. *"Die Liebe, die uns immer zur Hemmung wurde . . .": Weibliche Identitätsproblematik zwischen Expressionismus und Neuer Sachlichkeit am Beispiel der Prosa Claire Golls*, vol. 31. Studien zur Deutschen und Europäischen Literatur des 19. und 20. Jahrhunderts. Frankfurt am Main: Peter Lang, 1996.

Plato. *Phaedrus*. Translated and introduction by Walter Hamilton. Harmondsworth: Penguin, 1973.

Robertson, Eric, and Robert Vilain, eds. *Yvan Goll—Claire Goll: Texts and Contexts*. IFAVL 23. Amsterdam: Rodopi, 1997.

Studer, Claire. *Mitwelt*. Der Rote Hahn, nr. 20. Berlin, Wilmersdorf: Verlag *Die Aktion*, 1918.

———. *Der gläserne Garten. Zwei Novellen*. Munich: Roland Verlag Albert Mundt, 1919.

From the Ear to the Eye: Perceptions of Language in the Fictions of Laurence Sterne

ALEXIS TADIÉ

> When words cease to be vocalised in reading, they become images.
> —D. F. McKenzie

*T*RISTRAM SHANDY IS A COMPLEX ARTEFACT. WE HAVE LEARNED TO regard it as a famous novel of the eighteenth century, as a great textbook for modernists and postmodernists alike, as essential inspiration for Denis Diderot's *Jacques le Fataliste* or Salman Rushdie's *Midnight's Children*. But it is also a physical object, with an interesting history. Famously, it introduces in the midst of the printed words, blank pages, marbled pages, drawings and sundry lines, making of this creation of the print culture, a heterogeneous text. It was variously reprinted, throughout the centuries, with or without the visual paraphernalia, with or without all the episodes (*The Beauties of Sterne*, for instance, deliberately omits all the ugliness, that is, the nonsentimental moments[1]), with or without illustrations. The mutability of the text was of course programmed from the beginning, for there is not, and cannot be, one *original* text of *Tristram Shandy*.

This novel must further be seen as a hybrid object if we think of the ways in which Sterne himself used it, and organized its promotion. He devoted much energy to having the first two volumes read and circulated. He devised a complicated ploy, via Catherine Fourmantel, to secure Garrick's support for the book. He also applied to Richard Berenger, to bring Hogarth to illustrate scenes: "I would give both my Ears (If I was not to loose my Credit by it) for no more than ten Strokes of *Howgarth's* witty

Chissel, to clap at the Front of my next Edition of *Shandy*—."[2] Both ploys worked rather well since he obtained, for the second edition, illustrations of Trim reading the sermon and of Tristram's christening, and he developed a friendship with David Garrick as well. We also find him, in France, using his book to gain access to the salons of the learned society; he writes to Garrick: "Tristram was almost as much known here as in London, at least among your men of condition and learning, and has got me introduced into so many circles ('tis comme a Londres.)."[3] So that Sterne's book participates in the author's strategy of self-promotion. This is emphasized by his habit of entertaining a sense of confusion over his name, using "Yorick" or "Tristram" as frequently as "Laurence Sterne." Again to David Garrick: "have converted many unto Shandeism—for be it known I Shandy it away fifty times more than I was ever wont, talk more nonsense than ever you heard me talk in your days—and to all sorts of people. *Qui le diable est cet homme là*—said Choiseul, t'other day—ce Chevalier Shandy—You'll think me as vain as a devil, was I to tell you the rest of the dialogue—whether the bearer knows it or no, I know not."[4] Sterne would model his behavior on the language of his book, and use the novel in order to fashion his social reputation. This points to the complexities of saying what a book exactly is, and of defining its place within a culture. Although Sterne did not originally belong to the circles he wished to penetrate, his book helped him achieve this social goal.[5]

Books generate, within cultures, diverse ways of looking at them, of using them, of reading them. *Tristram Shandy* is a particularly interesting case of the heterogeneity of the reading practice which relies on social codes, as well as on culturally determined modes of perceiving and understanding language. It is caught in cultural habits, in socially determined modes of perception, and in a historical process which is marked by the movement from orality to literacy, and embodied in the forms of the printed book. Within the matrix of Sterne's books considered as *objects* as well as *works*, one may detect the hybridity of the reading experience, appealing to the eye as well as to the ear. The printed book bears the marks of, indeed commands, the differing ways of perceiving the language of the text.

Eighteenth-century theory seems to have been more concerned with eyes and ears than with the other senses; Priestley, not untypically, writes: "the only inlets of [the pleasures of the imagination] are, as Lord Kaims observes, the *eye* and the *ear*, and . . . the other senses have nothing to do with them"; and a little later: "feeling, tasting, and smelling are considered as sensations of a grosser kind, and seeing and hearing as something of a much more refined and spiritual nature. The former we cannot perceive without having at the same time an idea of the corporeal instruments by which they are conveyed to us; whereas we contemplate ideas of the latter kind, as if we were wholly abstracted from the body."[6] This ideal suppression of the body in perception can be regarded as one of the dominant changes in the representation of language in that period, one that has been linked, by Michel de Certeau among others, to the epistemological shift from orality to literacy, from the voice (and hence the ear) to the written word (and hence the eye): "While the perceived object is writerly, and consistent with the linearities of the meaning expressed and the space constructed, *the voice* creates a gap in the text, brings the body back into the reading experience."[7] This does not mean, as Greuze's painting of the young woman rapturously reading *Heloise et Abelard* reminds us, that the body is altogether absent from the reading experience,[8] but that the forms of the text tend to suppress it. This smoothing over which the written, or better, the printed text, generates, is, to an extent, the subject of this essay; I hope to suggest ways in which the heterogeneity of the reading practice is preserved by Sterne, in an age when conceptions of language were moving away from the oral to the written.

Books and Orality

The printed text changed radically the modes of verbal communication, replacing the audience, previously organized into a circle around the storyteller, with the isolated, private reader.[9] Specifically, around the eighteenth century, reading aloud was giving way to silent reading. Of course, the possibility of reading aloud always remains, as Joyceans around the world on the sixteenth of June remind us every year, but this does not constitute an oral experience, nor did, on the publication of *Paradis*, Sollers's broadcast of the text, twenty-four hours a day, in a Saint-Germain-des-Prés public place.[10] Even in Joyce's well-known reliance on Irish oral culture, the interaction with print is essential. The same is both true and not true of *Tristram Shandy* and *A Sentimental Journey*. Sterne's novels are irrevocably locked into the print culture, but I would suggest that one may detect traces of orality which point both to its heterogeneity as a written artefact, and to changing modes of verbal communication in the eighteenth century. This in turn affects reading.

The actualization of the text, which Michel de Certeau termed the *effectuation*, calls at times for oralization.[11] The text develops and investigates soundscapes that rely on a physical perception of language on the part of the reader. Sounds and musical tunes are constantly heard in his novels; the attention of the reader is drawn towards the variations in tone with which the human voice delivers words and sentences. Musical fragments reach the reader, none more famous than Uncle Toby's *Lillabullero*—various editors and publishers of *Tristram Shandy* even thought it necessary to include the musical score with the text. At times, this leads to a form of polyphonic irony, as when Slop reads the text of the *excommunicatio*, while Toby whistles his favorite piece: "Here my uncle *Toby* taking the advantage of a *minim* in the second barr of his tune, kept whistling one continual note to the end of the sentence———Dr. *Slop* with his division of curses moving under him, like a running bass all the way."[12]

These soundscapes connect with the various musical moments of the book. The conversation between musicians, which Michael Nyman once used as the starting point of a planned opera composed on a libretto derived from *Tristram Shandy*,[13] appeals directly to the ear of the reader, who hears a bad fiddle being played on, and who cringes at the sounds it produces. These sounds, which are transcribed by the narrator, demand that they be analyzed as aural signs, the variations on the vowels and consonants reproducing as many differences in acoustic images: "—Twaddle diddle, tweddle diddle,—twiddle diddle,—twoddle diddle;—twuddle diddle,—pruttrut—krish—krash—krush" (5. 15. 444).

Voices obey the same principle of presentation, and Tristram characterizes their delivery, identifying meaning in various tones. Musicality may be regarded as an essential requirement for the utterance of the *argumentum ad hominem*, that "soft and irresistible *piano* of voice" (1. 19. 59). The sweetest modulations often appear as the necessary condition to a distinct and clear utterance or to a moving message. Yorick, on his sentimental journey, is arrested by a voice which he first identifies as that of a child but discovers on inquiry to belong to a starling; he is as touched by the sight of the bird imprisoned in his cage, as he is by the true tune with which it complains of being unable to get out.

Keen attention to sounds also makes for moments of sheer comedy which are exclusively aural, such as the episode of the abbess of Andoüillets and Margarita, whose noise-making only provokes a release of air on the part of the mule that had stopped them in their journey:

>   ——Wh——ysh——ysh——cried Margarita.
>   Sh——a——shu-u——shu-u——sh——aw——shaw'd the abbess.
>   ——Whu—v—w——whew—w—w—whuv'd Margarita, pursing up her sweet lips betwixt a hoot and a whistle.
>   Thump—thump—thump—obstreperated the abbess of Andoüillets.
>   ——The old mule let a f—(7. 22. 407)

The emphasis on sounds suggests that the reader must be aware of the materiality of the word and of its acoustic properties; thus the description of speech may convey a sense of its music. The ears of the reader, one might want to say, are initially appealed to, and her or his necessary attention to the inflections of the voices, and to the sound environment staged by the novels, define, at least partially, the reading experience. The transcription of these elements is crucial, since they call for the reader's conversion of the printed sign into its oral counterpart. Specifically, the reason why such elements convey the oral dimension of language, the reason why the written text does not hinder the perception of other elements, is that Sterne's culture is still by and large oral, and that it relies on conversation as one of the dominant forms of communication.

Conversations in the eighteenth century, both in theory and practice, take place in a circle, a community of participants which guarantees proper intercourse. When books (conduct or otherwise) define rules for conversation, they do not lay out language rules, but they spell out principles of sociability. To converse, as now obsolete meanings of the word reveal, is to be part of a group, of a society, to *belong*. The salon embodies this most obviously, but genres of painting characteristic of the eighteenth century, such as the "conversation piece," point equally to the relationship between verbal communication and its social dimension. When Tristram insists on identifying conversation and writing, Sterne is acknowledging the sense of community implied by the practice of conversation, thus defining a place for the reader. Conversational undertakings must in this context be understood in several ways.

The perception of the characters' conversations by the reader operates against the background of conversational practice, the characters' failure to communicate through verbal interaction of this kind later suggesting the inadequacy of language in grounding and guaranteeing sociability. Further, the reading experience does not differ radically from conversing, or listening to conversations. In this sense, it may be said that the novel is born out of salon conversation.[14] Although this is not necessarily true of all novels, I think that Sterne's practice builds the text into a place of exchange where the reader, who remains free to ride his own hobbyhorse at will, is allocated a place within the conversational procedure. Interestingly, the novel itself generated for Sterne, as he was going around various salons, a verbal style derived from his narration, where, reversing Tristram's famous pronouncement, conversation might be said to be another name for writing: "I Shandy it away fifty times more than I was ever wont, talk more nonsense than ever you heard me talk in your days—and to all sorts of people."[15]

The interaction between conversation and writing is a complex one because Sterne's position rests on a paradox. As Walter J. Ong has shown, the relationship between both activities is based on opposition rather than similarity: "Reading, one might say, is always a preterite activity. It deals with something which is finished. Texts come out of past time. They are things, not events. Conversation is never a preterite activity. It is an event, not a thing."[16] Although the narrator tries to build the text into a place of exchange, into a moment when the constraints of the text may be counterbalanced by the freedom of the reader, into a social unit where the interaction between the reader and the text might be conceived of along the lines of conversational practice, such exchange can only point ironically to its own impossibility. So that Tristram/Sterne tempts the reader, through a reliance on oral practice, into the illusion of belonging to the text, into turning the printed book, the thing, into an event. In this sense, perception hints at an aural and physical dimension of language, before retreating, by essence, into the fixity of the printed word.

Orality in *Tristram Shandy* must therefore be considered in two ways. First, it is a residual element depending on a cultural practice which, at the time when Sterne was writing, was disappearing; the novel insists, both in its representation of soundscapes and of conversations, on the importance of such cultural schemes. Then, it is an obsolete element, one which, because it belongs to a printed text, can only be present as a trace of the heterogeneity of language practices, and of their changing modes. The reader's position, I would therefore argue, relies on the recognition of this double dimension, on the necessary elusiveness of the oral dimension of print. He or she is both made aware of the necessary perception of language through the ear, and of the impossibility of relying on it exclusively. Tristram's constant and fictitious appeals to male and female readers point to the necessary audience on which the oral tradition lived, as well as to the recognition of its disappearance.

BOOKS AND VISUALITY[17]

The matter may yet be more complicated. Although Sterne's novels are born out of the gradual replacement of an oral culture with a print culture in the eighteenth century, they display more signs of the materiality of language than the simple perusal of the words on the page might imply. Conversations require indeed a presence of the body which his texts always acknowledge. Precise descriptions of gestures and body language flourish; the characters may be perceived as if they were actors on a stage (the theater metaphor, indeed, runs through *Tristram Shandy* and, to an extent, through *A Sentimental Journey*). The gestures must be understood against a complex background of theoretical writings about body language, which includes rhetorical treatises as well as writings on the theater. Further, they must be seen as well as read, which means that they are to be perceived directly by the reader. How is this possible? Treatises on acting or on rhetorical performance offer a curious and interesting case of interaction between the printed word and the oral and physical dimension of language, for they imply that the text be converted into body action. In this sense, the words of the text are not pure words, but they are, potentially at least, a compound of words and gestures.[18] Further, these texts rely on images, using visual representations of the correct postures that an actor or a public speaker should strike, giving precise instructions on the angles that the body, the hand, or the head ought to adopt in the utterance of discourse.

Eighteenth-century theoreticians, when they rely on images for accurate descriptions of gestures, do not simply generate their own perceptions of body language, but draw as well on visual references. The circulation of attitudes between painting, drama, public speaking, oratory, and other forms of performance, characterizes a culture which relies on sight in the representation of language. The pictures one finds in treatises suggest that words need to be converted into images so as to aid the understanding; they also imply a mutual translatability from one medium to the other. An equivalence between text and image is thus established, so that reading about a particular gesture, or seeing its visual representation, appears as one and the same experience. This means that the distinction between reading and seeing may not hold as firmly as one may have grown accustomed to regard it. For theoreticians of gesture, but perhaps also for writers in the eighteenth century, reading a description of a gesture, and seeing that gesture performed, do not constitute radically opposed performances.

In this context, the use of, and the allusions to, gestures in the texts of both *Tristram Shandy* and *A Sentimental Journey* can be analyzed as resting on habits which would integrate seeing as an essential feature of the reading practice. First, accounts of reading suggest that readers might visualize the actions through the words of the text. Diderot for instance praised Richardson in part because he was directly affected by the movements of his heroes and could *see* their gestures. Conversely, some treatises on acting might derive their examples from Richardson's novels.[19]

Secondly, because of the dominance of the theater as a literary and indeed a social genre, readers were led to perceive language as if they were spectators at a play, be it because of widespread theories of acting, or because of accounts of dramatic performances; these used a visual vocabulary derived from painting and trained the reader to visualize bodies through language.[20] In this sense, Sterne's many descriptions of body movement could be perceived against such a cultural background.

Lastly, the importance of vision in the perception of language rests on a widespread theory, derived in part from Locke but which owes its popularity in art and literary criticism in the eighteenth century to *The Spectator*, according to which language generates lively and accurate images. Addison's position was echoed later on by Scottish thinkers such as Hugh Blair who derived their inspiration partly from the essays of "The Pleasures of the Imagination." Blair writes: "Of all the means which human ingenuity has contrived for recalling the image of real objects, and awakening, by representation, similar emotions to those which are raised by the original, none is so full and extensive as that which is executed by words and writing."²¹

Yorick's description of his encounter with the monk in Calais prompts such visualization. The mention of a painter whose works might be known to the reader creates a context: "It was one of those heads, which Guido has often painted—mild, pale—penetrating."²² The religious, allegorical paintings of Guido Reni suggest both a perception and a characterization of the monk, which is confirmed by the rest of the portrait: "The rest of his outline may be given in a few strokes; one might put it into the hands of any one to design, for 'twas neither elegant or otherwise, but as character and expression made it so: it was a thin, spare form, something above the common size, if it lost not the distinction by a bend forwards in the figure—but it was the attitude of Intreaty; and as it now stands presented to my imagination, it gain'd more than it lost by it" (72). The references to painting create more than a metaphor here because of the extensive, if not excessive, use of terms borrowed from the visual arts and because this portrait is one painted for the imagination.²³ We find in this scene a perfect example of Addison's emphasis on verbal image and a distinct reliance on vision in narration and language.

Although writing displaces the image, giving birth to an antipictorialist tradition apparent in the theories of Lessing for instance, such antipictorialism is all but absent from Sterne's culture. Burke, Lessing, the Romantics will insist on a firm distinction between the verbal and the visual, on "generic boundaries between the arts of eye and ear, space and time, image and word."²⁴ We frequently tend to consider language and images within this perspective, which indeed has shaped our "modern" understanding. Going back beyond the end of the eighteenth century, the links between words and images, between visuality and textuality, are much more intricate. Sterne's texts, as the example of the monk quoted above shows clearly, display constantly the heterogeneity of representations and therefore of perceptions. The reader is a listener and a seer.

This heterogeneity is itself the sign of a transitory phase. In this account of the representations of gestures, vision is linked to the presence of the body, to the physical nature of language performance. But if we consider an important treatise on acting, written at the turn of the nineteenth century (it was in fact published in 1806), vision connects with absence rather than with presence. Gilbert Austin's treatise, *Chironomia*,²⁵ invites further consideration of the relationship between words and image because he attempted to introduce a system of notation of gestures, inspired no doubt by treatises on dancing, that he regarded as a significant step forward for public speakers, actors, and painters. On the one hand, he used engravings to support the written word and to clarify the message, on the other, the written system he devised would help painters, who usually rely on deficient recollections, providing them with a logical mode of representation of gestures. The code he established translates the materiality of body language into written signs, thereby creating an equivalence between both; Austin insisted that the visual dimension of gestures could be adequately represented thanks to a written cypher. The perception of gestures, through the eye, was therefore turned into a perception of the written sign, through the eye as well, and such a shift converted the materiality of the body into the materiality of the printed sign. So that one of the epistemological changes which are taking place in the eighteenth century is, I think, nicely articulated in Austin's system through the notation of gestures. He exemplifies a movement away from directly visual, aural, and material perceptions of language, towards an emphasis on the written sign, which, in attempting to provide an equivalent for the diversity and heterogeneity of linguistic communication, eliminates the body from the sphere of language.

Books and Print

To read is to see (through) the words. The printed book embodies this characteristic, imposing its order, its "platonizing power,"[26] on the reader, to which he may or may not submit (choosing, for instance, to skim rather than to read from cover to cover). The "esprit de système" (systematic nature) of the printed book,[27] mocked by Pope in *The Dunciad*, embodies the fixity of writing and contributes to the definition of analytical cognitive devices characteristic of such verbal instances. Thus the forms of the text participate in the definition of its meanings. Sterne plays with the fixity of print and elaborates paradoxes that both reveal an acute awareness of its nature and power, and show how the inscription of the text on the page contributes visually to the meaning. The marbled page for instance, which is to be seen, looked at, and touched perhaps, by the disbelieving academic at least, so as to determine its nature and texture, turns, through the appeal to the eye, the physical object into textual presence (the margins are in place, the page is numbered). Considered as the "motly emblem" (3. 36. 268) of Tristram's/Sterne's work, the page introduces the unequivocal presence of the forms of printing within the text, of the book which demands to be read,[28] but, at the same time, this page subverts the fixity of print. Not only does it lack the regularity of the white and black marks, but in the original edition of the novel, each side was different from the reverse, and each marbled page was different, from copy to copy.[29] This meant that the invocation of the system, of the inalterable materiality of the object, led paradoxically to the very denial of it, through an assertion of the essential variability of the text, or rather of the book considered as an object. There cannot be one original edition of *Tristram Shandy*, one type, of which all other editions would be tokens, for all texts are materially, by essence, different. The inability of modern editions to reproduce this feature, including the most accurate ones such as the Florida edition,[30] underline further the irony and the paradox of it all. In the age of mechanical reproduction, a text which is so obviously a product of this age, resists all forms of reproduction.[31]

Corporal Trim's flourish of the cane provides an extreme example of the ways in which, through print, seeing is woven into the text. This drawing, perhaps the most famous in the history of the written text, transcends words. First, the gesture appears as more efficient in advocating celibacy and freedom than "A thousand of my father's most subtle syllogisms" (9. 4. 491), thereby emphasizing the partial inadequacy of words to convey ideas clearly. Then, the visual dimension of the gesture is converted for the benefit of the reader into a graphic equivalent; the reader sees this movement as it is performed on the page (the praise of freedom implies a direction of reading, from bottom to top). Although the black line does not represent words, but a gesture, it is only made possible through print. This representation cannot be translated into words, but it exists as *text*, within the clear confines of the page.

Rather than introduce here a disjunction between reading and seeing,[32] we should insist on the link between print and vision, between the form of the book and the perceptions of the reader. The apparent opposition between words and vision is unified, thanks to the eye, within the print system of *Tristram Shandy*. In preventing any form of oralization of the passage (although the text clearly invites the reader to do so at other moments), the episode of the cane defines the extreme position of the solitary, silent reader generated, according to Walter J. Ong and others, by the print culture: "Reading is a special kind of activity and cannot be understood as simply an activity parallel to listening."[33] This does not preclude the possibility that the written text be, at times, converted into oral manifestations, but the nature of the reading experience is by and large silent. Michel de Certeau writes: "Reading has become, over the past three centuries, a visual poem. It is no longer accompanied, as it used to be, by the murmur of a vocal articulation or by the movement of a muscular manducation. To read without uttering the words aloud or at least mumbling them is a 'modern' experience."[34] In this sense, Corporal Trim's flourish on the page constitutes the essence of the modern text, for it defines the silence of reading as the silence of vision.

The white page, finally, suggests ironically the reader's position as one of arch-seer. Although it purports to provide him with the greatest moment of freedom, it also embodies one of the moments of greater constraint, when the male reader comes to realize that he has been tricked into believing he could draw on this white page. The impossibility for him to do so without affecting the universal potentialities of such representations, or rather, the impossibility for his particular drawing to affect these potentialities, must lead to the recognition of the order of the book and of the defining powers of print on the reader. The further paradox on which the blank page is based belongs to the very nature of books. As historians have shown,[35] the changes in the visual presentation of the printed page between the sixteenth and the eighteenth centuries were considerable, and involved, among other elements, the leaving of the reader, literally, on the margins of the text; there, he remained free to interfere and to introduce comments where the text would originally have displayed shoulder notes. The blank page, like the blank space provided for swearing purposes, tempts the reader into (bookish) participation, at the same time as it denies him any kind of participation. These features prolong the paradox of conversational practice which I alluded to earlier; they both represent a participatory (nowadays, we would say interactive) conception of narration and of the book and reveal its very impossibility within a print culture, constraining freedom as soon as it suggests it.

The important modifications in the art of printing in the eighteenth century led to Sterne's recognition of the importance of books as objects and to his emphasis on vision, on *seeing* the text, on perceiving its materiality in order to generate meanings. The manuscript which Sterne prepared for the printing of *A Sentimental Journey* confirms this feature. Although the second half of it is now lost, Sterne's copy of the manuscript for the first volume reveals interesting aspects of the author's engagement with the form of the book.[36] Apart from a well-known interest of Sterne's for the final appearance of his text, which probably led him to introduce corrections in the proofs,[37] one can detect in the arrangement of the text on the page the author's distinct consciousness of the requirements of typography. The instructions for italics or capitals are integrated into the manuscript through the usual system of underlining; the lengthy dashes which most modern editions, to the exception of Gardner D. Stout's, do not reproduce, must be converted into equally lengthy dashes on the printed page; the polite address at the end of "The Letter" is arranged on the page following letter-writing practices.[38] Sterne, furthermore, indicated the divisions between paragraphs, the blanks that separate them, and he restarted the chapters on new pages, which created a blank space between each. This feature, absent from most modern editions, is essential, for it isolates each unit and confers on the chapters a certain autonomy, as if they were different scenes in a play. The lines which frame the titles contribute to this overall creation of a rhythm of reading which echoes the singularity of movements and pulsations as they circulate between the pen and the heart of the sentimental traveler. The typographical elements, the ordering of words and blanks on the page, thus define a component of meaning which is not to be found solely in the *text* considered as an abstract entity. Meaning, in Sterne's novels, elicits a perception of language grounded in the diversity of the senses, on the ear and the eye, on aural and visual characteristics, on hearing and vision as the varying modes of understanding, of, literally, *making sense*.

Conclusion

One may therefore emphasize several points in the analysis of the relationship between reading, hearing, and seeing. The various uses of the book, the various ways of relating to the novels of Laurence Sterne are, in part, culturally determined by habits of perception and of reading. Although it is sometimes inscribed in its very words, the oralization of the text is a practice which has tended to disappear over the last two centuries or has changed significantly. (Such commercial events as writers reading from their books, with varying degrees of competence and success, seem to indicate that it survives in places.) Its last sanctuary is perhaps the academic conference.

The visualization of the action, the representation of the scenes in the reader's fancy is likewise grounded in historical as well as cognitive factors. The importance of vision and images in our conceptual framework, emphasized by philosophers like Daniel Dennett, the treatment of information both linguistically and visually, determines the modes of reading. Current research in the domain of reading and visualization seems to indicate that there is still wide debate over the question of imaging during reading. Significantly, imaging may be culturally determined: "Whether or not the reader decides imaging is an appropriate and effective response depends on the particular cultural norm that the reader accepts."[39]

But reading is a form of seeing, as Sterne's novels remind us at times, and a text cannot be identified purely with its message, the physical arrangement of the words on the page contributing in no insignificant manner to the general meaning of the book. The movement from orality to literacy which characterizes the eighteenth century, the growing appeal to the eye over the ear in the perceptions of language, find in Sterne's novels echoes that account for the fundamental heterogeneity of the texts. Ultimately, the eye has won, being the sole organizer of those black marks, which cover at times the whole page, leave others blank, draw lines reminiscent of Hogarth's line of beauty, and outline, more often than not, these funny signs called words.

NOTES

1. *The Beauties of Sterne: Including all his Pathetic Tales and Most Distinguished Observations on Life. Selected for the Heart of Sensibility.* A new edition (London: Printed for T. Davies, J. Ridley, W. Flexney, J. Sewel, and G. Kearsley, 1782). Signed by W. H. This edition carries a quote from *A Sentimental Journey* on the first page: "Dear Sensibility! source inexhausted of all that's precious in our joys, or costly in our sorrows! thou chainest thy martyr down upon his bed of straw!—and 'tis thou who lifts him up to HEAVEN!—Eternal fountain of our feelings! 'tis here I trace thee."

2. To Richard Berenger, 8 March 1760, *Letters of Laurence Sterne*, ed. Lewis Perry Curtis (Oxford: Clarendon Press, 1935), 99.

3. To David Garrick, 31 Jan. 1762, *Letters*, 151.

4. To David Garrick, 19 March 1762, *Letters*, 157.

5. On Sterne's promotion of his book, see Arthur Cash, *Laurence Sterne: The Later Years* (London: Routledge, 1993). See also Frank Donoghue, *The Fame Machine* (Stanford, Calif.: Stanford University Press, 1996).

6. John Priestley, *A Course of Lectures on Oratory and Criticism* (London: Printed for J. Johnson, 1777), 125–26.

7. Michel de Certeau, *L'Ecriture de l'histoire* (Paris: Gallimard, 1975), 246.

8. See also, as a more contemporary example, the opening of Italo Calvino's *If on a Winter Night a Traveller* (London: Everyman's Library, 1993).

9. See Walter Benjamin, "The Story-Teller," in *Illuminations* (London: Cape, 1970), 83–110.

10. In fact, it was exactly the opposite of one and reproduced an essential feature of the experience of reading, namely the ability to drift in and out of a book, to resume it at leisure, whereas oral tales do not provide this kind of freedom. Closer to it perhaps is the common practice for writers of reading extracts from their books in public places, but these events constitute essentially a marketing ploy.

11. See D. F. McKenzie, "Typography and Meaning: The Case of William Congreve," in Giles Barber and Bernhard Fabian, eds., *Buch und Buchhandel in Europa im achtzehnten Jahrhunder* (Hamburg: Dr. Ernst Hauswedell and Co., 1981), 82: "The book itself is an expressive means. To the eye its pages offer an aggregation of meanings both verbal and typographic for translation to the ear; but we must learn to see that its shape in the hand also speaks to us from the past."

12. Laurence Sterne, *The Life and Opinions of Tristram Shandy, Gentleman*, ed. Joan and Melvyn New, 3 vols. (Gainsville: University of Florida Press, 1978) vol. 3, chapter 11, 207–8. Subsequent quotations from this work are cited parenthetically in the text under the form (3. 11. 207–8).

13. *I'll Stake My Cremona to a Jew's Trump* is a variation on chap. 15, vol. 5, of the novel.

14. See Marc Fumaroli, *Le genre des genres littéraires français : la conversation* (Oxford: Clarendon Press, 1992).

15. To David Garrick, 19 March 1762, *Letters*, 157.

16. Walter J. Ong, "Reading, Technology, and the Nature of Man: An Interpretation," *Yearbook of English Studies* 10 (1980): 134.

17. On the notion of visuality and its complexities in the eighteenth century, see Peter de Bolla, "The Visibility of Visuality," in T. Brennan and M. Jay, eds., *Vision in Context* (London: Routledge, 1996), 63–81.

18. See Roger Chartier, *The Order of Books*, trans. Lydia G. Cochrane (Stanford, Calif.: Stanford University Press, 1994), 20: "To take first the way in which writing and gesture mixed: not only was the written word at the centre of urban festivities such as religious ceremonies, but a number of texts were intended to cancel themselves out as discourse and to produce practical results in behaviour recognized as being in conformity with social or religious norms. This was the case with the civility books, which aimed at teaching the rules of polite social intercourse or Christian propriety."

19. See for example Engel's famous treatise which was adapted into English by Henry Siddons: Henry Siddons, *Practical Illustrations of Rhetorical Gesture and Action, Adapted to the English Drama* (London, 1807).

20. See Shearer West, *The Image of the Actor: Verbal and Visual Representation in the Age of Garrick and Kemble* (New York: St. Martin's Press, 1991).

21. Hugh Blair, *Lectures on Rhetoric and Belles Lettres* (Edinburgh: 1773), 1, 93.

22. Laurence Sterne, *A Sentimental Journey through France and Italy. By Mr Yorick*, ed. Gardner D. Stout Jr. (Berkeley: University of California Press, 1967), 71. Subsequent quotations from this work are cited parenthetically in the text.

23. Cf. "I have his figure this moment before my eyes" (*SJ*, 70).

24. W. J. T. Mitchell, *Picture Theory* (Chicago: University of Chicago Press, 1994), 114.

25. Gilbert Austin, *Chironomia; or a treatise on Rhetorical Delivery: comprehending many precepts, both ancient and modern, for the proper regulation of the voice, the coutenance, and gesture. Together with an investigation of the elements of gesture, and a new method for the notation thereof; illustrated by many figures* (London: printed for T. Cadell and W. Davies, by W. Bulmer, 1806).

26. Alvin Kernan, *Samuel Johnson and the Impact of Printing* (Stanford, Calif.: Stanford University Press, 1987), 165.

27. The phrase was coined by E. Eisenstein and is quoted by Kernan, *Samuel Johnson*, 12.

28. "Read, read, read, read, my unlearned reader! read,—or by the knowledge of the great saint Paraleipomenon—I tell you before-hand, you had better throw down the book at once; for without much reading, by which you reverence knows, I mean much knowledge, you will no more be able to penetrate the moral of the next marbled page (motly emblem of my work!) than the world with all its sagacity has been able to unravel the many opinions, transactions and truths which still lie mystically hid under the dark veil of the black one" (3. 36. 268).

29. It was in fact printed separately and later sewn into the text with the page number added in different type.

30. It includes a photographic reproduction of one of the marbled leaves.

31. This appears further in the torn chapter. The so-called torn chapter is again based on a paradox linked to the form of the book. Indeed, because there is a chasm of "ten pages" (4. 25. 372) original editions restarted with right-hand side pages numbered with even figures. Thus, the left page, in the first edition, reads page 146 and the right one page 156. This feature runs to the end of the volume. The paradox is obviously that such a feature is impossible because one may only physically tear out of a book an even number of pages, but Sterne's strategy, again, must be seen as both awareness of, and resistance to, the order of books. The insistence on the form of the book is apparent in Tristram's comments: "but the book-binder is neither a fool, or a knave, or a puppy—nor is the book a jot more imperfect, (at least upon that score)—but, on the contrary, *the book is more perfect and complete by wanting the chapter, than having it*, as I shall demonstrate to your reverences in this manner—" (4. 25. 372; my emphasis). Interestingly enough, the most recent scientific editions, be it Ian Campbell Ross's edition for World's Classics or Melvyn New's edition, fail to reproduce this feature.

32. The opposition between word and image is one that often translates into an opposition between reading words and seeing images. But the two activities rely obviously on the eye. Recent theoretical work on the subject seems to take this phenomenon into account, whether it be the semiotic approach of Norman Bryson, the deconstructionist analyses of Peter Wagner, or the more philosoph-

ical inquiries of W. J. T. Mitchell. For the relationship of seeing to reading, see Ellen Esrock, *The Reader's Eye: Visual Imaging as Reader Response* (Baltimore and London: Johns Hopkins University Press, 1994).

33. Walter J. Ong, "Reading, Technology, and the Nature of Man," 133.

34. Michel de Certeau, *L'Invention du quotidien* (Paris: Gallimard, 1980), 253.

35. See for instance Henri-Jean Martin and Roger Chartier, eds., *Histoire de l'édition française* (Paris: Promodis, 1982–86). See also Nicholas Barker, "Typography and the Meaning of Words: The Revolution in the Layout of Books in the Eighteenth Century," in Giles Barber and Bernhard Fabian, eds., *Buch und Buchhandel in Europa im achtzehnten Jahrhundert* (Hamburg: Dr. Ernst Hauswedell and Co., 1981), 127–65.

36. British Museum, MS Egerton 1610.

37. For example, the word *Literata* becomes in the printed version *precieuse*.

38. This feature, which is to be found as well in the first edition, has disappeared from most modern editions.

39. Esrock, *The Reader's Eye*, 180.

Works Cited

Austin, Gilbert. *Chironomia; or a treatise on Rhetorical Delivery: comprehending many precepts, both ancient and modern, for the proper regulation of the voice, the coutenance, and gesture. Together with an investigation of the elements of gesture, and a new method for the notation thereof; illustrated by many figures*. London: printed for T. Cadell and W. Davies, by W. Bulmer, 1806.

Barker, Nicholas. "Typography and the Meaning of Words: The Revolution in the Layout of Books in the Eighteenth Century." In *Buch und Buchhandel in Europa im achtzehnten Jahrhundert*. Edited by Giles Barber and Bernhard Fabian. Hamburg: Dr. Ernst Hauswedell and Co., 1981, 127–65

Benjamin, Walter. "The Story-Teller." In *Illuminations*, 83–110. (London: Cape, 1970).

Blair, Hugh. *Lectures on Rhetoric and Belles Lettres*. Edinburgh, 1773.

Bolla, Peter de. "The Visibility of Visuality." In *Vision in Context*. Edited by T. Brennan and M. Jay, London: Routledge, 1996, 63–81.

Cash, Arthur. *Laurence Sterne: The Later Years*. London: Routledge, 1993.

Certeau, Michel de. *L'Ecriture de l'histoire*. Paris: Gallimard, 1975.

———. *L'Invention du quotidien*. Paris: Gallimard, 1980.

Chartier, Roger. *The Order of Books*. Translated by Lydia G. Cochrane. Stanford, Calif.: Stanford University Press, 1994.

Donoghue, Frank. *The Fame Machine*. Stanford, Calif.: Stanford University Press, 1996.

Esrock, Ellen. *The Reader's Eye: Visual Imaging as Reader Response*. Baltimore and London: Johns Hopkins University Press, 1994.

Fumaroli, Marc. *Le genre des genres littéraires français: la conversation*. Oxford: Clarendon Press, 1992.

Kernan, Alvin. *Samuel Johnson and the Impact of Printing.* Stanford, Calif.: Stanford University Press, 1987.

Martin, Henri-Jean, and Roger Chartier, eds. *Histoire de l'édition française.* Paris: Promodis, 1982–86.

McKenzie, D. F. "Typography and Meaning: The Case of William Congreve." In *Buch und Buchhandel in Europa im achtzehnten Jahrhunder.* Edited by Giles Barber and Bernhard Fabian. Hamburg: Dr. Ernst Hauswedell and Co., 1981.

Mitchell, W. J. T. *Picture Theory.* Chicago: University of Chicago Press, 1994.

Ong, Walter J. "Reading, Technology, and the Nature of Man: An Interpretation." *Yearbook of English Studies* 10 (1980).

Priestley, John. *A Course of Lectures on Oratory and Criticism.* London: Printed for J. Johnson, 1777.

Siddons, Henry. *Practical Illustrations of Rhetorical Gesture and Action, Adapted to the English Drama.* London, 1807.

Sterne, Laurence. *Letters of Laurence Sterne.* Edited by Lewis Perry Curtis. Oxford: Clarendon Press, 1935.

———. *The Life and Opinions of Tristram Shandy, Gentleman*, 2 vols. Edited by Joan and Melvyn New. Gainsville: University of Florida Press, 1978.

———. *A Sentimental Journey through France and Italy. By Mr Yorick.* Edited by Gardner D. Stout Jr. Berkeley: University of California Press, 1967.

West, Shearer. *The Image of the Actor: Verbal and Visual Representation in the Age of Garrick and Kemble.* New York: St. Martin's Press, 1991.

III
EYES

Language, Color, and the Enigma of Everydayness
MICHAEL SHERINGHAM

THE LINKS BETWEEN COLOR AND EVERYDAY LIFE WERE UNDERLINED in a spectacular way in spring 1996, when Pepsi Cola decided to make a change of color—the can, not the drink—central to a change of image. The opening moves in one of the most expensive advertising campaigns ever launched included a transatlantic flight by a Concorde painted blue, with André Agassi, Claudia Schiffer, and sundry other celebrities aboard, all decked out in the new shade, and, on the same day, an edition of the London *Daily Mirror* printed on blue paper. This was followed by a poster campaign featuring everyday objects and icons strongly associated with the color red—Labour Party rosette, Royal Mail post box, Heinz ketchup, Swiss army knife—that all suddenly turned blue and were accompanied by the legend "Change the script!"

It is too soon to say whether, in Britain at least, people like having their color conventions tampered with, or if blue is an appropriate color for other aspects of the Pepsi image. Yet these issues were aired when, on Pepsi Day, BBC Radio 4 News ran an item featuring a surprising range of experts on color, demonstrating wide-ranging and complex links between color, science, and culture. A public relations consultant spoke about dress codes and image make-overs, a psychologist discussed moods, physiology, and such questions as whether blue really is a cool color, while another expert stressed the complex cultural history of color symbolism and the culturally variable associations colors possess, despite strong evidence that the central nervous system responds fairly universally to color difference. Then an art historian explained the Purkinje shift (after the Bohemian physiologist J. E. Purkinje who first described it in 1815) whereby, in a defined context such as a room, blue grows on the eye to the extent that, after twenty minutes or so, it supersedes red and dominates the perceptual environment, an effect often observed in Italian churches where the Virgin's blue mantle progressively stands out with a magical radiance. Then came internationally patented Yves Klein Blue, abstract expressionism, color field painting, and so on and so forth. Subsequently, a series of short programs on BBC Radio 3 explored the connotations of individual colors, covering, in an amusing and anecdotal way, the kind of ground surveyed in John Gage's magisterial 1993 text *Color and Culture*, which has a wealth of information concerning the development of dies and pigments, esoteric color symbolisms in heraldry and alchemy, mosaics and stained glass, and much else besides.

In the United States, enthusiasm for discussions of color can be gauged by the success of Alexander Theroux's *Primary Colors*, a witty, stylish, but ultimately somewhat tedious compendium of snippets of information illustrating the multiple meanings that have accrued through history to red, blue, and yellow. Color is clearly central to everyday life, not just in modern industrial societies dominated by mass-produced objects, although Jean Baudrillard, devoting a substantial section to color in *Le Système des objets* [*The System of Objects*] underlines how recent the liberation of color has been. In nonindustrial societies the ability to interpret the changing colors of the natural world has a functional role, and the earliest art—polychrome cave paintings—points to connections between magic, color, and hunting. As is well known, some communities have a very subtle color vocabulary for utilitarian reasons, and this poses teasing questions for linguisticians about the order of priority between language and reality. Moreover, readers of Lévi-Strauss may recall the passage in *Tristes tropiques* where the anthropologist goes shopping on the Boulevard Sebastopol in search of appropriately colored articles to take as gifts to the Bororo Indians, for whom certain colors are infinitely prized while others are shunned.

If, in a general way, there is a clear link between color and everyday life, we may ask if the connection is still there when we seek to investigate more deeply the nature of everydayness. Can color lead us to the heart of our sense of the quotidian? What constructions of everydayness does color fit in with, and which aspects of the phenomenon of color are particularly relevant to it? The first thing to note is that those who have made the everyday, or the ordinary, a familiar category in recent thought—from Henri Lefebvre to Roland Barthes, Jean Baudrillard, Michel de

Certeau, Umberto Eco, and Stanley Cavell; from the surrealists to Raymond Queneau, Georges Perec, Jacques Réda or Michel Vinaver—consistently underline the deeply ambiguous and problematic nature of this notion.

Problematic, in the first place, because of its inherent evanescence and instability: Maurice Blanchot notes that "le quotidien est ce qu'il y a de plus difficile à découvrir" [the everyday is the most difficult thing to discover]. The everyday can only be located at the intersection, or in the overlaps and interstices, of different systems and orders—public and private, real and imaginary, regular and haphazard. The everyday is also ambiguous and ambivalent because, as Lefebvre's work shows again and again, it is a place of estrangement and alienation, but at the same time a zone of liberation, joy, and contentment. Unlike other more localized sectors of experience—the aesthetic, the political, the sexual—which have at least overt positive valuations, the everyday is not only capable of being lived through in different ways, but is inherently ambivalent. There are various ways in to this labyrinth. For example, we can follow the trail of the object, or that of daily practices or rituals, or we can track the everyday through trajectories and ways of traversing space, or in the organization of the day itself, or in spatial practices—the layout of rooms in a house or the streets of a city. In the discussion that follows, color will be seen as one of these trails, a route towards the enigma of the everyday.

To approach the question of how color might be pertinent to the everyday, we need initially to look at the ways in which it can be valorized. One way of celebrating color that might seem particularly relevant to the everyday sees it in terms of immediacy, affect, the prelinguistic. Historians of color and culture locate the valorization of color within a fundamental opposition between two poles conveniently represented by Newton and Goethe. In a Newtonian perspective, color is a phenomenon to be understood in terms of the laws of optics and the physical nature of light. Goethe's theory of colors, on the other hand, elaborated in 1810, although based on experiment, exalts the subjective component in the perception of infinitely variegated hues. The Romantic investment of color as a mental phenomenon had been anticipated by many Renaissance proponents of *colore* as opposed to *disegno*, as well as in earlier theological distinctions between *lux* and *lumen*. But, directly and indirectly, Goethe's work heralded numerous investigations and classifications of the subjective dimension of color, and a wealth of often intensely poetic writing about its power, such as the famous section from Baudelaire's *Salon de 1846*, entitled "De la couleur" [Of Color], or the many reflections on color in the writings of Delacroix, Kandinsky, or Albers.

Common to these ecstatic evaluations of color is the emphasis on intensity, power, and communion, often supported by spirituality or a sense of the mystery of the universe. I wish, however, to focus on a tension within this radical privileging of color. This tension may exist within the discourse of a single proponent of color, and in its simplest form boils down to the question of whether what is valorized is the pure experience of a single color, a unified experience of one color at a time, or, on the other hand, the contrastive nature of color, the harmonies and resonances which colors can achieve in combination. Baudelaire, for example, may speak of "le rouge, cette couleur si obscure, si épaisse, plus difficile à pénétrer que les yeux d'un serpent" ("De la couleur," 446) [red, this color that is so dark, so dense, harder to penetrate than the eyes of a serpent], but essentially his approach to color, impassioned and wholehearted as it is, is rooted in the notion of "l'harmonie, la mélodie et le contre-point" [harmony, melody and counterpoint] (423). Color is an "hymne compliqué" [complex hymn] where "le rouge chante la gloire du vert; le noir—quand il y en a—zéro solitaire et insignifiant, intercède le secours du bleu ou du rouge" [red sings to the glory of green; black—when it exists—a solitary and insignificant zero—seeks the intercession of blue or red] (422). For all his enthusiasm for artifice, Baudelaire's championing of color is grounded in nature, in a

> bel espace de nature où tout verdoie, rougeoie, poudroie et chatoie en pleine liberté, où toutes choses diversement colorées suivant leur constitution moléculaire, changées de seconde en seconde par le déplacement de l'ombre et de la lumiére, et agitées par le travail intérieur du calorique, se trouvent en perpétuelle vibration
> [a lovely corner of nature where everything freely luxuriates, gleams, and glistens in its greenness or redness, where all things, diversely colored by dint of their molecular structure, changing second by second through the shifts of light and shadow, and activated within by the agency of heat, are to be found in perpetual vibration]
> (422)

By contrast, Kandinsky's enthusiasm for color, that he saw as a path along which artistic creation could free itself from enslavement to nature and attain spirituality, focuses on the intense material presence of pure color. An extraordinary passage in his autobiography describes a founding moment when, at the age of about fourteen, he bought a set of oil paints and saw the colors come to life as he squeezed them out of the tube:

> avec un profond sérieux, une pétillante espièglerie . . . une domination de soi opiniâtre . . . ces êtres étranges que l'on nomme couleurs venaient l'un après l'autre, vivants en soi et pour soi, autonomes, et dotés à chaque instant à leur future vie autonome, et, à chaque instant, prêts à se plier librement à de nouvelles combinaisons; à créer une infinité de mondes nouveaux
> [with a profound seriousness, a bubbling vivacity . . . a stubborn self-possession . . . these strange beings we call colors emerged one after the other, living beings both in and for themselves, autonomous, and endowed at every moment with their future autonomous life, and at each moment ready to lend themselves freely to new combinations, to create an infinite number of new worlds] (213)

Even when they enter into combination, colors retain their intense, sovereign, autonomy, a point Kandinsky emphasizes further on when he insists on the "forces fraîches" [fresh forces] of the newly emerged colors as they assert themselves against the background of the palette, creating chance combinations in a process he compares to both music and alchemy.

In a different vein, Ernst Jünger's remarkable meditations on color in *Das Abenteuerliche Herz* [*The Adventurous Heart*] also underline the immediacy and specificity of individual colors, over and above the combinations and juxtapositions which maximize their power. Very much in the German Romantic tradition, and following Goethe and Baudelaire, Jünger's stimulus is always color in nature, but his observations lead away from the familiar towards mysterious laws of metamorphosis and participation reflected in a wide range of contexts. A number of texts center on the mystery of redness, a "fundamental substance" associated with the life force in its intensity. For Jünger, red is both the color of the earth's core—Mother Earth is red—and of the human body, and particularly the inner organs:

> We are the little sparrows that Mother Earth catches with the color red. Deepest matter is red, even when it hides under green robes; under the white lace of glaciers, under the grey frills with which the ocean decks out its shores . . . the living matter of which we are made is red; we are totally enveloped in this color. That is why it is so close to us, so close that between us and it there is no room for thought.

> Red is the color of pure presence; under its sign we commune without words. (216)

The notion of color as presence and intensity is central to the aesthetic theory of Georges Duthuit and led him to write influential studies of Byzantine art and of the fauves. By contrast with Greek art, color in Byzantine icons, murals, and mosaics comes alive, becomes a celebration of place and moment. As for the fauves—Matisse, early Derain, anticipated by Cézanne—they fulfill the broken promise of impressionist art which, while ostensibly liberating color, had in fact kept it subordinate to design and classical space. By freeing color from perspective and reference, the fauves had allowed art to become an act in which the immediacy of sensation and affective experience is externalized. For Duthuit, as for Kandinsky, there is something eruptive, transgressive, and violent about color. But in Duthuit's case the experience of color is essentially immanent: what it apprehends, and in its way potentially divinizes, is the pure moment, the here and now. Color does not point in the direction of a harmony revealed through contrast and combination but becomes pure event, associated with the act of painting.

The kind of tension we are concerned with is reflected in psychoanalytical accounts of color. For the analyst Christian David, it is self-evident that what is at stake when color enters the psychological arena is an investment, and generally an overinvestment, in pure affect. The cult of color reflects a desire to escape the hegemony of language, the aspiration to an oceanic state without clear limits. Color is a sublime realm beyond conflict in which one seeks to immerse oneself. For Muriel Gagnebin, on the other hand, color, in a psychoanalytical perspective, is not an absolute but an instrument of mediation, a transferential zone. If color is indeed linked to "the infinite range of emotions"—and thus with the affective order—what it offers is in fact tied to its essentially differential nature. If color is a zone of energies and vibrations, these are not so much occasioned by pure color as by incompatibilities, reciprocities, and juxtapositions. Seen this way, color is essentially agonistic and thus expressive of, rather than a haven from, conflict.

For Gagnebin, the essential parameters that define colors—position on the chromatic scale, saturation, brilliancy—taken together with the play of opposition to other colors, produces a space of infinite variety which can match the singular and specifically differential aspect of each moment of perception. The factor of intensity makes color capable of registering the work of unconscious drives, while the chromatic scale relates to the perception of difference. For Gagnebin, the ambiguity of color makes it a go-between from sensory experience to unconscious desire, and this allows it to signal the work of fantasy and repression: "Colors point to the active power of repression" (106). This tension can be formulated in the context of language and identity. On the one hand, color is seen as antithetical to language, articulation, sense, mimesis, and thus to ordinary selfhood. It offers a release from the grip of these agencies into a realm of pure event, experience, affect.

For Michel Corvin "the lack of meaning 'brings back' the figure in its excessiveness as image . . . posited this way, color represents an absolute that cannot be transcended: something of which nothing can be said, but which imposes itself through an excessive plenitude and presence that is impossible to refute" (82). Roland Barthes subscribes to this discourse when he writes in his autobiography, "serais-je peintre, je ne peindrai que des couleurs: ce champ me paraît libéré également de la Loi (pas d'imitation, pas d'Analogie) et de la Nature" [if I were a painter I'd paint nothing but colors: this field seems to me to be equally free of the Law (no imitation, no Analogy) and of Nature] (146). But Barthes's antinaturalism points to the ambivalence of this kind of release which, even if it is linked to the rhythms of the body, can seem to have connotations of emptiness, in the Buddhist sense, rather than plenitude.

Equally, however, the other side of our polarity—the sense that color harmonies are compatible with, indeed analogous to, language—is also marked by ambivalence. The features of color reference which have fascinated philosophers, most notably Wittgenstein—for example the huge disparity between the very restricted number of basic colors: the primaries, or those of the spectrum, or just red, blue, and green, and the hundreds and thousands of nuances which even an untutored eye can discriminate—encourage talk of the language of color (a notion also linked to color symbolism). Yet if this can be used to underwrite a sense of the profound affinity between color range and the subtleties of individual psychology, the linkage of color and language, hue and cry, can also sponsor classifications which, even as they attempt to tie color to mood or humor, end up being immensely abstract and conceptual.

At this point, Maurice Merleau-Ponty's discussions of color in his writings on perception become an indispensable point of reference. Color is both incidental and fundamental to Merleau-Ponty's accounts of the human subject's "mélange avec le monde" [mingling with the world], the two-way processes, designated by such terms as *l'entrelacs* [the intertwining] or *le chiasme* [the chiasm], or concepts such as "la chair du monde" [the world's flesh] and "le corps interposé" [the interposed body] that mark out perception not as the work of one agency or another but as communion or synergy, a mutual participation in an open totality. Incidental, because although painting, and particularly the work of Cézanne, was a constant source of meditation for Merleau-Ponty, his concern is not with color itself. Fundamental, nonetheless, because, as is testified by frequent references in *La Phénoménologie de la perception* [*The Phenomenology of Perception*], *Le Visible et l'invisible* [*The Visible and the Invisible*], and *L'Oeil et l'esprit* [*Eye and Mind*], color had a particular relevance to Merleau-Ponty's concerns, a pertinence that is very revealing for our concern with the everyday because it is connected with one of color's inherent dualities. As a type of sense-datum associated with physical phenomena, color can be linked with a materialist and empiricist viewpoint where mind receives the imprint of matter. Conversely, a quality dependent on light, it can be seen as an abstraction, the product of a mental operation effected by a subject separate from the world. Since he sought to overturn both these perspectives, and the false duality they imply, it is not surprising that Merleau-Ponty often focuses on color.

My discussion will center principally on one passage from *Le Visible et l'invisible* [*The Visible and the Invisible*], but I will first outline briefly what I want to draw from the way Merleau-Ponty uses color in his attempts to render the difference between thinking about the world and living in it, and to characterize our inclusion in the visible, the way perception interrogates the world. The points I want to stress have to do with three related areas: immediacy, identity, and language. Already central to the discussion of *le sentir* [feeling] in the *Phénoménologie* is the insistence that sensation is never just of the here and now but incorporates the past: "sensation presupposes in me the sedimentation from an earlier process" (240). Nonetheless, there is something profoundly anonymous about it: "Every perception takes place in a climate of generality and presents itself to us as anonymous.... I ought to say that there is perception going on in me and not that I perceive. Every sensation comprises an element of dreaming or of depersonalisation" (242).

In its singularity, each sensation is always the first and last of its kind and invokes the response not of a subject who makes decisions but "another self who has already espoused the world." *Le Visible et l'invisible* extends the discussion of what it is like to be a subject of perception and, as the title indicates, this work emphasizes that the visible is rooted in the invisible—in what the subject brings to the process of perception. Language, far from being alien, an agent of severance, is seen to be potentially integral with it. Both seeing and speaking, according to Merleau-Ponty, if we seek to grasp them concretely rather than discursively, can be what he calls "experiences [that are] both irrefutable and enigmatic" (130).

Near the beginning of the book's last chapter, titled "L'Entrelacs—le chiasme" [The Intertwining—The Chiasm], Merleau-Ponty uses color to explore a central paradox, the way seeing involves both proximity and distance, absorption and separation. How can it be, he asks, that the apparently seamless quality of visual experience does not constitute either a total takeover of the object by the subject or conversely of our mind by the object? What magic property must the visible have—"What is this talisman of color, this singular virtue of the visible" (131)—that we can apprehend it so totally, while at the same time it retains its sovereignty? If the structure of vision is chiastic, and seeing involves a crossing over into the realm of things—a movement outwards, but at the same time an internalization, an invasion by the outside—why do subject and object not simply fuse, or coincide absolutely, or cancel one another out? Because, in a metaphor Merleau-Ponty develops extensively, they are of the same flesh: "The gaze itself envelops things, clothes them with its own flesh" (131). Vision marshals in things a dimension which is other than the thing in itself, which inheres in our apprehension of them, but which is nevertheless not simply our projection, because, reciprocally, vision marshals in us a dimension which does not preexist this chiastic exchange or intertwining "the world and I are within one another" (123). Crucial here is the fact that vision is a bodily experience by dint of the fact that seeing is a kind of touching: "tout visible est taillé dans le tangible" [every visible is cut out in the tangible] (134). The act of vision enlists our body, through which we are "pris dans le tissu des choses" [caught up in the fabric of things] (135).

To illustrate this, Merleau-Ponty develops the example of color: a shade of red that catches my eye is seen to be not one thing that I relate to all at once, but a layered and variegated phenomenon which implicates widely different orders of experience:

> We must first understand that this red under my eyes is not, as is always said, a quale, a pellicle of being without thickness, a message at the same time indecipherable and evident, which one has or has not received, but of which, if one has received it, one knows all there is to know, and of which in the end there is nothing to say. It requires a focusing, however brief; it emerges from a less precise, more general redness, in which my gaze was caught, into which it sank, before—as we put it so aptly—fixing it. And, now that I have fixed it, if my eyes penetrate into it, into its fixed structure, or if they start to wander round about again, the quale resumes its atmospheric existence. Its precise form is bound up with a certain woolly, metallic, or porous configuration or texture, and the quale itself counts for very little compared with these participations. (131–32)

"Participations" is a key word here. Talking about a particular shade of redness, Merleau-Ponty seeks to show that our rapport with it is engendered not by its fixed character, as a pure quality, but by the fact that it belongs simultaneously to different orders. First, my way of attending to it is physical, mobile—"it requires a focusing": I need to locate its specificity in the way it is not just red, but this red. And to do this I scan it and feel it with my eyes. The particular quality of redness does not just stand still. A work of differentiation takes place. A second dimension is situational—the relation between this red and other contiguous shades of red, or other colors and colored things in the same environment. This red is not an isolated phenomenon but "a certain node in the woof of the simultaneous and the successive. It is a concretion of visibility, it is not an atom" (132). Thirdly, and most importantly, with regard to the chiastic relationship of viewer and viewed, this red's participation in "the fabric of the visible" also locates it in a "tissu d'être invisible" [a fabric of invisible being] (132):

> The red dress a fortiori holds with all its fibers onto the fabric of the visible, and thereby onto a fabric of invisible being. A punctuation in the field of red things, which includes the tiles of roof tops, the flags of gatekeepers and of the Revolution, certain terrains near Aix or in Madagascar, it is also a punctuation in the field of red garments, which includes, along with the dresses of women, robes of professors, bishops, and advocate generals, and also in the field of adornments and that of uniforms. (132)

Take a red dress. Its redness punctuates "the field of red things"—roof tiles, flags, landscapes tinged with ochre: this red has a place in a constellation of reds I have seen before, reds I remember, as well as other reds in its immediate environment. These absent reds make up one level of invisibility. But this red dress worn by a woman fits not only into a constellation of other red costumes—associated with particular officers: teachers, bishops, judges—but with uniforms generally. And the red of this particular dress differs according to which constellation I fit it into:

> and its red literally is not the same as it appears in one constellation or in the other, as the pure essence of the Revolution of 1917 precipitates in it, or that of the eternal feminine, or that of the public prosecutor, or that of the gypsies dressed like Hussars who reigned twenty-five years ago over an inn on the Champs-Elysées. (132)

Finally, a given red also belongs to an imaginary constellation: it is "a fossil drawn up from the depths of imaginary worlds." This vivid series of enumerations leads into a crucial general statement summarizing what Merleau-Ponty is saying about colors, and how they represent visible things in general. If we take into account all these orders of belonging, "these participations," then:

> A naked color, and in general a visible one, is not a chunk of absolutely hard, indivisible being, offered all naked to a vision which could be only total or null, but is rather a sort of strait between exterior horizons and interior horizons ever gaping open, something that comes to touch lightly and makes diverse regions of the colored or visible world resound at the distances, a certain differentiation, an ephemeral modulation of this world—less a color or a thing, therefore, than a difference between things and colors, a momentary crystallization of colored being or of visibility. (132)

So a color is not a thing, one and indivisible, to be apprehended or not, but a kind of narrow strait between an outer horizon—other visible reds—and an inner one—other invisible reds. To attend to a color is not to home in on some pure quality or essence but to enter a field of resonances embracing various domains in the world of the visible. But if this means moving away from the color itself, the trajectory is not away from the particular but paradoxically towards the specificity of a particular moment, "a certain differentiation, an ephemeral modulation of this world."

The move is not towards the generic character of the color or thing, but towards its difference from other colors or things, or the same colors and things perceived in other circumstances. To attend to an occasion with regard to the dimension of color is to attend to what makes it this occasion and not another.

At this point let us bring language back into the picture. One of the factors that is precious about Merleau-Ponty's way of thinking about color is that it has explicit parallels with what he has to say about language and particularly a dimension of language he calls "la parole opérante" [operative speech]. Just as a perception of color is not a one-off thing but draws on a hinterland of other perceptions going to make up "the fabric of our experience," so "univocal signification is but one part of the signification of the word, . . . beyond it there is always a halo of signification that manifests itself in new and unexpected modes of use" (96). And just as the field of our experience comprises "this immense latent content of the past," and is not constituted by indivisible entities or essences but rather by "a time and a space that exist by piling up, by proliferation, by encroachment, by promiscuity—a perpetual pregnancy, perpetual parturition, generativity and generality" (115), so language partakes of this: "like the flesh of the visible, speech is a total part of the significations [. . .] there is solidarity and intertwining [. . .] speech prolongs into the invisible, extends unto the semantic operations, the belongingness of the body to being" (118). Within the linguistic field "operative speech" is "a way of making things themselves speak" (125).

Here language is not being used instrumentally; words combine according to the "natural intertwining of their meaning, through the occult trading of metaphor" (125). What counts is not the manifest meaning of words, "but the lateral relations, the kinships that are implicated in their transfers and their exchanges" (125). In the context of lived experience, language does not mask or conceal Being. Rather, "if one knows how to grasp it with all its roots and all its foliation" (126), it is "the most valuable witness to Being" (126). This reasoned confidence in language, and its connection with the domain of color, lead naturally in the direction of poetry, a frequent point of reference for Merleau-Ponty, as well as towards painting.

Connections between color, language, and everyday experience play an important role in contemporary French poetry, and I wish now to focus on two contrasting approaches in the work of

Yves Bonnefoy and Philippe Jaccottet. Bonnefoy is well known for his writings on art, from his studies of Poussin and Roman baroque to the many essays on modern artists including a fine monograph on Giacometti, but Bonnefoy's concerns are the same whether he is thinking about poetry, writing poems, or seeking to understand an artist's work, and meditations on color feature in all three areas. Bonnefoy's central theme is what he calls "la présence" [presence], an experience of Being in the context of the everyday world, particularly associated with language, landscape, and love. In all these fields his writing investigates how human desire, articulated through the imaginary, propitiates or thwarts the approach to presence. Is the realm of the image, generically speaking, an arena for presence or not? To the extent that the imaginary may involve a confiscation of the real, of presence, a substitution of something else in its place, should authentic art and poetry constitute "une guerre contre l'image" [a war against the image], a repudiation of form, concept, ornament, beauty, or is there a "good" way of way of dealing with images, a way of lucidly contesting the negative features of the image within the imaging process itself?

These are the kinds of issues on the horizon when Bonnefoy talks about color. In three books published in 1977, color features in three different kinds of context. First, a section of his long poem *Dans le leurre du seuil* [*In the Threshold's Lure*] is entitled "Deux couleurs" [Two Colors]. The colors allude to a series of paintings by Poussin on the subject of Moses in the bulrushes, but more importantly they instigate what will be a recurrent motif: the notion of two colors working in contrapuntal fashion, with and against one another, each contesting and relativizing the proposition of the other, and through this interplay opening up another dimension. Subsequent poems by Bonnefoy, most notably "Dedham, vu de Langham" [Dedham, seen from Langham], which concerns the landscapes of Constable, will also be concerned with color. Secondly, a number of essays in *Le Nuage rouge* [*The Red Cloud*] involve interrogations of color. The title essay refers to a painting by Mondrian, predating his turn to pure abstraction, depicting a landscape near the sea and a single large red cloud in the sky. Bonnefoy pays close attention to all the colors in the painting, in the context of which the red cloud—compared at one point to the burning bush—is read as a profoundly ambivalent sign, because it represents at the same time an aspiration to a transcendent order and the questioning or checking of that impulse to achieve transcendence through the affirmation of what Bonnefoy calls "l'hétérogène à jamais qui dresse la présence contre l'image, la faille qui revendique ce que nulle écriture ne saurait jamais accepter . . . un ici . . . un lieu . . . une durée" [the eternally heterogeneous which confronts the image with its sheer presence, the gap which lays claim to what no writing can ever accept . . . a here . . . a place . . . a duration] (123).

The ambivalence of color, or its capacity to incarnate ambivalence, is at the center of essays on Georges Duthuit—"Un Ennemi des images" [An Enemy of the Image]—and on the nudes of Claude Garache, who uses only one color, red. In his discussion of Garache, as Richard Stamelman has underlined, Bonnefoy considers the way color has often represented a desire for immediacy in artists ranging from Titian and Rubens, to Delacroix or Van Gogh. Demonstrating how immediacy is in fact negated by the purely formal character of color harmonies, color being in some respects simply another language, a system of mediation, Bonnefoy points to ways in which, in brief passages, the closed order or system of color language can be evaded, and how tonal values can suddenly engender presence: "Loin de vouer la perception sensorielle aux apories du médiat [. . .] les valeurs [. . .] replantent autour de nous, l'apparence fermant sa roue, toutes les belles plumes de la présence du monde" [Far from condemning sensory perception to the aporias of mediation (. . .) tonal values (. . .) restore around us, appearance having closed its peacock's tail, all the fine scattered feathers of the world's presence] (325). Third, 1977 also saw the publication of a work entitled *Trois remarques sur la couleur* [*Three Remarks on Color*] consisting not of an essay but of three enigmatic prose texts, similar in character to another series brought together the same year under the general title *Rue Traversière* [*Cross Street*].

When, ten years later, Bonnefoy brought the two sets of texts together, along with others written in the meantime, Bonnefoy gave them the generic label "récits en rêve" [dreaming narratives]. Bonnefoy's "récits en rêve" can be seen as a cross between the "poème en prose" [prose poem], the "récit de rêve" [dream narrative], the lyrical or meditative essay, and the parable or metaphysical tale in the manner of Borges. They generally feature a fictional narrator, often a traveler, but the oneiric aspect does not usually involve a markedly dreamlike atmosphere and consists more, as the phrase "récits en rêve" suggests, in the way the narratives develop, often switching abruptly from one time and place to another. In fact, most of the texts involve two or three scenes linked by a commentary, as well as fleeting dialogues between the narrator-traveler and the people he observes or encounters.

When these texts were incorporated as a section in the larger volume, *Récits en rêve*, a number of new ones were added under the rubric "Remarques sur la couleur," but interestingly two of the original three had in fact migrated to join another cluster entitled "L'Origine de la parole" [The Origin of Speech]. This underlines the close connection between color and language which is a consistent feature of these texts, several of which feature imaginary communities, generally islands, where the conventions regarding the names of colors, or the relation between colors and things, differ from those with which we are familiar. In "Deux et d'autres couleurs" [Two and Other Colors], for example, the traveler encounters three different ways of thinking about color, or rather three ways in which an attitude to color can bespeak an attitude to, or understanding of, human reality.

In the first part, he is told that the local language uses two color names to designate a single color, and conversely a single color term to designate something that is of two colors, though it is also possible to designate the latter by two pairs of names corresponding to the two constituent colors. So a green and white ferry can be referred to as red or, alternatively, as yellow, blue, black, and red since green can be designated as yellow and blue, and green as red and black. The aim of this system is to remedy the poverty of ordinary language, which does not even begin to render the richness of reality, by the creation of a "second degré de la parole" [second degree of speech], a language of proliferation and surprise which aims to circumvent the limits of "la dénomination abusive" [inappropriate designation]: "Défaire la dénomination abusive, lever par ce levier, l'infini, l'arbitraire triste du signe, mais c'est laver la face du monde, mon ami, c'est se retrouver respirant dans la respiration de tout, silencieuse! Nous avons inventé le second degré de la parole!" [To rectify inappropriate designation, to abrogate by this means, the infinite, sad arbitrariness of signs, why, this is to wipe clean the face of the earth, my friend, it's to recover one's breath, in the silent breathing of all things! We have invented the second degree of speech!] (81).

This fantasy of using language to go beyond language leaves the traveler sceptical, and on his journey to various islands on the ferry he will encounter another kind of potential link between color and presence. As the ship leaves its various ports of call, he notices that colored streamers maintain, for a while at least, until they drop or break, a link between departing passengers and those they leave behind. The flashes of color, which stand out against the purple sea-mist, figure the intermittent, unpredictable, snatches of shared experience or communal presence which, for a while at least, provide a vital link, a line of communication between human beings: "Certains rubans cassient, assez vite, et retombaient dans l'écume, y salissant et trouant, le bleu, le vert ou le rouge. Mais d'autres duraient, improbables, miraculeux, dans les cris de bonheur ou le silence attentif" [Some ribbons broke fairly quickly, and fell back into the spray, puncturing and dirtying the blue, the green or the red. But others kept aloft, improbably, miraculously, amid cries of joy or attentive silence] (83).

In the third part of the text the traveler, back in the port where he had started, encounters the man he had spoken to earlier. He now dismisses, as no more than an image, the linguistic theories he had expounded, but, while apparently confirming what the traveler had understood by the strips of ribbon, and the moments of joy and grief enshrined in momentary flashes of color, he urges him to witness another spectacle the next day. Go to the temple on the mountainside, he says, and look at the grey earthenware jars half buried in the garden behind. Once a year they are filled with different colored powders which when lit create a vast flame where the colors both fuse together and remain distinct:

> C'est phosphorescent, c'est changeant, c'est un et multiple à la fois, c'est indéchiffrable comme la vie, c'est immatériel comme elle, on peut dire, je crois, qu'il s'agit là d'une couleur autre, dont la terre ne savait rien avant que l'on eût compris que l'on meurt, et naît, et renaît, et renaît encore.
> [It's phosphorescent, it's changing, it's one and multiple at the same time, it's indecipherable as life, and as immaterial, one can say, I think, that we have here another color, of which the earth knew nothing before people understood that we die, and are born, and are born again, and yet again.] (85)

As I suggested earlier, in this text and others like it, Bonnefoy uses color as an idiom or key in which to explore allegorically questions of language, ethics, and aesthetics. Another piece, "La Résurrection," juxtaposes three elements, W. B. Yeats's play *Resurrection*, which Bonnefoy had translated, the paintings of Bram van Velde, which involve variations on three or four basic colors, and the death of the narrator's mother. Initially the meditation establishes a parallel between the play, where three characters incarnate three ways of understanding Christ's resurrection, and thus three different visions of the world, and the colors in van Velde's paintings which can be seen to figure different "modes d'être" [ways of being], and, in their combination, like different colored flames in a single hearth, to signify "les vérités diverses de la raison, du coeur, du corps que le sang remue, ou la contemplation qui l'apaise" [the diverse truths of reason, of the heart, and of the body animated by blood, or by contemplation which restores its peace] (140).

Seen this way, color is "une spéculation tendue à l'extrême de soi, donc instable, ouverte aux contradictions, militante" [a tense speculation at the self's extremity, hence unstable, open to contradictions, militant] (141). But suddenly this vision collapses and gives way to a different perception of van Velde's colors, Their combinations are now seen as "sans cause, sans finalité" [without cause, without aim]; their beauty is that of the void, the timeless; they turn everything into absolutes. And perhaps the same is true of Yeats's play. At any rate, at the end of the text the notion of resurrection is applied to someone known, and the narrator wonders whether, were his mother to be resurrected with the look she bore when she had been loved most intensely—perhaps the day she met his father—he would be able to recognize her at all (144).

In two further texts, colors incarnate antithetical extremes: on one hand, total stability, on the other, total mutability. "Au Mont Aso" describes a mountainside, in an Eastern country, perhaps Japan, renowned for its uniform greenness, where visitors find that the experience of "la simplicité de la perception" [the simplicity of perception] has a powerful effect on their relation to language: "car c'est la notion même de différence qui se dissipe ici [. . .] Et avec elle s'efface le vain désir de nommer ou plutôt [. . .] s'atténue cette sorte de houle dont les vocables, cette intempérance de la couleur, enveloppent et brisent ce qu'ils nomment" [for it's the very notion of difference that dissolves here. . . . And with it the vain desire to name is effaced, or rather . . . that kind swell with which speech, that intemperance of color, envelops and destroys what it names] (87). But this experience is seen in fact to dispel the enigma of experience, and the narrator's subsequent vision of two streaks of color in the sky, and then his memory of a tomb made out of red clay, and finally his recollection of being told of one moment in the year when

Mount Aso does slightly change its shade of green, and that in this period of mists people go in groups and hold picnics where ribald jokes are told and couples are formed, serve to dispel the Oriental perfection of pure experience without language.

In "Le Crépuscule des mots" [The Twilight of Words], on the other hand, the narrator visits a land where the meaning of words is subject to sudden changes and shifts, in response to the ever-changing nature of reality. But while at any given time there may be a word not only for this type of boat but for the impression a boat gives as it approaches the harbor, or for the aura which surrounds a newly arrived passenger, people on street corners endlessly debate the meanings of utterances. Colors are repeatedly invoked as the narrator reports his debates with the local inhabitants and expresses his doubts about this linguistic regime. Does it not imply a sacrifice of communality and disregard for certain elemental realities? He conveys the delight of gliding in a world of metamorphosis where "l'univers n'est plus qu'une esplanade infinie" [the universe is no more than an infinite esplanade] (98) and concedes that in the realm of color the infinite nuances of tone and shade occur within the framework of seven basic colors which preside and unify. But he wonders, nonetheless, if it is not precisely the mission of poetry to preserve meanings rather than to dispel them, and at the end of the text there is still a sense that the debate remains open, that perhaps the issue is not one of adjudicating between color and language, but exploring under what conditions both these domains can open up rather than close off an encounter with the world.

In general, the drift of Bonnefoy's meditations about colors, which are always meditations on ways of living in the world and on the ethics of representation, is away from the sovereign beauty of pure color towards contrast, juxtaposition, change, and mutability. In a series of reflections on the paintings of Miklos Bokor, he stresses the sudden emergence of colors in Bokor's works which he sees as a kind of germination or crystallization, a process reflecting inner change:

> Couleurs, non, l'expérience du monde, du destin que la couleur a permise.... D'année en année ... la musique des yeux pénètre plus avant l'apparence ... c'est la passion qui se fait en lui couleur, ombres de couleur, afin de se clarifier, se musicaliser.
> [Colors, no, the experience of the world, of a destiny that color has facilitated.... Year after year ... the music of the eyes penetrates further into appearance.... It's passion which in him is transmuted

into color, colored shadows, in order to become clarity, to become music.] (101)

And in a text from a more recent collection, *La Vie errante* [*The Wandering Life*] "L'alchimiste de la couleur" [The Alchemist of Color] the alchemist, having spent years trying to transmute colors into gold, pure light, endlessly mixing them on his palette but producing only grey, suddenly sees two stains of different colors. Possessed now by this contrast, he juxtaposes colors and begins to see fields, branches, and birds. In the end, the parable suggests, colors take us back to where we are, they are the earth, and the true alchemist is the landscape painter whose art constitutes a revelation of the real (25).

I want now to turn to the work of Philippe Jaccottet, in which landscape is also a central preoccupation. Though originally Swiss-French, Jaccottet has lived since the 1950s at Grignan in northern Provence, and the greater part of his work in various forms, including collections of poems, an ongoing poetic diary or log-book, *La Semaison* [*Sowings*], several volumes of prose pieces, and some mixing of all three forms, originates in his contemplation of the landscape in which he lives. Observations and meditations regarding color can be found in all aspects and periods of his work, but I will base my remarks on three prose texts from a recent book, *Cahier de verdure* [*Green Diary*] (1990), which in fact contains both poems and prose texts, combining them in a way which, as the title of the volume suggests, adds up to a sort of notebook or ongoing register. It is worth noting that a number of Jaccottet's earlier prose texts, including *Paysages avec figures absentes* [*Lanscapes with Absent Figures*] and *A travers un verger* [*Through an Orchard*], were collected together under the title *Des histoires de passage* [*Stories of Passage*]. Most of them have a narrative element, like Bonnefoy's "récits en rêve," but here the autobiographical dimension is totally explicit and there is no fictionalization, even if the development of the text, sometimes referred to as a reverie, is often engendered by associations, images, and memories which emerge in a way reminiscent of dreams. The word *passage* relates to the fact that the starting point for most of these autobiographical reveries or meditations, which often reconstruct a past event in great detail, sometimes relating it to other events, is generally something that has been observed in passing, generally on one of Jaccottet's daily walks around Grignan, but sometimes also on journeys elsewhere.

So these "histoires" are closely linked to contingent moments, to chance and accident, but also to everyday experience, to the repetitions and rituals of the everyday. In seeking to home in on and to understand retrospectively something that has moved or surprised him, galvanized his attention, or roused him from a state of indifference or dejection into a mood of celebration or reflection that makes him want to investigate his own experience, Jaccottet may follow a number of paths. As a rule, what prompts him to reflect and write is a natural phenomenon, the impression made by a tree, a mountain, a vista; and very often one of the things which may be central to the initial experience is color.

This is the case in the three texts I want to discuss from *Cahier de verdure*. In the first, "Le Cerisier" [The Cherry Tree], it is the sight of a cherry tree at nightfall which he seeks to explore, and particularly the impression conveyed by the redness of the cherries in conjunction with the dark green of the foliage. In the second, "Blason vert et blanc" [Green and White Emblem], it is a small orchard of quince trees, and in the third, "Apparition des fleurs" [Apparition of the Flowers], it is the conjunction in the same place of three flowers, each a different color—blue, yellow, and white. In none of these cases is it color itself, independently of the rest, that is paramount. But on each occasion, both in the initial event, and its exploration in words, the question of color, of what the colors meant, of what they contributed, is absolutely central. In many ways Jaccottet's texts can be seen to exemplify perfectly the account of what it means to be arrested by and to explore a color impression put forward by Merleau-Ponty in the passage commented on earlier. What Jaccottet investigates are the various orders of "participation" to which the color seems to belong, ranging from other elements in the same context, to the subject's own personal associations and experiences, often rooted in the distant past, to the cultural associations of the colors and color combinations concerned. In doing so, and although he constantly registers his sense of failure and dissatisfaction in this regard, Jaccottet is not favoring color over language, but trying to exploit the "parole opérante" [operative speech] of poetry, trying to register and match the work of perception with the work of language.

Although he writes in prose, Jaccottet exploits to the full the resources of diction, assonance, rhythm, repetition, and metaphor and composes his text in a series of fragments, each consisting of one or more paragraphs, separated by a double space. As in the case of Bonnefoy, color has a place in Jaccottet's concerns not just because of a delight in the visual, and indeed in painting, but because the process of attending to color, particularly in the context of the natural world, seems to involve not an escape from the real but a profound engagement with it, at a level and in a manner which raises questions about language, about experience, and about everydayness. The sense of beauty, and the ecstasy of looking, are in fact central insofar as for Jaccottet, as for Bonnefoy, the beauty of the world maintains the possibility—to be set against abundant incitements to despair—of some sort of harmony.

In each of the texts from *Cahier de verdure*, the initial experience is one of being stunned by the beauty of what has been seen, but if this inspires a desire to reflect and understand, it is in response to what is experienced as a kind of duty, an ethical demand solicited by the experience of looking. In "Le Cerisier," for example, Jaccottet refers several times to the feeling of responding to something akin to the light pressure of a hand gently inciting him to change his direction: "Cette fois, il s'agissait d'un cerisier" [This time, it was a cherry tree] (9). The opening passage reconstructs the very specific circumstances—time of day, lay of the land, elements of the scene, initial on-the-spot feelings—but also draws out and embroiders various threads of association relating to night, metamorphosis, apparitions. Then there is the description of the one particular cherry tree:

> Ses fruits étaient comme une longue grappe de rouge, une coulée de rouge, dans du vert sombre; des fruits dans un berceau ou une corbeille de feuilles; du rouge dans du vert, à l'heure du glissement des choses les unes dans les autres, à l'heure d'une lente et silencieuse métamorphose, à l'heure de l'apparition, presque, d'un autre monde. [Its fruit were like a long cluster of red, a flow of red, in dark green; fruit in a cradle or basket of leaves; some red in some green, at the hour when everything flows into everything else, at the hour of a slow and silent metamorphosis, at the hour of the apparition, almost, of another world.] (12)

In the following paragraph Jaccottet addresses himself to why this particular quality of redness, in its conjunction with the green, should have prompted such a response in him, why it should have had so much the quality of an apparition and to have suggested images of gentle metamorphosis: "Que pouvait être ce rouge pour me surprendre, me réjouir à ce point?" [What could this red have been to surprise me, to delight me so much?] (12). It suggested neither blood nor flames. (A long parenthesis conjures up, with great accuracy and immediacy, the recent, contrasting, experience of staring at flames in a bonfire. This contrast emphasizes the differential quality of the phenomenon under consideration—the redness of the cherries.) The recollection that the cherries seemed to flow links them to wine, and he ends up settling for the notion of a "feu suspendu . . . une grappe de feu apprivoisé, marié à de l'eau nocturne" [suspended fire . . . a cluster of tamed fire, married to nocturnal water] (13). And in subsequent paragraphs this will lead to the idea of seeing the cherries as a kind of votive offering, and then to seeing them as somehow "couvés" [watched over] by the green foliage, and thus as representing past experiences held in suspension, allowed to ripen under the protection of the green.

In the second text, "Blason vert et blanc," prompted by the glimpse of quince-blossom through a steamed-up car window, the conjunction of white and green, and of the words "vert et blanc," becomes the emblem of the experience which is pursued almost exclusively in terms of color, through the question of what the conjunction of colors intimated. Yet here the path of association does not involve other things of the same color, but rather literary and cultural references. The particular character of this blossom, this mode of "floraison," different from cherries and apples, on this particular occasion of passage, prompts a welter of feelings and impressions to do with calm, simplicity, or self-sufficiency, which seem to be epitomized most satisfactorily in the conjunction of green and white. Having established that "Vert et blanc. C'est le blason de ce verger" [Green and white. The emblem of this orchard] the meditation, "rêvant, réfléchisssant à ces deux couleurs" [dreaming, thinking about these two colors] (26) explores the resonances of the colors, through Dante's Vita nova, Hölderlin's Hyperion, Botticelli's Flora, Verlaine's Gaspard Hauser, and so forth. The summary of the qualities of the two colors together elicits the notion of enveloping femininity, and this engenders a further cultural reference—to Mozart's Zerlina—which then leads into the idea of rustic ceremonies and well-ordered spaces, conjuring up a country church where all is ready for the wedding. Then, partly via the waxy whiteness of candles, we are introduced to further ways of rendering the sense of security and gentle solidity exuded by these colors, "couleurs fermes, opaques et tranquilles; rien qui frémisse. . . . Comme si le mouvement n'existait plus" [colors that are firm, opaque and tranquil; nothing brusque . . . As if movement no longer existed] until the meditation ends a few pages further on.

The third text also relates to something in the natural world that arrests the writer's attention, but the decision to explore this "apparition" is prompted by a repercussion it had already had in Jaccottet's writing when, at the end of a dark poem inspired by the death or serious illness of several friends, the names of three flowers had represented the universe's response to the poet's sardonic desire for some sort of explanation: "Pour réponse, au bord du chemin: seneçon, berce, chicorée" [For reply, at the side of the path, groundsel, hogweed, chicory] (69). To try and understand what it was about them that had brought these flowers to mind, Jaccottet goes back to the occasion when their unusual conjunction in a field, during the summer when one friend of his was dying, had overwhelmed him with wonder and joy. In fact, the investigation will not prove very satisfactory. Although Jaccottet perceives that the three colors are vital, and that "ces couleurs devaient donc bien 'donner sur' autre chose" [these colors, it was clear, "gave onto" something else], and although he has no difficulty in pursuing the resonance of the three particular shades, he feels nonetheless that "ces couleurs m'échappaient" [these colors eluded me], or rather that what it was that had enabled them to appear for a moment "comme des clefs de ce monde" [like keys to this world] still eluded him. "Je ne comprenais donc toujours rien" [Clearly, I still hadn't understood anything] (72). To some extent, Jaccottet's dissatisfaction stems from the contradiction between the basic simplicity of the experience, and indeed the simple, unsophisticated quality of both the flowers and their colors, and the elaborateness of his poetic investigation, the endless comparisons and relays through which he seeks to pin them down.

In the end, perhaps, he comes closest to defining the crucial quality in the experience which made it seem to hold out a response to the terrible doubts cast by the shadow of suffering and death, when he shifts away from the colors and comes back to the flowers themselves, and particularly to their associations with Persephone, who was condemned to the underworld for picking flowers in the meadow, or when he focuses on the notion of "surgissement" [sudden appearance], the sudden "apparition" of the flowers which seem all at once to appear out of nowhere. But this in no way alters the pertinence of colors to Jaccottet's project or the validity of color as a pathway towards a deeper understanding of his experience.

By way of conclusion, I will sum up what seems to be involved in Jaccottet's preoccupation with color, and in doing so link it to some of the main strands of my argument. First, the general links between color and subjectivity must be reiterated. We are concerned here with a phenomenologically constructed subjectivity, inseparable from the subject's engagement with the world of things and others, and moreover a dimension of subjective experience that comes close to being anonymous or impersonal, to being everybody's experience. As a cardinal dimension of perceptual and sensual experience, color manifests the way sensation is both highly individualized, something that happens to this subject in this time and place, and at the same time depersonalized. Being contingent on atmospheric conditions, on available light, and on a whole range of other situational factors, color also links subjectivity to temporal process, to the momentary but also to duration, and thus to the unfolding rhythm of the day. All Jaccottet's passages occur at a particular time of day, often a transitional one like morning or evening, and as such they manifest something more general about the connection between colors and everydayness. In most contexts color is only one component of a phenomenon or occasion, often seemingly an inessential or trivial one, yet it can present itself as the key in which a certain experience is lived through and thus, in another sense of the word, as the key to its wider significance.

Like Merleau-Ponty, Jaccottet shows that to follow the trace of color is to attend to an occasion in a particular way, that may lead in many directions, but keeps the experience in play, deepening our sense of its possible bearings. In this respect, the peripheral nature of color turns out to be a strength since it does not prejudge the order of gravity or significance the perception may turn out to have. Merleau-Ponty compares colors which grab our attention to screen-memories which are often put together out of various occasions, and in which what initially seems incidental may turn out to be fundamental, and vice versa. Colors are the receptacles of desire, but as Bonnefoy's "récits en rêve" consistently show, colors lend themselves to being the vehicles of desire sublimated into ethical, metaphysical, or ecological concerns. Color is always difference, but difference in a narrow compass. There are far more nuances and combinations of colors than words to describe them, but where the proliferation of language can seem to threaten the bond of language and experience, the endless nuances of tone are held in place and ordered by their primordial relationship to a very small number of basic colors. What is more, colors are universal even if the way they are perceived is culturally relative. If I have said little about the numerous kinds of color symbolism, and the function of certain esoteric ways of thought such as heraldry and alchemy, it is because these are always ways of pinning color down, of extolling its riches but at the same time curtailing its infinity. Yet of course all ways of organizing colors pay tribute to the boundlessness of nuance.

However compellingly it may address us, color is always an enigmatic feature of any phenomenon. Physically, chemically, functionally, color is a side effect rather than the main point. It often seems gratuitous, even frivolous; generally nonutilitarian, color has no particular job to do, far less than other physical qualities such as shape or size. Nevertheless one of the enigmas of color is that it can seem to be the soul of an object or occasion. And this means that to say of something that it is this color or that, to present a passage of experience in terms of what color things were, can seem to be saying very little, or, on the contrary to say a great deal, but a great deal about that particular moment, about your participation in it. Colors are physical but also doubly immaterial. We apprehend them by dint of our capacities as physical organisms capable of acts of perception. Colors address us through our senses, through our bodily presence in the world (Merleau-Ponty), but at the same time they involve us in a mental process of discrimination and deciphering which both resists and solicits language. Colors provoke desire and deliver us from fixity, but at the same time they stir up the archives of our identity. If color offers us one way of grasping everydayness, it is perhaps because of the type of fascination it exerts and the kind of attention it requires, a mode of attention attuned to the mysterious reciprocities of self and world, and to a realm where everything is always changing, and yet much remains the same.

Works Cited

Where no English-language edition is listed translations are my own.

Barthes, Roland. *Roland Barthes by Roland Barthes* [1975]. Translated by Richard Howard. New York: Hill and Wang, 1977.
Baudelaire, Charles. "Salon de 1846." In *Œuvres complètes*, vol. 1. Edited by C. Pichois. Paris: Gallimard, 1974.

Blanchot, Maurice. "Everyday Speech" [1963]. In *Everyday Life*. Edited by Alice Kaplan and Kristin Ross. *Yale French Studies*, no. 73 (1987).
Bonnefoy, Yves. *Dans le leurre du seuil*. Paris: Mercure de France, 1977.
———. *Le Nuage rouge*. Paris, Mercure de France, 1977.
———. *Rue Traversière et autres récits en rêve*. Paris: Gallimard "Poésie," 1992.
———. *La Vie errante*. Paris: Mercure de France, 1993.
Corvin, Michel. "La Passion des mots." In *Des Mots et des couleurs*, vol. 2. Lille: Presses universitaires de Lille, 1986.
David, Christian. "Iris au service d'Eros: remarques sur le pouvoir expressif des couleurs." In *Questions de couleurs*. Rencontres psychanalytiques d'Aix-en-Provence. Edited by C. David et al. Paris: Les Belles Lettres, 1991.
Duthuit, Georges. *Représentation et Présence*. Paris: Flammarion, 1974.
Gagnebin, Muriel. "Chromatique et herméneutique." in *Questions de couleurs* (see above).
Jaccottet, Philippe. *Cahier de Verdure*. Paris: Gallimard, 1990.
Jünger, Ernst. *Le Coeur aventureux* [*Das Abenteuerliche Herz*, 1929]. Translated by Henri Thomas. Paris: Gallimard, 1979.
Kandinsky, Wassily. *Regards sur le passé* [1912], quoted in P. Choulet, "L'Esprit de la couleur chez Kandinsky," In *La Couleur*. Edited by L. Coulonbaritsis and J-J Wuneburger. Bruxelles: Editions Ousia, 1993, 205–28.
Merleau-Ponty, Maurice. *The Phenomenology of Perception* [1945]. London: Routledge, 1992.
———. *The Visible and the Invisible* [1964]. Translated by Alphonso Lingis. Evanston, Ill.: Northwestern University Press, 1968.
Stamelman, Richard. "Transfigurings of Red: Color, Representation, and Being in Yves Bonnefoy and Claude Garache." *The Comparatist* (May 1986): 90–106.

Reading *La Lectrice*
PAUL SUTTON

THE FILM *LA LECTRICE*, AS ITS VERY TITLE MIGHT SUGGEST, CAN BE read as a film about reading: reading, however, in a number of different guises.[1] It is, at its most obvious, a reading (and adaptation) of a novel by Raymond Jean similarly entitled *La Lectrice*.[2] It is also a film that is concerned with the physicality or vocality of reading, *lecture à haute voix*, reading aloud. Conversely the physical is itself subject to reading, thus in *La Lectrice* the body is textualized, and sexualized, both in and through reading. This is a body manifested in, and read by, the senses (a body determined by the visual, vocal, and aural; a body that exceeds the very containment the term suggests). The film, in presenting reading as an object for reading (or viewing), thus both represents and enacts reading, reading as performance, but also as will become evident, performative reading.[3]

This chapter proposes to perform a reading of Michel Deville's film through the readings the film itself enacts. It will demonstrate through these readings that both textual and cinematic reading can be usefully theorized as sensual, although at this stage one might refer more properly to an evocation rather than to a theorization.[4] Before undertaking these readings, it will be necessary to briefly summarize the film's diegetic structure, which in many ways mirrors the configuration of readings just described. It should be noted that this chapter represents a relatively tentative and circumspect intervention on the subject of sensual reading and is, in the context of a brief study, forced to overlook much that is both interesting and problematic in the film. It touches, therefore, only upon particular examples and does so in a highly strategic manner.

Thus *La Lectrice*, rather than simply reading or adapting the novel, could be said to be more properly staging or performing it, for it begins beyond the novel, *hors texte*, opening with a shot of Philippe, in bed, reading Raymond Jean's *La Lectrice*. Complaining that his eyes hurt he asks his partner, who "reads well and has a very pretty voice," to read to him. She begins, "My friend Françoise told me: 'Marie, you have a lovely voice,' " breaking off to remark to Philippe, " 'Just like me.' "[5] Thus the *lectrice* of the film, who shall be referred to, for the sake of simplicity, as Constance, is aligned with the *lectrice* of the novel, Marie, an alignment of what Peter Brooks might call the "outer narrator" with the "inner narrator."[6] It should be noted here that the novel begins: "Let me introduce myself: Marie-Constance," and that the film refers to this same narrator as Marie.[7] The outer narrator is never named in the film and if anything can only be referred to as Marie. Reviewers of the film, in order, it would seem, to facilitate a comfortable and coherent reading of the film, split the novel's Marie-Constance, designating Constance the "outer narrator." Interestingly, then, the film's reading of the novel has already split the unproblematic subjectivity of the novel's protagonist, and ironically rendered her, despite her visibility, more vocal. (The potential effects of this division will be explored later in the chapter.) From this point onwards, the film, narrated by Constance, charts the developing career of Marie, who, on account of her "lovely voice" has decided to advertize in the local newspaper and set herself up as a *lectrice* or reader, an activity that soon comes to be regarded as a threat to the stability of the community. It is upon this career, or more specifically, upon readings in that career that this chapter will now concentrate.

Marie's first client is Eric, a wheelchair-bound teenager, to whom, at their first encounter, she reads Guy de Maupassant's famous story of male fetishism and obsession *La Chevelure* (*The Braid*), a text that in the film supplants the reading of *La Main* (*The Hand*) that takes place in the novel.[8] The scene in which Marie reads this text requires close textual and shot analysis, as both the film and short story become increasingly inseparable. It will be necessary, therefore, to offer a description of and running commentary on the scene, reading both the cinematic and literary texts simultaneously. In traditional shot/reverse shot format, Marie reads and Eric listens. Marie begins:

> One sunny morning I was wandering in Paris. . . . Suddenly I noticed, in an antique dealer's, a very rare and extremely beautiful 18th century inlaid writing desk. What a remarkable thing temptation is! A need for possession creeps over you, at first gentle, almost bashful, but a need which soon heightens, becoming violent and irrestible.[9]

At this point there is a cut-in to an extreme close-up of Marie's legs, revealing, as she continues to read, a band of flesh between the tops of her stockings and the folds of her skirt: "I purchased this piece of furniture and . . . placed it in my bedroom." A brief reverse back to Eric aligns the cinematic spectator with his gaze at Marie's legs, the Maupassant text appearing to confirm Marie's objectification and commodification. Marie's reading continues: "One evening, I noticed whilst testing the thickness of a panel [reverse from Eric looking, back to Marie], that there must have been a hiding place there . . . and I spent the night searching for this secret. . . . I discovered it the next morning by sticking a blade into a crack in the panelling."

Another reverse shot back to Eric, looking and listening, is followed by a medium shot of both Marie and Eric. Marie says to herself, "Everything is going well; he's listening to me and what's more he seems to be enjoying this reading." She continues with the Maupassant: "I noticed, spread out on a background of black velvet, a wonderful braid of woman's hair. Yes, a braid, an enormous plait of blond hair, almost red, . . . and bound by a gold cord." There is a cut here back to Eric, his gaze transfixed upon Marie's thighs. Meanwhile her reading continues: "I remained stupefied, trembling, perturbed! I picked it up gently, almost religiously." There is a further cut-in to an extreme close-up of Marie's thighs, and as she continues to read the camera pans up her body coming to rest on a close-up of her face: "Immediately, the braid unfurled, spilling its gilded locks which fell to the ground, thick and light, supple and brilliant, like the fiery tail of a comet. I was overcome by a strange emotion." Here Marie looks up at Eric, seen in reverse shot, who appears tense and somewhat distressed. As the camera cuts back to Marie, she says to herself, "Strange boy. Well, I'm enjoying this. I'll continue." She takes up her reading once more: "The intense thought of the braid was to never leave me. . . . In my hands and my heart I had a remarkable, sensual, endless need to plunge [again a reverse shot of Eric, now more distressed] my fingers into this delightful stream . . . when I had finished caressing it and shut it away in the desk . . . I once again had the pressing need to pick it up once more, to finger it, to excite myself to the point of faintness."

During the previous shot the camera has panned up to Eric's face, which is now presented in extreme close-up, so close in fact, that it appears to consciously foreground the eyes, ears, nose and mouth, which fill the entire screen. There follows a further sequence of shot/reverse shots in extreme close-up: from Eric to Marie and back to Eric, whose open mouth appears to utter a silent cry. Panning downwards, Eric's fist can be seen gripping the side of his wheelchair, and cutting back to Marie, we hear her scream and drop the book from which she was reading. Eric's mother rushes into the room and, tending to a now apparently unconscious Eric, she asks Marie what she was doing. Marie responds, "I was only reading."

This "innocent" reading produces effects in the listener, Eric, that are similar to those produced on the narrator of the Maupassant story; it is, in a sense, performative. The sensuality that relates to the braid is transferred to the reading. Marie's reading is portrayed as both erotic and as sensual, of the senses—it is visual and vocal—as is Eric's reading of both the Maupassant text and of Marie herself. It is also possible that just as the narrator of *La Chevelure* constructs a fantasy woman based upon the fetishized trichological remnant, a kind of fetishism in reverse, so Eric also constructs a fantasy, or perhaps one should say, produces a reading. Robert Stoller famously asserted that a fetish is a story masquerading as an object; thus here one might assert that Eric's reading of *La Chevelure*, through the reading of Marie, is a fetishization of Marie; and certainly the camera's gaze during that scene would seem to confirm such a reading.[10] One might also speak of a certain kind of vocal fetishization that functions prior to the predominantly visual concept of the fetish, where Marie's voice represents perhaps, the female voice as maternal fantasy, for there is no doubt that Marie's voice is continually stressed in the film ("jolie voix," "voix merveilleuse," "votre voix, votre voix, tout vient de votre voix, je n'ai jamais entendu une voix comme la vôtre" ["Lovely voice," "wonderful voice," "your voice, your voice, your voice is everything, I've never heard a voice like yours"]).[11]

Another scene of reading presents itself through a rather knowing conjunction. On the occasion of his birthday, Eric's mother makes a homemade gift to Marie of a *liseuse*, which while being the term for the bed jacket she receives, also refers to a "reader" and thus would appear to have a connection with the Barthesian notion of the text as braid.[12] Here the *liseuse* has been knitted by Eric's mother in an activity similar to that of braiding, which ties in with Barthes's notion of the text as an intertwining of voices and to his discussion of the Freudian symbolism of the braid, seen as originating in "the labour of a woman braiding her pubic hairs to form the absent penis."[13] Barthes argues that: "The text, in short, is a fetish; and to reduce it to the unity of meaning, by a deceptively univocal reading, is to cut the braid, to sketch the castrating gesture" (*S/Z*, 160). Marie, the *lectrice*, in putting on the *liseuse* becomes the braid, the textual site of intertwined readings, a fetish.[14] This is confirmed by the metaphoric collapsing of the *toison d'or*, golden fleece, referred to by Eric at a later "reading," with his gaze at Marie's crotch, her "golden fleece."[15] In this scene Eric asks Marie what the *toison* or fleece is. She replies that it is the *toison d'or* or the golden fleece and that in order to win it one must embark upon a long journey. Eric immediately asks, "What about me, Madame, when will I leave on such a journey?" Marie's response is to stand and lift her skirt, revealing her underwear to Eric, who requests that the next time she wear none at all. Each reading to Eric, from *La Chevelure* onwards, has involved a degree of unveiling, a *dévoilement* that seems uncannily reminiscent of Barthes's famous description of textual pleasure as synonymous with that of the striptease. Having proposed that "the most erotic place of a body [is] there where the clothing gapes," he suggests that in the striptease, "all the excitement is concentrated on the hope of seeing the genitals (the schoolboy's dream) or of knowing the end of the story (the novelistic satisfaction)" (Brooks, 31). Eric would appear to be this very schoolboy, along with, it would seem, Barthes, Brooks, and Deville, who are all reading from a position that is both masculine and heterosexual.

This film, then, directed by a man, based upon a novel also written by a man, about a woman reader, a *lectrice*, is arguably both masculinist and heterosexual; it lends itself to the kinds of readings proposed by Barthes, Brooks, Eric, and Deville, and while it focuses on a woman reader, she is caught up in this masculinist and heterosexist economy. A film that offers a somewhat different and potentially more progressive reading position for its protagonist is Peter Greenaway's *The Pillow Book* (1996), a film that is also concerned with reading, writing, and fetishism. In Greenaway's film Nagiko shifts from being a simple reader of the texts inscribed upon her own body and becomes a *scriptible* or "writerly" reader herself. Nagiko moves from inscribed to inscriber. It is the performative, reiterative aspect of a *scriptible* reading that might be aligned with a similar kind of spectatorial performativity, as will become apparent later in this chapter.

The importance of fetishism for the film extends beyond the readings and representations it contains to include the film's title. Generally, the title to a film represents a singular moment of reading, for it is that which a spectator must always read (which is not to say, of course that one cannot watch a film if one hasn't read the title, but to simply assert that it is always conspicuously textual), and it is also that which functions to organize any reading or viewing of that film. The title, *La Lectrice*, refers to a woman reader who reads texts out loud, who performs texts. This title might also, of course, refer to a woman reader, who "consumes" texts as a woman. The English subtitle for *La Lectrice* is unable to translate the gender specificity of the French and in referring to "The Reader" names a universal reader, and universality tends, of course, to collapse into masculinity. Thus for an English-speaking audience reading both the French and English title, this film is perhaps most challenging at the moment of its most singular "double" reading. Returning to the Maupassant story, it might be argued that the sensuality of the text (itself a reading of fetishism), combined with the sensuality of Marie's articulation of it (Marie as textual fetish made flesh), produce a direct effect upon the body of Eric. Through a kind of sensory overload, Eric temporarily loses consciousness, literally loses himself. Eric falls into a kind of trance, similar perhaps to what Freud and Breuer called a "hypnoid state" (a concept which will be returned to shortly, as it has a particular resonance in relation to cinematic spectatorship).

This scene of reading has been described and analyzed in some detail because this text, read by Marie, enacts almost, displays, sensually (visually and vocally) reading itself.[16] It stages reading as a process of sensual probing, reading as what Peter Brooks punningly calls, "forepleasure," describing it as a concept that

> would include the notion of both delay and advance in the textual dynamic, the creation of that "dilatory space" . . . through which we seek to advance towards the discharge of the end, yet all the while perversely delaying, returning backwards in order to put off the promised end, and perhaps to assure its greater significance. (29–30)

Such an articulation links forepleasure to fetishism, one of the Freudian "deviations in respect of the sexual aim," where to cite Brooks again, fetishism invokes "the interesting threat of being waylaid by some element along the way to the "proper" end and, taking some displaced substitute or simulacrum for the thing itself" (30). Forepleasure, then, refers to the perverse. It refers to an economy that values expenditure over profit, an economy wherein disunity and flux are the only structuring terms, an economy ultimately of the polymorphously perverse. Such an economy allows for the possibility of a text that, according to Brooks "would delay, displace, and deviate terminal discharge to an extent that it becomes nonexistent—as, perhaps, in the textual practice of the 'writeable text' (*texte scriptible*)" (33).

Jean-François Lyotard speaks of cinema in similar terms, proposing the term "acinema" and suggesting that film is inherently polymorphously perverse and that it is the dictates of capitalist economy and the Freudian libidinal economy that require it to conform to profit motives and narrative coherence. Thus he points out:

> Just as the libido must renounce its perverse outflow to propagate the species through a normal genital sexuality allowing the constitution of a "sexual body" having that sole end, so the film [. . .] springs from the effort to eliminate aberrant movements, useless expenditures, differences of pure consumption.[17]

Lyotard further suggests:

> The *film*, strange formation, reputed to be normal, is no more normal than the *society* or the *organism*. All of these so-called objects are the result of the imposition and hope for an accomplished totality. They are supposed to realise the reasonable goal *par excellence*, the subordination of all partial drives, all sterile and divergent movements to the unity of an organic body. (176)

Lyotard questions the notion that the cinematic screen functions as a unifying, "orthopedic" mirror; he refers explicitly to Lacan's mirror stage, and that as such, it provides the site/sight for a perceived bodily unity and coherent subjectivity. Lyotard's anti-Bazinian reading of cinema positions him as a potentially sensual reader of film.

Developing this idea, it might be argued that the film *La Lectrice*, as a reading of the novel of the same name, is itself what one might call a "sensual reading," the premise being that the cinematic experience is a fundamentally sensual one (despite attempts to channel and regulate this sensuality). This is to positively valorize the descent into the realm of the imaginary (or "of the senses") that psychoanalytic film theory tends to denigrate. For it is precisely in this too-closeness, this intimacy between screen and spectator that the sensual is foregrounded. As Steven Shaviro remarks in *The Cinematic Body*:

> Sitting in the dark, watching the play of images across a screen, any detachment from "raw phenomena," from the immediacy of sensa-

tion or from the speeds and delays of temporal duration, is radically impossible. Cinema invites me, or forces me, to stay within the orbit of the senses. I am confronted and assaulted by a flux of sensations that I can neither attach to physical presences, nor translate into systematised abstractions. I am violently, viscerally affected by this image and this sound, without being able to have recourse to any frame of reference, any form of transcendental reflection, or any Symbolic order. No longer does a signifying structure anticipate every possible perception; instead, the continual metamorphoses of sensation pre-empt, slip and slide beneath, and threaten to dislodge all the comforts and stabilities of meaning.[18]

A return to the infantile domain of component instincts and polymorphous perversity, a period marked by its lack of genital organization, where the economic imperative of value is negated, where "aberrant movements" and "useless expenditures" are validated. The spectator occupies a kind of inverse position in respect of the Lacanian mirror/screen, a position of temporal anteriority, before the projection of the ego-ideal, where the body is not experienced as a unity but rather as a site of fragmented zones of pleasure, fragments experienced sensually. It is no longer a question of identification and mastery. The spectator no longer appears to control the image but simply responds sensually to it. The cinematic experience can thus be seen to radically undermine the notion of stable subjectivity, rather than being the site of its reinforcement. Such a "loss," rather than being mourned negatively as loss, might in fact offer, as Shaviro proposes, "a new approach to the dynamics of film viewing: one that is masochistic, mimetic, tactile, and corporeal, in contrast to the reigning psychoanalytic paradigm's emphasis on sadism and separation" (56).

The work of Celia Lury suggests just such an approach to film viewing. Lury argues that the body in its interaction with visual technology loses coherence and unity. In what she calls "prosthetic culture," subjectivity results from a mimetic and sensual relationship with the visual. Lury develops her argument with reference to Roland Barthes's notion of the photographic *punctum*, stressing the physicality of the *punctum*/viewer relation. The *punctum* is seen to describe a violent and visceral moment, a moment that is multiplied (twenty-four times a second) in Shaviro's description of the cinematic experience. Working with a definition of mimesis as "both a copying or imitation *and* a palpable, sensuous connection between the very body of the perceiver and the perceived, copy *and* contact, coincidence and metamorphosis," Lury proceeds to articulate a concept of "seeing photographically."[19] This mode of vision, Lury suggests, has a double function. It facilitates "a dissociation of the senses that disturbs the coherence of the individual" (5), while at the same time enabling a process of transformation or "self-extension" (3). Developed in relation to a concept of "prosthetic biography," this self-extension is conceived of in terms of performativity. Identity is performative in relation to a process of reenvisioning or remaking, occurring as a result of, and subsequent to, the "trauma" of the sensual encounter with the photographic or cinematic image (Barthes's *punctum* or Shaviro's "cinematic 'invitation' "). Thus Lury argues:

> In adopting/adapting a prosthesis, the person creates (or is created by) a self-identity that is no longer defined by the edict "I think, therefore I am"; rather, he or she is constituted in the relation "I can, therefore I am." In the mediated extension of capability that ensues, the relations between consciousness, memory and the body that had defined the possessive individual as a legal personality are experimentally dis- and re-assembled. (3)

Perhaps the spectator envisioned here escapes the heterosexual, masculinist position that *La Lectrice* seems to offer its viewers. In a spectatorial relation that is performative, that requires dis- and reassembly, it is perhaps possible for the spectator to renarrate the film in ways that move beyond the inadequacies of the reading that *La Lectrice* appears to promote. Through mimesis and reiteration, the spectator can open up a space for a new self-identity, a novel spectatorial position.[20] Constance's performace here becomes performative, especially given the Constance/Marie split referred to earlier. Ultimately, Constance's performance forms part of her "prosthetic biography," a self-identity based upon mimesis and reiteration, upon performativity. Thus as the final shot of the film affirms, Constance in her relationship with Marie, articulated via "sensual reading," has adopted a new identity, an identity that potentially reverses the problematic positioning of Marie.

To conclude, and further stress the sensuality of the cinematic experience, one might usefully refer to the concept of the "hypnoid state" mentioned earlier in the context of Eric's loss of consciousness after listening to the Maupassant short story. This concept was important in the early development of psychoanalysis and, despite its subsequent rejection by Freud, was nonetheless instrumental in the genesis of psychoanalytic free association. Catharsis, the "talking cure," required that the patient be in an "hypnoid state" in order that the recovery and replay of the traumatic memories, believed to cause hysteria, might take place. The "hypnoid state," then, referred to a condition analogous to that achieved under hypnosis and occurred either, as Freud and Breuer argued, "during positively abnormal psychical states, such as the semi-hypnotic twilight state of daydreaming" or during a state of "severely paralysing affects" or intense emotion.[21] They further remark that "[hypnoid states] often, it would seem, grow out of the day-dreams which are so common even in healthy people and to which needlework and similar occupations render women especially prone" (64).

Aside from Freud's gender stereotyping, one might remark upon his fortuitous reference to needlework, an activity that recalls, on the one hand the knitted *liseuse* given to Marie, and on the other, Barthes's reference to the literary text as constituting "a braid (text, fabric, braid: the same thing)" (160). Ironically, in the case of Eric, it is he, who as the reader of Marie's vocalization of Maupassant's textual braid, metaphorically knits and thus becomes "especially prone" to the "hypnoid state." Barthes, in his short essay "Upon Leaving the Movie Theatre," likens the silent, melancholic moment experienced as one emerges from a cinema to the hypnoid state. Entry into the "movie theater" is aligned with the daydream, the "crepuscular reverie" of the "cinematic condition."[22] This state of being appears to result from a certain communion with the cinematic image, with cinematic sound, a too-closeness that has resulted from a state of intense textual "knitting" or reading, a reading that is radically sensual in its immediacy. In this condition, identity (despite the possible play of identifications experienced relative to the film or perhaps because of the very fluidity of identificatory positions), is momentarily erased. Subjectivity, the body—these self-articulations are shattered in a claustrophobic moment of sensual excess.

"Reading *La Lectrice*" refers to this brief moment and suggests that the film might be described as a sensual reading of the novel, in that it articulates a reading of that novel, sensually. It transforms what is already perhaps a sensual reading into a medium that functions wholly in the domain of sight and sound (at the very least). In terms of the spectator, it is no doubt true that some films produce readings that are more or less "sensual" than others, for some films rely more on (or at least make a greater appeal to) visual and aural stimulation than others. One such film, *Mission: Impossible*, was described by the critic José Arroyo as a film that "assaults the senses," a film "so thrilling that even hermeneutics are left behind for a while."[23] Positively valorizing the film for this quality, despite its status as a "popcorn movie," one might concur with Arroyo's response to *Mission: Impossible* and even, perhaps, go so far as to argue that all films are ultimately sensual and that therefore all cinematic readings are sensual readings.

Notes

1. *La Lectrice*, dir. Michel Deville, 1988, France. Originally delivered as an oral conference paper, the introduction to this article noted the various ironies inherent in reading aloud a paper on the subject of reading at a conference entitled "Sensual Reading." The very act of sensual reading was foregrounded through a discussion of Roland Barthes's concept of *écriture vocale* (vocal writing) or *l'écriture à haute voix* (writing aloud). Barthes's suggestion that the objective of vocal writing was not the clarity of the message but the physicality of the utterance, was taken up in relation to the article's genesis and its performace. It was stressed, of course, that the article nonetheless sought both hermeneutical clarity and corporeal or sensual articulation. See Roland Barthes, *Le Plaisir du texte* (Paris: Editions du Seuil, 1973).

2. Raymond Jean, *La Lectrice* (Paris: Actes Sud, 1986).

3. Reading as performance is stressed in the film *La Lectrice*, for example when the "lectrice" herself notes, after a particularly difficult reading, "My voice neither wavered, nor weakened. I didn't falter" (transcribed from the film, my translation). This aspect of reading was also foregrounded in relation to the article's original oral presentation.

4. Evocation refers to the Platonic idea of "the calling to mind or recollection of knowledge acquired in a previous state of existence." From this specific definition comes the more general notion of evocation as "the action or act of calling into existence or activity something non-existent or latent; something that brings to mind a specified memory, image or feeling." *New Shorter Oxford English Dictionary* (Oxford: Clarendon Press, 1993).

5. The French is "C'est exactement moi," which could mean either "That's me" or "Just like mine."

6. See Peter Brooks, *Psychoanalysis and Storytelling* (Oxford: Blackwell, 1994), 90–91. Subsequent quotations from this work are cited parenthetically in the text.

7. Jean, *La Lectrice*, 5.

8. It should be pointed out that non-French-speaking viewers of the film are required to literally read this text by means of the film's subtitles. There is a film version of Maupassant's short story, entitled *The Golden Braid*, dir. Paul Cox, 1990, Australia.

9. Unless otherwise specified, all translations from the French are my own.

10. "[A]n object . . . becomes a fetish when it stands for—condenses in itself—meanings that are, wholly or in crucial parts of the text, unconscious: a

fetish is a story masquerading as an object." Robert Stoller, *Observing the Erotic Imagination* (New Haven and London: Yale University Press, 1985), 155.

11. For a detailed discussion of this concept, see Kaja Silverman, *The Acoustic Mirror: The Female Voice in Psychoanalysis and Cinema* (Bloomington and Indianapolis: Indiana University Press), 1988, particularly chap. 3 and 4.

12. A *liseuse* is also a book cover, which, of course further emphasizes Marie's status as object, in this instance, to be read.

13. Roland Barthes, *S/Z*, trans. Richard Miller (New York: Hill and Wang, 1974), 160. Subsequent quotations from this work are cited parenthetically in the text.

14. She also, in a sense, becomes a book for, as noted earlier, a *liseuse* is also a book cover.

15. Freud remarked that "fur and velvet—as has long been suspected—are a fixation of the sight of the pubic hair, which should have been followed by the longed-for sight of the female member." Sigmund Freud, "Fetishism," in *On Sexuality*, Pelican Freud Library, trans. James Strachey, ed. Angela Richards, vol. 7, (London: Penguin, 1987 [1977]), 354. It should be noted also that in the myth of the golden fleece, the fleece functions as a fetish; Jason requires the fleece in order that he may claim legitimate inheritance of his grandfather's throne. Golden fleece, golden phallus?

16. This text was, of course, also read aloud as part of the article's original conference performance.

17. Jean-François Lyotard, "Acinema," in *The Lyotard Reader*, ed. Andrew Benjamin, (Oxford: Blackwell, 1989), 169–80; 172. Subsequent quotations from this work are cited parenthetically in the text.

18. Steven Shaviro, *The Cinematic Body* (Minneapolis and London: Minnesota University Press, 1993), 32–33. Subsequent quotations from this work are cited parenthetically in the text.

19. Celia Lury, *Prosthetic Culture: Photography, Memory, and Identity* (London: Routledge, 1998), 91. Subsequent quotations from this work are cited parenthetically in the text.

20. For an extended discussion of these issues, particularly in relation to the Freudian concept of deferred action as a paradigmatic structure for cinematic spectatorship, see Paul Sutton, "Remaking the Remake: Olivier Assayas' *Irma Vep* (1996)," in *French Film in the 1990s: Continuity and Difference*, ed. Phil Powrie (Oxford: Oxford University Press, 1999).

21. Sigmund Freud and Joseph Breuer, *Studies on Hysteria*, Pelican Freud Library, trans. James Strachey, ed. Angela Richards, vol. 3, (London, Penguin, 1991 [1974]), 61. Subsequent quotations from this work are cited parenthetically in the text.

22. Roland Barthes, "Upon Leaving the Movie Theater," in *Cinematographic Apparatus: Selected Writings*, ed. Theresa Hak Kyung Cha (New York: Tanam Press, 1980), 1.

23. José Arroyo, "Mission: Sublime," *Sight and Sound* 6.7 (July 1996): 18–21; 21.

Works Cited

Arroyo, José. "Mission: Sublime," *Sight and Sound* 6.7 (July 1996): 18–21.
Barthes, Roland. *Le Plaisir du texte*. Paris: Editions du Seuil, 1973.

———. *S/Z*. Translated by Richard Miller. New York: Hill and Wang, 1974.

———. "Upon Leaving the Movie Theater," in *Cinematographic Apparatus: Selected Writings*. Edited by Theresa Hak Kyung Cha. New York: Tanam Press, 1980.

Benjamin, Andrew, ed. *The Lyotard Reader*. Oxford: Blackwell, 1989.

Brooks, Peter. *Psychoanalysis and Storytelling*. Oxford: Blackwell, 1994.

Cha, Theresa Hak Kyung, ed. *Cinematographic Apparatus: Selected Writings*. New York: Tanam Press, 1980.

Freud, Sigmund. *On Sexuality*, Pelican Freud Library, vol. 7. 7th ed. Translated by James Strachey. Edited by Angela Richards. London: Penguin, 1987.

Freud, Sigmund and Joseph Breuer. *Studies on Hysteria*, Pelican Freud Library, vol. 3. 2d ed. Translated by James Strachey. Edited by Angela Richards, London: Penguin, 1991.

Jean, Raymond. *La Lectrice*. Paris: Actes du Sud, 1986.

Lury, Celia. *Prosthetic Culture: Photography, Memory, and Identity*. London: Routledge, 1998.

Lyotard, Jean-François. "Acinema." In *The Lyotard Reader*. Edited by Andrew Benjamin. Oxford: Blackwell, 1989.

Powrie, Phil. *French Film in the 1990s: Continuity and Difference*. Oxford: Oxford University Press, 1999.

Shaviro, Steven. *The Cinematic Body*. Minneapolis and London: Minnesota University Press, 1993.

Silverman, Kaja. *The Acoustic Mirror: The Female Voice in Psychoanalysis and Cinema*. Bloomington and Indianapolis: Indiana University Press, 1988.

Stoller, Robert. *Observing the Erotic Imagination*. New Haven and London: Yale University Press, 1985.

Sutton, Paul. "Remaking the Remake: Olivier Assayas' *Irma Vep*." In *French Film in the 1990s: Continuity and Difference*. Edited by Phil Powrie. Oxford: Oxford University Press, 1999.

The Metamorphosis of Vision in the Surrealist Text: José María Hinojosa's "Granadas de fuego"

JACQUELINE RATTRAY

ACCORDING TO PIERRE REVERDY, WHOM ANDRÉ BRETON CITES IN the "First Manifesto of Surrealism":

The image is a pure creation of the mind.
   It cannot be born from a comparison but from a juxtaposition of two more or less distant realities.
   The more the relationship between the two juxtaposed realities is distant and true, the stronger the image will be—the greater its emotional power and poetic reality.... (Pierre Reverdy, *Nord-Sur*, March 1918).[1]

In poetic terms, metaphor, meaning literally "to carry over," is one obvious way in which the transformative power of the poetic image is conveyed. The "vehicle" of the metaphor generates a type of intellectual movement for the reader by transporting one concept onto another. For Reverdy, the tension created by juxtaposition and distance is what fuels the dynamic force of the poetic image.[2] The intellectual movement which this force requires of the reader is relative to the degree to which the metaphor stretches the immediate limits of reason. As Louis Aragon notes in his *Treatise on Style*, "in reality, all poetry is surrealist in its movement."[3]

Starting from an analysis of the image based upon a classical model of mimesis, the reader finds that the distance to be crossed is deliberately kept to a decorous proximity, for, as Aristotle has signaled in his *Poetics*, "the ability to use metaphor well implies a perception of resemblances."[4] Objections to this view have been raised throughout the course of literary history.[5] When the use of metaphor is kept under such careful control, the potential force of language itself is curtailed and the creative drive of words denied. In addition, Aristotelian rules regard "ambiguity" as "vice," and "clarity" as language's sought-after "virtue," which quickly stalls any generative and procreative function of language made possible through exploiting polysemy. In demanding the necessity of "resemblance" between the component parts of the metaphor, the image which is envisioned becomes bound by reason and anchored to its original, etymological meaning of "imago," that is to say, a copy or duplicate.[6] This constraint of language allocates words a purely referential role by regarding them as transparent truths depicting external reality. The brakes are quickly put on a creative or poetic use of language by directing the construction of literary images, in predominantly visual depiction, under the "despotism" of the eye.

Such a restrictive employment of language is analyzed by Martin Jay in accounting for the rise of "ocularcentrism" in Western culture. This ocularcentrism constrains the potential power of the poetic image by presenting the reader with an already complete and easily recognizable concept. However, as Jay goes on to note, "the liberation of language from its alleged mimetic function led to a burst of creative energy in which the relations between vision and text were boldly explored."[7] The potential creative energy of the imagination has been famously theorized by Coleridge under the term, "esemplastic power."[8] Meaning literally "to shape into one," this drive comes into play when there is not an obvious resemblance between the component parts of the metaphor, the "tenor" and the "vehicle," and the imagination is required to complete the image.

Shifting our attention to an analysis of the surrealist use of language, the reader finds that the distance has been stretched even further between the component parts of the metaphor. The surrealist image, although often breaking the limits of reason, does not, however, become reducible to the merely absurd. As Reverdy observes, the relationship between the two juxtaposed components of the metaphor must be "true" as well as "distant" to ignite the emotive power of the image. In order for the poetic image to maintain a "surreality" (a realizable possible state of reality above this one), there must still be some recognizable degree of coherence. A revolutionary trait of surrealism is indicated here through the power of this poetic reality which seeks to provoke a "re-vision" of the world as habitually depicted through conventional language. As soon as the reader makes the necessary mental switching between diverse concepts in order to visualize the surrealist image, a type of Wittgensteinian "aspect-dawning" is experienced.⁹ Breton refers to this illuminating effect as "the light of the image," continuing in a type of ignition analogy by stating that "the value of the image depends upon the beauty of the spark obtained; it is, consequently, a function of the difference of potential between the two conductors."¹⁰

One surrealist use of language which notably accelerates the dynamic process in visualizing metaphors is achieved in such devices as the surrealist extended metaphor. Michael Riffaterre defines this concept, seen particularly in the "automatism-effect" text, as being "in fact a series of metaphors semantically tied together by syntax and meaning. They belong to a single sentence or to a single narrative or descriptive structure. Each expresses a particular aspect of the whole, be it a thing or a concept, represented by the first metaphor in the series."¹¹ The initial process of transformation which accompanies the reading of any metaphor or trope is turned over and over by means of a series of signifieds which the starting image had originally sparked off. The extended metaphor then generates frantic hermeneutic activity from the reader by carrying the mind off with the string of images which now floods the reading process.¹² Breton relives the dynamic experience brought on by these hurtling images, commenting that "the Surrealist atmosphere created by automatic writing [. . .] is especially conducive to the production of the most beautiful images. One can even go so far as to say that in this dizzying race the images appear like the only guideposts of the mind."¹³

An analogy for the dynamic force of intellectual movement generated by the surrealist extended metaphor is depicted in surrealist art through Salvador Dalí's use of the paranoia-critical method.¹⁴ In a painting such as *Impressions of Africa* (1938),¹⁵ when the spectator allows the eye to follow the metamorphosis of images in the top, left-hand corner of the canvas, an extended experience of the Wittgensteinian "aspect dawning" is observed. In referring to the artist's experience while "sitting in the driver's seat" to create the work, Dalí describes how "the double image [. . .] may be extended, continuing the paranoiac advance, and then the presence of another dominant idea is enough to make a third appear [. . .], and so on, until there is a number of images limited only by the mind's degree of paranoiac capacity."¹⁶ The viewer's experience, when faced with one of these paintings, is one where rapid shifts in perspective accompany each realization that what is depicted on the canvas with near photographic quality is in fact constantly evading any singular or fixed form. An early example of Dalí's paranoia-critique is seen in his work *The Invisible Man*, a painting which he was working on while visiting the Malagan group of poets in Torremolinos.[17] One of these was the surrealist writer José María Hinojosa, whose work will often reveal the tracks left by the presence of surrealist painting and cinema.

"Granadas de fuego"[18] [Granadas of fire] is one of Hinojosa's poems which immediately presents itself to the reader as a linguistic example of paranoia-critical activity, powered by the potential ambiguity of words rather than plastic forms. Although Hinojosa's poem derives its energy from linguistic as opposed to optical ambiguity, both the reader of the poem and the viewer of the paranoia-critique painting are steered down a parallel route of continually metamorphosing images.[19] Dalí had defined the method of paranoia-critique as embodying "such a representation of an object that it is also, without the slightest physical or anatomical change, the representation of another entirely different object, the second representation being equally devoid of any deformation or abnormality betraying arrangement."[20] Likewise, the particular form of linguistic paranoia-critique evident in Hinojosa's poem may be seen to involve "such a signification of one object that it is also the signifier of another object, the visualising of the second being equally devoid of any break in the conceptualising process whilst reading." One word prevails upon the whole of Hinojosa's poem to steer the metamorphosing images. This word is "granada," which, in Spanish, signifies a pomegranate, a hand grenade, and Granada the city. To hold down the meaning of the poem, the reader frantically attempts to visualize what the language is seeking to convey. But, a lack of punctuation hinders the reader's attempts to compartmentalize these different possible images, for just at the moment when one concept of "granada" has been grasped, it slips through the reader's fingers and the next image comes to impose itself upon the reading process.[21]

The very title of the poem initiates the visualization process by inviting the reader to grasp one image before the metamorphosis sets in. The reader would most commonly understand "Granada de fuego" to signify the hand grenade of warfare. However, the use of the plural in the title, "Granadas," already indicates that this poem will be dealing with more than one "granada." Multiple images are suggested here, and these will then be seen constantly fading in and out of the imagery of the poem, as is made evident from the very outset of the first verse.

> *Esta granada abierta que está entre nuestros manos*
> *tiene dientes de sangre y carne de ballena*
> *y ahora conserva intacta su agria arquitectura*
> *porque fue desertora de las últimas guerras.*
> [This opened *granada* that is between our hands
> has teeth of blood and whale's flesh
> and now it maintains its acrid architecture
> because it was a deserter in the last wars.]²²

By opening with an initial demonstrative deictic the reader feels compelled to grasp at a concrete visualization of what "this granada" is pointing to. However, not one but all three concepts of "granada" can potentially be pictured here; the image of war is evoked through the open hand grenade with the pin removed ready to be hurled. The image of Granada the city, close at hand to Hinojosa's hometown of Málaga, is a further possible view. However, the image of the pomegranate is perhaps the most dominant as this fruit bursts open when ripe or it can be cut open in order to eat the fleshy red seeds inside. This last image gains strength in the second line, but the unusually violent language used to describe the seeds inside the fruit blurs the reader's perception. The third line continues to focus on the physical appearance of the opened pomegranate through the structure of the distasteful yellow pith that encases the red seeds. However, an echo of the bitterness associated with war and death can also be heard here, linking this image to the destructive effects of the exploding hand grenade's sculpted shell. The reference to architecture additionally brings the image of Granada the city into view, with its skyline dominated by the ancient fortress of the Alhambra, its high walls constructing a defensive shell against attack. The final line of the verse, opening with a causative and then making explicit reference to war, appears to offer clarification for the reader. However, as "fue" can signify "s/he" or "it was," the possibility of ambiguity is still retained as the reader moves into the following verse.

The second verse opens with an image that blurs together two possible signifieds of "granada"; making reference to a city at war.

> *Entre vallados negros de gemidos y olas*
> *sus granos desgranados iluminan la tierra*
> *rompiendo oscuridades con su roja sonrisa*
> *en el perfil agudo del agua sin conciencia.*
> [Between black ramparts of groans and waves

THE METAMORPHOSIS OF VISION IN THE SURREALIST TEXT 171

>   its shelled seeds illuminate the ground
>   breaking the darkness with their red smiles
>   in the sharp profile of the water without conscience.]

The reader is aware that there are black ramparts, which might bring to mind once again the defensive fortress of the Alhambra. This same image might also evoke a depiction of trench warfare, the horrors of the First World War still being very much alive in people's thoughts at the time the poem was written. This imagery of warfare overflows into the second line of the second verse, but the words that evoke the image of "granada," the exploding grenade, are full of additional associations. The language used here provokes a metamorphosis in the reader's vision by depicting the hand grenades as seeds removed from a fruit. Moreover, there is a further metamorphosis for the reader to deal with through the close visual and phonetic connection between the words "desgranado," meaning having the seeds removed from something, and "desangrado," having lost a lot of blood.

The fluctuation of images in this verse, and indeed in the poem as a whole, is a recognizable surrealist practice. When the reader focuses on this second verse, but takes a figurative approach, the surrealist attributes which have helped shape the text through its very writing become even more pronounced. For example, in the first line of the second verse the word "olas" also evokes the idea of waves of thought, with this link between fluidity and the subconscious being reinforced in the image of consciousless water in the final line. Although it is problematic for the reader to visualize water with a physical quality of sharpness, in continuing the analogy with surrealist writing, this sharp outline gains visual coherence when the reader imagines the poet in the actual process of shaping words upon the paper with the point of his pen. In this instance, the creative element of the reader's imagination is seen to switch to a different mode in order to grasp at associations suggested by words that constantly insist upon playing hide and seek with her.[23] The amusement that this game-playing element arouses in the poem brings forth the red smile of the stanza's third line.

In the next verse, the opening oxymoron appears to be a clear reference to Granada the city:

>   *Con sus ascuas de nieve calcina la alegría*
>   *sobre un piso de mármol de alguna ciudad eterna*
>   *para dejar desnudas verdades en pirámides*

> *de tempestad y miedo ondear sus banderas.*
> [With its embers of snow it burns happiness
> on a marble floor of some eternal city
> to leave naked truths in pyramids
> of storm and fear to wave their flags.]

The extremes of cold and heat are redolent of this Andalucian city, situated on a snow-covered mountain range in the heat of southern Spain. A reader unfamiliar with the physical aspects of Granada and its surrounds might not realize this, however, until the following line makes additional reference, via the marbled floors, to the ancient moorish architecture of the Alhambra palace. However, even though the poem has now seemingly made direct reference to this "eternal city" of Granada, the image of "granada," the hand grenade, is still to be seen lurking in the picture. Reversing, in order to reread from the first line, the reader can turn the focus to the image of reducing happiness to ashes. The predominant signified of "granada" here now evokes the destructive potential of warfare, an image which is reinforced in the final two lines of the verse. The horrific reality of war, the image of naked truths left behind, can quickly bring to mind the sight of piles of charred bodies. This chilling note that such a view brings to this verse is echoed in the final image of flags being hoisted to wave, not in victory, but in the winds of storm and fear.

Although this third verse focuses particularly on two of the three signifieds of "granada," the concluding verse blurs the reader's perception by provoking a triple vision from the word "granada."

> *Esta granada abierta no es el fruto de un árbol*
> *que se engendró en el vientre de mares y de selvas;*
> *en su cáscara amarga tiene amplitud de cielo*
> *y en sus entrañas pican las aves y las fieras.*
> [This opened *granada* is not the fruit of a tree
> that was begotten in the womb of seas and forests;
> in its bitter shell it has an abundance of sky
> and in its entrails the birds and wild beasts pick away.]

Immediately, an echo is heard with the very first line of the poem to evoke the image of the pomegranate once again. And yet, this signified is simultaneously negated by the statement that what the poem has been dealing with is *not* the fruit of a tree. The following line maintains the confusion, as the reader is told that neither is this "granada" that which is begotten in the womb of seas and forests. This image, although continuing the link with nature, and therefore with the fruit, also includes an allusion to the image of Granada the city and its geographical location. With the negation of "granada" the pomegranate and Granada the city, this would logically leave the third signified of "granada" the hand grenade as being the definitive one. However, the third line of the stanza reintroduces the image of all three "granadas," which "stay in the picture" like a frozen frame to end the poem. The concluding image of the poem maintains this triple imagery of all three granadas: the fruit on the tree, with its outer shell removed and its inner red flesh being eaten by the wild animals of the forest; the casualties of war, with their bodies stripped of their flesh by scavenging beasts; and, thirdly, the stray animals that roam around the deserted alleyways at the heart of the city.

In negating the image that was initially constructed by the reader in the first verse, the whole poem "Granadas de fuego" exhibits a further kinship with surrealist painting, seen in the example of Magritte's *The Treason of Images* (1928–29), more popularly known as *This is not a Pipe*. In Magritte's painting, even though the statement underneath serves to negate the image of the very pipe which dominates the picture, the object of the pipe still persists for the viewer.[24] Likewise, in Hinojosa's poem, the denial of "granada" the fruit in the final verse does not eliminate the image of "granada" the pomegranate in the poem. The "granada" of Hinojosa's poem remains all three "granadas," as well as not any single one, with all three signifieds present within the poem but in a state of continual metamorphosis. In "Granadas de fuego," words and images do not serve passively to depict, but rather it is language itself that steers the visualizing of the text, presenting images to the reader and then transforming them into further images before the eyes. Just as Magritte's painting laughs mockingly at the spectator who treats the canvas as a window looking on to external reality, "Granadas de fuego" likewise mocks the reader who understands the text merely through a process of painting mental pictures through what its words depict. In truth, "this opened granada" is not the fruit, but neither is it the hand grenade nor the city of southern Spain. For what is *really* between our hands is an opened book in which we read this poem.

Notes

1. André Breton, *Manifestoes of Surrealism*, trans. Richard Seaver and Helen R. Lane (Ann Arbor: University of Michigan, 1969), 20.

2. For a detailed exploration within the context of Reverdy's quote on poetic language, see Graham Dunstan Martin's "A Measure of Distance: The Rhetoric of the Surrealist Adjective," in *Surrealism and Language*, ed. Ian Higgins (Edinburgh: Scottish Academic Press, 1986), 12–25.

3. Louis Aragon, *Treatise on Style*, trans. Alyson Waters (London and Lincoln: University of Nebraska Press, 1991), 95.

4. *Aristotle, Horace, Longinus: Classical Literary Criticism*, trans. T. S. Dorsch (Harmondsworth: Penguin, 1965), 65.

5. Martin Jay has examined the predominant changes towards the domination of vision in artistic representation through the ages. These changes are listed particularly in his introduction and first chapter to *Downcast Eyes* (Berkeley: University of California Press, 1993), 1–82.

6. This one word, *image*, has come to embody a whole range of signifieds. For an analysis of the different meanings, see W. J. T. Mitchell, "What is an Image?" in *Iconology: Image, Text, Ideology* (Chicago: University of Chicago Press, 1986).

7. Jay, *Downcast Eyes*, 173.

8. See the chapter on "Imagination and Fancy," in I. A. Richards, *Coleridge on Imagination* (London: Kegan Paul, Trench, Trubner and Co., 1934), 72–99 (76).

9. For a definition of this phenomenon, see Stephen Mulhall, *On Being in the World: Wittgenstein and Heidegger on Seeing Aspects* (London: Routledge, 1990), 6–15.

10. Breton, *Manifestoes*, 37

11. Michael Riffaterre, "The Extended Metaphor in Surrealist Poetry" in his *Text Production*, trans. Terese Lyons (New York: Columbia University Press, 1983), 202–20 (203).

12. In the experience of reading the automatic text, J. Gratton writes that "To participate in a surrealist poem is to consent to its movement, to surrender one's totalizing impulse to the very spur of writing's moment." See "Runaway: Textual Dynamics in the Surrealist Poetry of André Breton," in Ian Higgins, ed., *Surrealism and Language*, 30–45 (31).

13. Breton, *Manifestoes*, 37.

14. Although Dalí has come to epitomize this method of painting and, indeed, he was the artist who famously classified it under the term "paranoia-critique," by no means should he be accredited with being its inventor because, in reality, examples of paranoia-critique have always existed. Dalí himself has remarked that the influence for many of his paintings came from the double-images which could be discerned in the rocks of Cadaqués.

15. A reproduction of this painting with a close-up of the multiple imagery accompanies a chapter on Dalí's paranoia-critical method in Dawn Ades, *Dalí* (London: Thames and Hudson, [1982] 1992), 91–149 (131, 138).

16. Dalí, "The Stinking Ass," in *Surrealists on Art*, ed. Lucy R. Lippard (Englewood Cliffs, New Jersey: Prentice-Hall, 1970), 97–100 (98).

17. The episode in Torremolinos is recounted in a number of sources, among them: "1930: Salvador Dalí, en Torremolinos. Como se frustra—y por qué—la aparición de una revista del Surrealismo español en Málaga" by Alfonso Sán-

chez Rodríguez in *Treinta años de vanguardia española*, ed. Gabrielle Morelli (Seville: El carro de la Nieve, 1991), 193–204.

18. "Granadas de fuego" can be found reproduced in facsimile in José María Hinojosa's *Poesías completas*, vol. 2 (Torremolinos: Litoral, 1983), 106–7. *Obra Completa* (Seville: Fundacion Genesian, 1998), re-edited by Alfonso Sánchez Rodríguez.

19. In reference to Dalí, the critic Ignacio Gómez de Liaño notes the process which actually generates this visual energy: "La imagen doble es, en la obra daliana, el vehículo fundamental de los fantasmas; un vehículo que atraviesa los territorios del destrozamiento y la reunificación, de la decomposición y la recomposición" [In Dalí's work, the double-image is the fundamental vehicle for apparitions; a vehicle which crosses territories of destruction and reunification, of decomposition and recomposition.] Ignacio Gómez de Liaño, *Dalí* (Barcelona: Polígrafa, 1982), 15. (Translation my own.)

20. Dalí, "The Stinking Ass," 98.

21. In the First Manifesto, Breton describes surrealist poetry as possessing a fluid effect and notes that "the fact still remains that punctuation no doubt resists the absolute continuity of the flow with which we are concerned." Higgins, ed., *Surrealism and Language*.

22. The translation which accompanies Hinojosa's "Granadas de fuego" is my own.

23. The ludic is an essential element of the avant-garde for the surrealists, one which has been famously likened to a game by the Spanish philosopher José Ortega y Gasset in *La Deshumanización de art*. See José Ortega y Gasset, *Obras completas*, vol. 3 (Madrid: Alianza, 1983), 353–86 (360).

24. Michel Foucault has examined the reaction from the spectator-reader when confronted with Magritte's painting: "This is not a pipe, but a drawing of a pipe," "This is not a pipe but a sentence saying that this is not a pipe," "The sentence 'this is not a pipe' is not a pipe," "In the sentence 'this is not a pipe,' this is not a pipe": the painting, written sentence, drawing of a pipe—all this is not a pipe." Negations multiply themselves, the voice is confused and choked." Michel Foucault, *This is not a Pipe* (Berkeley: University of California Press, 1983), 30.

Works Cited

Ades, Dawn. *Dalí*. London: Thames and Hudson, 1982.

Aragon, Louis. *Treatise on Style*. Translated by Alyson Waters. London & Lincoln: University of Nebraska Press, 1991.

Aristotle, Horace, Longinus: *Classical Literary Criticism*. Translated by T. S. Dorsch. Harmondsworth: Penguin, 1965.

Breton, André. *Manifestoes of Surrealism*. Translated by Richard Seaver & Helen R. Lane Ann Arbor: University of Michigan, 1969.

———. *Surrealism and Language*. Edited by Ian Higgins. Edinburgh: Scottish Academic Press, 1986.

Foucault, Michel. *This is not a Pipe*. Berkeley: University of California Press, 1983.

Gasset, José Ortega y. *Obras completas. Tomo III*. Madrid: Alianza, 1983.

Hinojosa, José María. *Poesías completas. Tomo II*. Torremolinos: Litoral, 1983.
Jay, Martin. *Downcast Eyes*. Berkeley: University of California Press, 1993.
Lippard. Lucy R., ed. *Surrealists on Art*. New Jersey: Prentice-Hall, 1970.
Mitchell, W. J. T. "What is an Image?" in *Iconology: Image, Text, Ideology*. Chicago: University of Chicago Press, 1986.
Morelli Gabrielle ed.. *Treinta años de vanguardia española*, Seville: El carro de la Nieve, 1991.
Mulhall, Stephen. *On Being in the World: Wittgenstein and Heidegger on Seeing Aspects*. London: Routledge, 1990.
Richards, I. A. *Coleridge on Imagination*. London: Kegan Paul, Trench, Trubner & Co., 1934.
Rifaterre, Michael. *Text Production*. Translated by Terese Lyons. New York: Columbia University Press, 1983.

IV
TEXTUAL FEASTS

"Promnesia" (Remembering Forward) in *Midnight's Children*; or Rushdie's Chutney versus Proust's *Madeleine*
LAURENT MILESI

FROM THE "SOLITARY, UNIQUE, AND [. . .] RECHERCHÉ BISCUIT" which Lenehan awards Corley for his crafty seduction maneuvers in Joyce's short story "Two Gallants"[1] to the grandfather's *pain grillé* or *biscotte* in Proust's preface to his *Contre Sainte-Beuve*, the earlier prosier avatar of the famous *madeleine* in *A la recherche du temps perdu*,[2] modern(ist) literature has provided all manners of grist to our critical mills—or, more accurately here, dough to our academic bread. In particular, Proust's all-time-hit, the sexually replete, religious-sounding *madeleine*, and its other (past or related) attendant bakery produce have been chewed to death, amidst a whole range of consumable goodies that, in Proust's oeuvre, constantly nourish desire and feed plot and narration alike (for example, besides the anamnesic catalyst of the *madeleine*, the near-ubiquitous *orangeade*, which on one occasion even triggers off Swann's decision to marry Odette, *Du côté de chez Swann*, 1:293–94).[3]

Since Jean-Pierre Richard's memorable *Proust et le monde sensible*[4] we have been able to taste the fuller "consistency" of the alimentary object in *A la recherche*, within the synaesthetic spectrum of the five senses. But my aim here is to investigate in what ways Rushdie's hors-d'oeuvre or accompanying delicacies of chutneys and pickles in *Midnight's Children*[5] (but also the pepper-and-spice base of *The Moor's Last Sigh*[6]) offer a politically resistant, "pepped-up" version of the modernists' bready or doughy staple and, more generally, of their aestheticization of munchies. I would like to compare the failure of even the emblematic *madeleine*, despite its sensual anamnesic force instrumental in first conjuring back the past (lost) time into the present as a transitory but necessary waystation onto the future of a *temps retrouvé*—not to mention other culinary favorites interspersed throughout Proust's seven-course treat—with what I shall later call the "promnesic" effect of Rushdie's chutnification as, perhaps, characteristic of the postmodern's, and in this case postcolonialist's, self-assumed "pickles" of (hi)story, in a gesture of "preservation" to be redefined. Put less appetizingly, yet arguably in more serviceable critical parlance: although Rushdie himself repeatedly documented his conception of fiction as a modernist act involving an apprenticeship in the traditional craft of oral storytelling, whose matter was then converted into a written narrative through a sort of "make it new" process,[7] this essay will hope to show how *Midnight's Children* (and, tangentially, *The Moor's Last Sigh*) goes beyond such an aesthetic project, in particular through a more successful culinary embodiment of history, memory, and time, amounting to a political gesture, which enabled Rushdie to leave behind the "initial" Proustian framework.[8]

As my argument will have to take as predigested over three thousand pages of Proust and a few good hundreds of Rushdie, I shall focus on the most eloquent vignettes, the choice "gobbets" in a comparative trajectory which will thus smack more of the unjustly legendary paucity of *nouvelle cuisine* (into which currying methods have been introduced relatively recently) than of Proust's protracted aristocratic *dîners*. Generous side-helpings from a range of other fictional dishes will be made available as argumentative fodder to this study whose larger critical horizon is the repositioning of modern, postmodern, and postcolonial temporalities along their respective culinary laws.

APERITIF: PREPARING THE TEXTUAL FEAST

> Although *apéritif* is an evocative word—in itself containing a vivid image of *luxe, calme et volupté*, a sense of life spaciously lived—my own preferred term for the alcoholic beverage consumed at the end of the working day is "sundowner."[9]

Stories, novels, their details and the language (or any number of these and other ingredients) can be salacious, unsavoury, even unpalatable, or, on the contrary, delicious, juicy, even meaty; or else they can be insipid, frankly distasteful, or just in need of some peppering or spicing up so as to compete with the obscene "conversational dishes" of *The Moor's Last Sigh* (*Moor*, 320; also

343: "garam-masala exclamations"). But what, then, if it is the fictional fiery family rag that is being chewed at some length?

> Family history, of course, has its proper dietary laws. One is supposed to swallow and digest only the permitted parts of it, the halal portions of the past, drained of their redness, their blood. Unfortunately, this makes the story less juicy; so I am about to become the first and only member of my family to flout the laws of halal. Letting no blood escape from the body of the tale, I arrive at the unspeakable part. (*MC*, 59[10])

In the mixed metaphorical moods of Rushdie's novel, storytelling is thus, in Christian terms, a word made flesh then sacrificially drained of its blood—just as its narrator Saleem Sinai will later be drained of all fluids, nasal or sexual, of hope and finally of life—or, according to the Oriental spirit, a reincarnation to be then disincarnated, "un-meated" in un-halal fashion. If one takes seriously Stuart Gilbert's following tongue-in-cheek comparison, in an essay on Joyce's *Work in Progress* (later to become *Finnegans Wake*) for the collection *Our Exagmination*, whose tone and topics were engineered by Joyce himself, the linguistic ingredient of a story is indeed a butcher's delicacy whose handling depends on national carving and, therefore, culinary habits:

> he [the Englishman—Edward Lear] cuts vertically through the meat of sound and the fat of common sense, with an eye only to the funny effect of the chunk removed; whereas the Irish writer [. . .] carves his *gigot* in the continental manner, that is to say, parallel to the etymological bone, following the way the muscles are naturally and anatomically set.[11]

And indeed, in the last of a series of "inartistic" self-portraits, in *Finnegans Wake*, 1.7, Joyce has the inquisitorial, bourgeois, nationalistic Shaun the Post, butcher by trade, denounce his twin artistic alter ego Shem the Penman, baker by profession, for preferring foreign, artificial, (al)chemical products, not unlike Joyce's own portmanteau idiom concocted from foreign parts of speech through the "*Art of Panning*,"[12] and only when the culinary delicacy is naturally, organically grown on foreign soil which has been domesticated through an imperialistic act of colonization is it valued over the "parochial" fare:

> Shem was a sham and a low sham and his lowness creeped out first via foodstuffs. So low was he that he preferred Gibsen's teatime

salmon tinned, as inexpensive as pleasing, to the plumpest roeheavy lax or the friskiest parr or smolt troutlet that ever was gaffed between Leixlip and Island Bridge and many was the time he repeated in his botulism that no junglegrown pineapple ever smacked like the whoppers you shook out of Ananias' cans, Findlater and Gladstone's, Corner House, England. None of your inchthick blueblooded Balaclava fried-at-belief-stakes or juicejelly legs of the Grex's molten mutton or greasilygristly grunters' goupons or slice upon slab of luscious goosebosom with lump after load of plumpudding stuffing all aswim in a swamp of bogoakgravy for that greekenhearted yude! Rosbif of Old Zealand! he could not attouch it. (*Finnegans Wake*, 170.25–171.02)

Of course our low hero [. . .] got up whatever is meant by a stourbridge clay kitchenette and [. . .], playing lallaryrook cookerynook [. . .], brooled and cocked and potched in an athanor, whites and yolks and yilks and whotes to the frulling fredonnance of *Mas blanca que la blanca hermana* and *Amarilla, muy bien*, with cinnamon and locusts and wild beeswax and liquorice and Carrageen moss [. . .], chanting [. . .] his cantraps of fermented words, abracadabra calubra culorum, (his oewfs à la Madame Gabrielle de l'Eglise, his avgs à la Mistress B. de B. Meinfelde, his eiers Usquadmala à la pomme de ciel, his uoves, oves and uves à la Sulphate de Soude, his ochiuri sowtay sowmmonay à la Monseigneur, his soufflosion of oogs with somekat on toyast à la Mère Puard, his Poggadovies alla Fenella, his Friedeggs à la Tricarême) [. . .] *Finnegans Wake*, 184.11–32[13])

The narrator-writer of *Midnight's Children* proclaims the (albeit rare, though not in the sense of "underdone") virtue of mastering "the multiple gifts of cookery and language" (*MC*, 37), if only because linguistic ingredients are used to "cook" history and dish it up to one's own taste, using a "mixture of condiment and oratory" (*MC*, 210) for persuasion, but also to fight against the ravages of time, as in the following excerpt whose context recalls the treatment of "clock time" in *Tristram Shandy*:

my chutneys and kasaundies are, after all, connected to my nocturnal scribblings—by day amongst the pickle-vats, by night within these sheets, I spend my time at the great work of preserving. Memory, as well as fruit, is being saved from the corruption of the clocks. *MC*, 38)

Always a potentially nefarious activity if not well practiced—as in the ominous question "what is cooking?" (compare with *Moor*, 177)—"cooking" becomes a crucial textual-historical skill whose mastery enables the successful reprocessing of the past towards the creation of a more relishable future for the community, just as the temporal unfolding of life-as-narration undoes the earlier fictional cookings of (hi)story:

> "Baba sahib, sit only and we will cook up the happy future. We will mash its spices and peel its garlic cloves, we will count out its cardamoms and chop its ginger, we will heat up the ghee of the future and fry its masala to release its flavour. [. . .] We will cook the past and present also, and from it tomorrow will come." (*Moor*, 273)

With its two-way emphasis on the fieriness of Indian (family) politics and the eco-politics of spices (for example *Moor*, 4–5, 42, 71, 73, etc.), *The Moor's Last Sigh* brings home the near-atavistic potency of cooking first explored in *Midnight's Children*.

Entrée: Aestheticization versus "Embodiment"

> Food, said Goethe, is the topmost taper on the golden candelabrum of existence.[14]

No matter what its virtues or impact may be in *A la recherche*, food is more a transcendable viand than one that permeates the whole fabric of the Proustian project, whose sheets of paper never go as far as "[smell] just a little of turmeric" (*MC*, 24) or chutney (*MC*, 37), since Rushdie's scenes of telling-writing are either a pickle factory (*Midnight's Children*) or a pepper-and-spice-trade-'n'-big-business whose "hot stuff" has infiltrated family politics, sex, and language (*Moor,* passim). Subtle aesthetic parallels between delicate dishes and characters in Proust, vindicated by centuries of good fare and literary-psychological metaphors, cannot rival with the potency of effects, based on ancestral culinary but also medicinal lore, unleashed by the spicy ingredients and concoctions from the Indian "sub-condiment" (*Moor*, 5).[15] One could weigh the equation between the flavor of the numerous virtues of Françoise and the succulent, tender aroma of her broiled chicken in *Du côté de chez Swann* (1:120), or even the glorious use of foodstuffs (*madeleine, orangeade*) as psychological trigger recalled earlier, against the disastrous action of diverse currying methods in *Midnight's Children*, almost redolent of medieval humours, or, more recently, against the insidious explosive power of the whole palette of Mexican food in Laura Esquivel's bestseller novel *Like Water for Choco-*

late, which narrates, in twelve chapter-months, each with its own crucial recipe, the frustration of the passion between Tita, the narrator's great-aunt, and Pedro by the family's ancestral matriarchal tradition, and its ultimate defeat through the culinary art's powers of domestic-political resistance, the "flavours, smells, textures and the effects they could have [. . .] beyond Mama Elena's iron command."[16] Thus Padma is angered by something "hot and vinegary" (*MC*, 24)—"we have red chillies in our veins," says Aurora Zogoiby in *The Moor's Last Sigh* (5)— and we are repeatedly privy to scenes of vengeance contrived through "the impregnation of food with emotions" (*MC*, 330):

> Amina began to feel the emotions of other people's food seeping into her—because Reverend Mother doled out the curries and meatballs of intransigence, dishes imbued with the personality of the creator; Amina ate the fish salans of stubbornness and the birianis of determination. [. . .] Mary's pickles had a partially counteractive effect— since she had stirred into them the guilt of her heart, and the fear of discovery, so that, good as they tasted, they had the power of making those who ate them subject to nameless uncertainties and dreams of accusing fingers. [. . .] (*MC*, 139)

> she [aunt Alia] fed us the birianis of dissension and the nargisi koftas of discord (*MC*, 330)

> the kormas of my aunt's vengeance—spiced with forebodings as well as cardamoms (*MC*, 332)

> "I told them, nobody makes achar-chutney like our Mary [. . .] because she puts her feelings inside them." (*MC*, 458)

Similarly, in Esquivel's novel—whose original English title, *Like Water for Hot Chocolate*, as the text explains, is the "active" yeastlike metaphor for an uncontrollable rage about to boil over[17]—the empire of food stretches beyond the placid nostalgia of Proustian remembrance (138) "smells have the power to evoke the past, bringing back sounds and even smells that have no match in the present" [13]), the comparisons dictated by the laws of social decorum ("how long ago it seemed that Tita had felt like a chilli in nut sauce left sitting on the platter out of etiquette, for not wanting to look greedy" [217]), and, more generally, beyond the aesthetic correlation of the poetic with the culinary ("Just as a poet plays with words, Tita juggled ingredients and quantities at will, obtaining phenomenal results" [64]), into the more deeply felt political effects of an eruptive psychosocial dynamics. Thus Tita's tears of sorrow and resentment that fell into the meringue peaks of the cake of her sister Rosaura's wedding to her own sweetheart distill their emetic venom into the guests' guts and wreak havoc on the social set-up:

> The moment they took their first bite of the cake, everyone was flooded with a great wave of longing. [. . .] But the weeping was just the first symptom of a strange intoxication—an acute attack of pain and frustration—that seized the guests and scattered them across the patio and the grounds and into the bathrooms, all of them wailing over lost love. (*Like Water for Chocolate*, 39)

Or else, in a passage describing how sexual communion is achieved through the consummate sensuality of the inspired cooking (and which can be tacitly compared with the aestheticizing slant of the Proustian "orangeade scene" referred to in note 3):

> It was as if a strange alchemical process had dissolved her entire being in the rose petal sauce, in the tender flesh of the quails, in the wine, in every one of the meal's aromas. (*Like Water for Chocolate*, 49)

> Tita knew through her own flesh how fire transforms the elements, how a lump of cornflour is changed into a tortilla, how a soul that hasn't been warmed by the fire of love is lifeless, like a useless ball of cornflour. (*Like Water for Chocolate*, 63)

> The anger she felt within her acted like yeast on bread dough. She felt its rapid rising, flowing into every last recess of her body; like yeast in a small bowl, it spilled over to the outside, escaping in the form of steam through her ears, nose and all her pores. (*Like Water for Chocolate*, 137)

> When Esperanza told Tita that when she felt Alex's eyes on her body, she felt like dough being plunged in boiling oil, Tita knew that Alex and Esperanza would be bound together for ever. (*Like Water for Chocolate*, 215)

Spanning four generations, from the fetal conditioning by onions of the great-aunt, whose salt from the oniony tears shed at birth was recycled for cooking, to the narrator who, via her mother, inherited the culinary torch of female resistance, the book ends on the legacy of Tita's nonpareil cookbook, "which tells in each of its recipes this story of a love interred" (221), the sole survivor from the holocaustic destruction of the family ranch following the climactic consummation of her passion with Pedro.

Nothing of the kind in Proust's more mellow saga; even Françoise's famous treat of *boeuf froid aux carottes*, which earns her the enviable label of "chef de tout premier ordre" from the connoisseur M. de Norpois amidst a lyrical description of the dish's excellence (*A l'ombre des jeunes filles en fleurs*, 1.1.449–50), is ultimately processed as a strategic token of conviviality, a truly "*conversational* dish" which elicits from the mouth-watered guest equally delectable tidbits or choice morsels of well-oiled gossip:

> M. de Norpois pour contribuer lui aussi à l'agrément du repas nous *servit* diverses histoires dont il *régalait* fréquemment ses collègues de carrière [. . .] (*A l'ombre des jeunes filles en fleur, I*, I:450; my emphases)
> [To add his own contribution to the pleasure of the repast, M. de Norpois entertained us with a number of the stories with which he was in the habit of regaling his diplomatic colleagues. [. . .] (*Within a Budding Grove*, 2:34)]

Or else, in the Guermantes' time-worn communal ritual of the postprandial *orangeade*, the exquisite drink, quintessentially distilled from the fruit and eked out by a carafe of cooked cherry or pear juice by Marcel, becomes the yardstick of his social power (*Le Côté de Guermantes*, 2.2.803). The chemical sublimation of color into taste is fictionalized through the aestheticizing power of writing-as-cooking; it can be counterpointed to Roland Barthes's mythology of "Ornamental Cookery," in which an aesthetics of gastronomy, its "magical" visions of unaffordable, therefore unpreparable, paradises of "rococo cookery" ("chiselled mushrooms, punctuation of cherries [. . .], arabesques of glacé fruit") served up to the working-class public of the more populist magazines like *Elle*, whose consumers "are entitled only to fiction," is opposed to an economics of culinary representation in journals like *L'Express*, which caters to an affluent, gourmet, middle-class readership and can thus afford "real" images of recipes.[18]

To put it in the words of the overall project of *A la recherche* conceived as a formal *oeuvre-cathédrale*,[19] social and aesthetic "palatability" ultimately presides over the architectural dressing of viands in Proust's *magnum opus*. Thus, Françoise's *boeuf-*

mode, a dignified statuary achievement "couché par le Michel-Ange de notre cuisine sur d'énormes cristaux de gelée pareils à des blocs de quartz transparent" (*A l'ombre des jeunes filles en fleur*, 1.1.449) [couched by the Michelangelo of our kitchen upon enormous crystals of aspic, like transparent blocks of quartz (*Within a Budding Grove*, 2:33)], is eventually recognized as the paragon of the prospective work, the symbiotic interpenetration of its textures and flavors providing a model for the uniform binding of writing (unlike the more coarsely blended *salade d'ananas et de truffe*): "ne ferais-je pas mon livre de la façon que Françoise faisait ce boeuf-mode [. . .] et dont tant de morceaux de viande ajoutés et choisis enrichissaient la gelée?" (*Le Temps retrouvé*, 4:612) ["I should be making my book in the same way that Françoise made that *boeuf à la mode* which M. de Norpois had found so delicious, just because she had enriched its jelly with so many carefully chosen pieces of meat" (*Time Regained*, 4:434)],[20] and one could bring up numerous other instances of the sustained parallel between food and architecture/statuary, which periodically prolong and recall the grand design: the description of aunt Léonie's bedrooom (1:49), the mouthing of the name of the cathedral town "Coutances" (1:381–2), the evocation of a cake's powerful structure (1:497; cf. also 2:257 quoted *infra*), the multifaceted monumentality of ice creams (3:636–37), and so on.

Indeed, consumables are made to run through the whole gamut of fine arts and artistic associations, which arguably raise the status of eating and cooking to aesthetic heights of *savoir vivre* and *savoir faire*, but they are equally subjected to the filter of personal evocation (rather than historical awareness; see *infra*)—one of the ways in which the shift from objective to mental reality is achieved, as in the following pairing of sweetmeats and sweethearts:

> Mes amies préféraient les sandwiches et s'étonnaient de me voir manger seulement un gâteau au chocolat *gothiquement historié* de sucre ou une tarte à l'abricot. C'est qu'avec les sandwiches au chester et à la salade, nourriture ignorante et nouvelle, je n'avais rien à dire. Mais les gâteaux étaient instruits, les tartes étaient bavardes. Il y avait dans les premiers des fadeurs de crème et dans les seconds des fraîcheurs de fruits qui en savaient long [. . .]. Ils me rappelaient ces assiettes à petits fours, des *Mille et Une Nuits*, qui distrayaient tant de leurs "sujets" ma tante Léonie [. . .], etc. (*A l'ombre des jeunes filles en fleurs*, 2.2.257; first emphasis mine)
> [My friends preferred the sandwiches, and were surprised to see me

eat only a single chocolate cake, sugared with Gothic tracery, or an apricot tart. This was because, with the sandwiches of cheese or salad, a form of food that was novel to me and was ignorant of the past, I had nothing in common. But the cakes understood, the tarts were talkative. There was in the former an insipid taste of cream, in the latter a fresh taste of fruit which knew all about Combray, and about Gilberte [. . .]. They reminded me of those cake-plates with the Arabian Nights pattern, the subjects on which so diverted my aunt Léonie. [. . .] (*Within a Budding Grove*, 2:559)]

Ultimately, Proust's *chef d'oeuvre*, from the "destruction des choses," initially evoked in relation to the crumbling away of the mnemonic mouthful of the *madeleine* (1:46), to the final musings over the "action destructrice du Temps" (4:508), is the product of an alchemical and "digesting" writing that aesthetically processes and assimilates so-called "consumables" for what they literally are, down to the aliment's quintessentials (compare with 3:136).[21] In this typical product of modernity's part-inheritance of a postsymbolist fin-de-siècle aesthetics, which found one of its most celebrated expressions in the black-monochrome menu composed by an overrefined Des Esseintes in Huysmans's cult novel *A Rebours*—itself echoed, amid Proustian and other literary aestheticizations of an impressive range of international culinary traditions, in John Lanchester's esculent *The Debt to Pleasure* (100–101)—we are a far cry from any sort of irreducibly physical embodiment of food, let alone of the kind perpetuated by Roger Mexico and Pig Bodine towards the end of *Gravity's Rainbow*, a "treat" out-Rabelaising the French Renaissance writer's own flamboyant literary orgies.

ENTREMETS: POSTMODERN DECADENCE VERSUS BELATED (MOCK-)MODERN AESTHETICISM

ENTREMETS
1.a. Side dishes.
2. *Antiq.* A spectacular entertainment between the courses of a banquet.
(*OED*)

Possibly prompted by the ghoulish presence of Brigadier Pudding, that connoisseur of indigestible delights who, in one of many S-and-M rituals, was seen earlier squatting below Katje and ingesting her shit, the following banquet of excretions is conjured up for purposes of sociopolitical disturbance: snot soup, pus pudding, scum soufflé "with a side of—*menstrual marmalade!*", "rich, meaty smegma stew," clot casserole, before being blown up to its fullest coprophagic effect:

> "We could plan a better meal than *this*," Roger waving the menu. "Start off with afterbirth appetizers, perhaps some clever little *scab sandwiches* with the crusts trimmed off of course . . . o-or booger biscuits! Mmm, yes, spread with mucus mayonnaise? and topped with a succulent bit of slime sausage. . . ."
> "Oh I see," sez Commando Connie, "it has to be alliterative. How about . . . um . . . *discharge dumplings?*"
> "We're doing the soup course, babe," sez cool Seaman Bodine, "so let me just suggest a canker consommé, or perhaps a barf bouillon."
> "Vomit vichyssoise," sez Connie.
> "You got it."
> "Cyst salad," Roger continues, "with little cherry-red squares of abortion aspic, tossed in a subtle dandruff dressing."[22]

And on through "fart fondue (skillfully placed bubbles of anal gas rising slowly through a rich cheese viscosity, yummm), boil blintzes, Vegetables Venereal in slobber sauce . . .", then wart waffles, puke pancakes with sweat syrup and spread with pinworm preserves, hemorrhoid hash, bowel burgers, gangrene goulash, scrumptious creamy-white leprosy loaf, fungus fricassee, carbuncle cutlets with groin gravy and ringworm relish—at this point one aptly named Hannibal Grunt-Gobbinette threatens "to bring the matter up in Parliament"—finally to dessert possibilities of crotch custard, phlegm fudge, mold muffins, and last but not least, after the performance of a "Disgusting Duo" featuring "Toe-jam tarts 'n' Diarrhea Dee-lite," announced by the black butler: "Pimple pie with filth frosting, gentlemen." One will readily concede that these heights of abjection are furthest, on the double scale of social and literary decorum, from the elegant, polite dinner parties à la Proust, even if, paradoxically, the nostalgic evocations of the rich socialized sensations from bygone days in *A la recherche* find an anamorphic counterpart in Pynchon's text in the characters' desperate protest against the paradoxical loss of the wartime economy of human relationships.

Starting on the acknowledgement that "This is not a conventional cookbook" (1) and structured as a seasonal culinary manual, John Lanchester's *The Debt to Pleasure*, subtitled "A Novel," claims to eschew the double vein of encyclopedism[23] and confession which sums up the classic example for its eclectically erudite and insufferably snobbish narrator, the Francophile Tarquin Winot, who elects as inspirational model for his own "gastro-historico-psycho-autobiographico-anthropico-philosophic lucubrations" (224) "the culino-philosophico-autobiographical volume *La Physiologie du Goût*" by Brillat-Savarin, the literary-culinary *chef d'oeuvre* from one of the most eminent *chefs* ever (2). Nurtured as a synergestic exchange between "savours and essence like some ideal *daube*" (4), *The Debt to Pleasure* is a deftly overwrought spoof on the *passé* postsymbolist epicure, replete with roll calls of (inter)national dishes and linguistic-etymological glosses, force-fed with umpteen literary allusions, literati's *bons mots* on food and (to put it in Joyce's Wakean idiom) "quashed quotatoes" (*Finnegans Wake*, 183.22), and, among other targets of reverential imitation that might include a Barthesian stint ("when you eat caviare you are partaking of this mysterious juxtaposition of the exquisite and the atavistic" [16]), on a gastronomized version of anamnesis (for example, 22) and on the Proustian paradox of the imperfect work beckoning to the true imaginary oeuvre to come: "the most important part of any artist's oeuvre is the work he knows it is no longer possible to attempt" (69).[24] The culinary aesthete's own belated modernity—both are associated in his mention of the availability of salad leaves in the depths of winter (40)—as well as his *outré* artificiality, ceaselessly blur the boundary between art and life (for example, 71), thus leaving out politics and the "real." Here are some choice vignettes from Winot's gourmet pages (the first excerpt is in the Huysmans mood of his self-styled "aesthetic period"):

> In my black room, dressed in black velvet, black silk cravat—no need to change the inherent colour of the single orchid in my button hole—I would arrange for meals consisting entirely of black food: truffles grated over squid-ink pasta, followed by *boudin noir* on a bed of fried black radicchio. For dessert, I wanted to emphasize the essential artificiality of the event, the fact that it was a celebration of art, whim, caprice, set over against the brutal facts of nature and death: so I served *crème brûlée*, dyed black. Naturally we drank Black Velvet, that very English confection, combining clubmanly propriety with nineties-ish, Café Royal-ish institutionalized aestheticism. (*The Debt to Pleasure*, 100–101)

> I borrowed W. H. Auden's technique of mixing the vermouth and gin at lunchtime (though the great poet himself used vodka) and leaving the mixture in the freezer to attain that wonderful jellified texture

of alcohol chilled to below the point at which water freezes. The absence of ice means that the Auden martini is not diluted in any way, and thus truly earns the drink its sobriquet "the silver bullet." In his autobiography the Spanish film director Luis Buñuel says that the correct way to make a martini is simply to allow the light to pass through the vermouth on the way to striking the gin, in a method analogous to the Immaculate Conception. [. . .]

While it is true that a dry martini should be served unbruised—i.e. still translucent, hence the traditional emphasis so self-consciously defied by James "Shaken Not Stirred" Bond—a vinaigrette should be lightly agitated with a fork until it becomes cloudy and emulsified, the work of a few seconds. (*The Debt to Pleasure*, 41)

A similar filtering aestheticization presides over the recolonialization of curries and spices as a cultural-national ingredient—despite Winot's later boast that his own curries appeal to the real, as opposed to the Orientalized, East (112). In a doctrinal prose whose style is more reminiscent of what Proust's adjectival self-indulgings would read like if soured by an overdose of cultural stereotypes than of the punch of Rushdie's "pepperpot revolution," these arguably Oriental staples are reclaimed (as is Champagne later [124–25]) as an inherent part of the national fiber rather than as a "nostalgic, retrogressive" legacy of the lost empire, replaced by "the street-corner tandoori house:"

> One might go as far as to say that a taste for spices is an ingredient (!) of the national character, an instinct comparable with the Welsh talent for singing, the German liking for forests, the Swiss knack for hotel-keeping, the Italian passion for motor-cars. [. . .] Thus the records of English spice consumption show a heroic commitment to (especially) overrated cinnamon; the even more overrated, not-far-short-of-actively-nasty clove; tasty, soporific nutmeg and its sibling, mace; aromatic allspice; flashy paprika; historic mustard seed; popular ginger; chilli [. . .]; warm-tasting, personal-favourite, beds-i'-the-east-are-soft cumin; evocatively Middle-Eastern coriander [. . .]; risky cardamom; unmistakable caraway; lurid turmeric—I could go on. (*The Debt to Pleasure*, 105–6)

Winot's "memories" (in his own double quotation marks) consist of literary *purple* patches ("certain passages in Rilke and Proust, certain poems of Leopardi and axioms of Lichtenberg" [196]) and painterly culinary flashbacks ("a certain bag of hot chestnuts eaten outside the Dominion Theatre on Tottenham Court Road two days before the winter solstice" [ibid.])—the former felicitously colored as our class-conscious, chromatically touchy aesthete abhors the color pink, a weakness for which is "an infallible sign of the defective taste one associates with certain groups and individuals: the British working classes, grand French restaurateurs, Indian street-poster designers and God, whose fatal susceptibility for the colour is so apparent in the most lavishly cinematic instances of his handiwork (sunsets, flamingoes)" (126). And, as a logical result, life and cooking are compared with or "translated" into textual tropes and elements of a decorous semantics (compare with passage on page 122, where the menu is compared to a sentence)—by a rhetorico-gastronomic process of culinary intertextuality or (to take a starchy leaf out of Winot's turgid book) "interculinarity" (as in the second of the four following extracts; compare also with phrases on page 50 about culinary translation and adaptation):

> Perhaps, just as every love stands in some relationship to our first love affair—a relation which holds only if one extends the possible nature of interdependency to include parody, inversion, quotation, pastiche, operatic recasting, as well as slavish and identical reduplication—no restaurant in later life comes entirely unaccompanied with some associations with our first restaurant. (*The Debt to Pleasure*, 45—another echo of *A la recherche*)

> one high-level criticism might be that the pastry-and-curd combination [of the lemon tart included in the *petits fours*] mimicked too closely, or quoted too narrowly, or created an unfortunate assonance with, the curd-and-pastry combination of the *tarte à la crème*. (*The Debt to Pleasure*, 140)

> A dish such as *volaille truffée au beurre d'asperge à la crème de patate "Elysée Palace"* exists in a realm which has managed to exceed the wildest imaginable reach of parody. (*The Debt to Pleasure*, 97—on the excessiveness of French cooking)

> One of the disappointing features of this pudding [the Queen of Puddings] is that it is almost impossible, in writing about or discussing it, to avoid the double genitive "of" that used so to upset Flaubert. (*The Debt to Pleasure*, 27)

As I suggested before, this epiphanic "crystallization" of food as a lifelong passion and artistic *modus vivendi* (compare to 47) leaves out politics altogether, which features only once it has been filtered through a culinary capriccio, as when the futurist Marinetti's battered and deep-fried *rose diaboliche* (diabolical roses) are evoked (137),[25] or when, as we unwittingly approach

Winot's vindicatory confession of his murderous megalomania, we are told that the deeper meaning behind Hitler the failed painter and Mao the failed poet is not that the megalomaniac is an *artiste manqué* but rather that the artist is a timid megalomaniac (226). And indeed, "In terms of our inner lives, our *real* lives, what effect, after all, is had by the result of the battle of Waterloo compared with the question of whether or not to put Tabasco sauce on one's oysters?" (195).

Our "connoisseur of chaos" ultimately makes a plea for an aesthetics of destruction—which we learn he first intimated when he rode his tricycle backwards and forwards over one of his brother's earliest compositions (197)—which finds its outlet in a series of murders as meticulously cooked up as they have been, we belatedly realize, discreetly hinted at throughout the novel and which, in blending with his aesthetic theory of the superiority of the incomplete or even unexecuted work of art, and of the absent memories (compare also on page 197: "I am more interested in the things I cannot remember, in absences, elisions, vacuities, negativities, voids, aporiae, nothingness"), eventually "murders" art itself. In his self-aggrandizing peroration on the two most important cultural figures in the modern world, the artist and the murderer, the superiority of the latter, i. e. himself, is justified as follows:

> The murderer [. . .] is better adapted to the reality and to the aesthetics of the modern world because instead of leaving a presence behind him—the achieved work, whether in the form of a painting or a book or a daubed signature—he leaves behind him something just as final and just as achieved: an absence. Where somebody used to be, now nobody is. What more irrefutable proof of one's having lived can there be than to have taken a human life and replaced it with nothingness, with a few fading memories? (*The Debt to Pleasure*, 25–26)

The mention of *The Arabian Nights*, in the last passage I quoted from *A la recherche*, a crucial intertext in both Proust and Rushdie—at the end of *Le Temps retrouvé* Scheherazade's oral cycle of tales is a possible literary model for the projected work (4:621)—is an apt reminder that the thrust of my argument at this stage bears on the contrastive roles of (culinary) anamnesis in two oeuvres and writers occasionally sharing a common literary lineage. But to that effect, a short detour via the general structure of time and memory in Proust and Rushdie is first needed.

First Course: Time, History and Memory in Proust and Rushdie

The critical focus and very nature of my argument should not be misconstrued as a vested interest in doing Proust's admirable project a slighting injustice; a few preliminary reflections on *A la recherche* are therefore called for at this point in order to dispel this impression.

There is no denying what I started praising in my introduction via Richard's revealing analyses: the irreducible materiality of food and wares in some purple patches, usually through the sexualization of recurrent motifs, like the asparagus[26] (compare with the cucumber in *Midnight's Children*), or—but it is significant—through the jarring or colorful intrusion of a "lower" life into the aristocratic fabric of *A la recherche*. Perhaps the most famous and lengthiest scene of this kind is to be found in *La Prisonnière*, where the popular onslaught of fish, fruit, and vegetable mongers crying their wares of *crevettes, merlans, maquereaux* and *moules* (3:633ff.—i.e. rent boys, ponces, pimps, and pussies respectively) is a climax in the Dionysiac treatment of fresh raw natural produce.

It is also true that the narrator's effort ultimately is not to take refuge in the past but to attempt to transform the past into the present and, when the deep hermeneutic significance of those "spots of resurrection"—the steeples of Martinville (1:177–78), the row of trees at Hudimesnil (2:76–77), the *petite phrase* of Vinteuil's sonata (passim), the unevenly adjusted flagstones of Guermantes (4:445 ff.), etc., usually leading to a recapitulative summoning (for example, 3:876–77) and to a deeper penetration into the essential significance of the experience —has been more fully digested in *Le Temps retrouvé*, equally to usher in the possibility of a future. As Deleuze neatly summed up in *Proust and Signs*, in an attempt to relativize the critical weight placed on involuntary memory and, hence, the view that the essential movement of Proust's *oeuvre* is towards the nostalgic past: "however important its role, memory intervenes only as the means of an apprenticeship which transcends recollection both by its goals and by its principles. The Search is oriented to the future, not to the past."[27] In what is still one of the most sensitive essays on the nature of Proust's experience of imaginary time, Maurice Blanchot had already given voice to the metamorphic structure of time as a two-stage ambidextrous process of retrospection and prospection—Deleuze's ambivalent "repetition" as both iteration of the past and rehearsal of the future:[28]

> As a metamorphosis of time, [Proust's experience of imaginary time] starts by transforming the present in which it seems to occur, drawing it into the indefinite depths where the "present" re-enacts the "past," but where the past opens onto the future which it mirrors, so that what is about to happen occurs again and yet again.[29]

And indeed various crucial "statements," that still somehow testify to the more essayistic mixed origin of *A la recherche*, periodically recall this to our attention if need be (of the following quotations, the first highlights the cumulative retroactive effect of the ecstatic "spots of anamnesis," and the second, from the prospective "last" book, relates backwards to the work as a whole):

> Aussi il ne faut pas ne redouter dans l'amour [. . .] que l'avenir, mais même le passé qui ne se réalise pour nous souvent qu'après l'avenir, et nous ne parlons pas seulement du passé que nous apprenons après coup, mais de celui que nous avons conservé depuis longtemps en nous et que tout d'un coup nous apprenons à lire. (*La Prisonnière*, 3:595)
> [And so we ought not to fear in love [. . .] the future alone, but even the past, which often comes to life for us only when the future has come and gone—and not only the past which we discover after the event but the past which we have long kept stored within ourselves and suddenly learn how to interpret. (*The Captive*, 5:91)]

> une oeuvre est à la fois le souvenir de nos amours passées et la prophétie de nos amours nouvelles. (*Le Temps retrouvé*, 4:486)
> [a work [is] at the same time a recollection of our past loves and a prophecy of our new ones. (*Time Regained*, 6:269)]

Georges Poulet meticulously teased out and analyzed these cross-currents of temporal (re)orientations in *A la recherche*; the initial impetus towards the past reveals itself to be the secondary (reversal) transformation and result of a more originary orientation towards the future,[30] but, as one progresses towards the end of the whole edifice (*Time Regained*)—while the reader's knowledge of the hero's completed experience remains suspended throughout until the end—this retrogressive movement within the work gives way to a third instant, a new perception of futurity as the dis-closure, completion, and belated recognition of an essential plenitude (333–34), of an artistic *mise en oeu-*

vre of a past no longer simply nostalgic but endowed with a future. Thus "Le grand roman de la rétrospection commence par la prospection" [The great novel of retrospection begins with prospection] (305) and "C'est cette prospectivité finale qui importe avant tout, encore qu'elle ne puisse être comprise que grâce à une vue régressive embrassant tout le passé du roman" [It is this final prospectiveness which matters most of all, although it can only be understood thanks to a regressive view which embraces the whole past of the novel] (335): "Sans doute, ce qui sera restitué en ce nouveau temps, en ce temps du futur, c'est seulement le passé; mais c'est un passé où l'on espère le futur, non un passé figé en sa passéité" [Without doubt, what will be restored in this new time, in this time of the future, is only the past; but it is a past in which one hopes for the future, not a past solidified in its pastness] (328).

The overall trajectory and effect is thus one of future perfect realization of one's life and works, partly on account of the loop back to the beginning taken in different ways both by Proust's oeuvre (for example *Jean Santeuil*, the earliest sketch, contains a narrative comparable to the narration of the final experience of *Le Temps retrouvé*)[31] and in Rushdie's near-cyclical "purging" of family genealogies. One is reminded of Lacan's shrewd observation in "The Function and Field of Speech and Language in Psychoanalysis," informed by a deft use of grammatical tenses, that "What is realized in my history is not the past definite of what was since it is no more, or even the present perfect of what has been in what I am, but the future anterior of what I shall have been for what I am in the process of becoming."[32] Still in "L'Expérience de Proust," Blanchot has emphasized the palimpsestic structure of *événements* and *avènement* that is so distinctive of Proust's masterpiece, a fourfold metamorphosis of time and subject (the real Proust, the writer, the narrator, the narrated character) so intricate that Proust himself "is incapable of telling [. . .] to which time the events he evokes belong, if they are taking place in the world of narration or if they happened in order that the point in the narration at which they happen may become actuality and truth."[33] The spiralling of the planes of temporality throughout the narrator's/Proust's *recherche* creates its dynamic movement and metamorphosis "qui n'est que le mouvement du livre vers l'oeuvre" [literally: "which is nothing but the movement from the book towards the work."][34] until the full disclosure of the narrator's calling, which "punctuates" (that is, crystallizes past-present-future into a point of coincidence

[Blanchot, "Proust," 70]) the whole of the narrated history of the *recherche* and opens it to its future (perfect) textual (re)enactment. The *Recherche*'s larger movement is from life to the work to come via the narration of the *recherche*—the ultimate point being the recognition in life of "the process of transformation through which it is directed towards the work [*oeuvre*] and towards the time of the work in which it will be achieved" (Blanchot, "Proust," 66; translation modified)—and its essential *désoeuvrement*[35] lies in the "unworking" of the book that is the condition of the movement of writing towards the disclosure of the future work.[36] Without this double pull of the retrospective and the prospective, Proust's essentializing synaesthetics of the lost and found (again) could not successfully take place. And with this retroactive effect of reading/writing—also noticeable in the discontinuous sequence of the last and first episodes/manuscripts of *The Moor's Last Sigh*—the work of anamnesis would seemingly open on to a more Lyotardian ana-mnesic process, in accordance with his conception of postmodern temporality as a process in ana- (rather than a mere process of flashback and repetition), whose grammatical tense, equally at work in the analytic "deferred action" or *Nachträglichkeit*, is the future perfect.[37] The nature of the Proustian "event" would thus lie in the power of the *moments bienheureux* to palliate lost time through the ana-chronic structure of their temporization.[38]

Blanchot's elegant conclusion that Proust "s'est donné le temps" ["gave himself time"] ("L'Expérience de Proust," 40)—a phrase which beautifully suggests that the valorization of idleness and dilatoriness (such as falling in love) in *A la recherche*, which takes the future artist's mind away from the active pursuit of the projected creation, is eventually sublated into a victorious (re)capturing of time—marks precisely the difference with the strictures of historical time in *Midnight's Children*, which far outweigh the staging of momentous events as a mere backdrop to the evolutions of Proust's characters and to Marcel's discontinuous work against time to turn life into art (with the exception of the Dreyfus affair, perhaps). If, as Blanchot also writes, "[i]t required the whole of real time to attain this unreal movement"("Proust," 71; translation modified), Proust's imaginary experience, even in the "Oriental marvellous" aspect it first takes on at the end of the *madeleine* episode through the cross between the Japanese game of immersing bits of paper which will then take on shape and life and the djinnlike conjuring up of a whole past world from the cup of tea, or through the final parallel with *The Arabian Nights* as a paragon of the future literary achievement, eventually runs counter to *Midnight's Children*'s resources of magical realism, the subversively inextricable mingling of fantasy and naturalism[39] as an act of politico-historical resistance through fictional allegorization in Latin American and several "postcolonial" countries. (During an interview in which he was asked about the comparison of his works with Garcia Marquez and magical realism, Rushdie pointed out that the Colombian writer's best-known novel, *One Hundred Years of Solitude*, was not thought of as fantasy but as realism in South America, just as in India people do not really treat *Midnight's Children* as a fabulous fiction: "The fantasy elements in it [. . .] are only enabling devices to talk about actuality."[40] And to come back to the Barthesian polarity in "Ornamental Cookery," the real and the magical here is the combination which, in Rushdie's writing and style, raises the ingredients of an aesthetics to the level of sociodomestic politics.) It is because, for Rushdie, "all description is itself a political act,"[41] rather than a novelist's compulsory rite of passage in the post-Balzacian tradition which "modern" writers like Proust were still contending with, that the culinary embodiment of the "pickles of [Indian] history" cannot ultimately be *reduced* to the purely stylistic or rhetorical trope of a literary aesthetics.

Plat de résistance: The *Madeleine* of Anamnesis versus the "Pickles of History"

Although Rushdie declared that "what I tried to do [. . .] was to make sure that the background, the bedrock of the book, was right—that Bombay was like Bombay, the cities were like the cities, the different dates were recognisably correct so that the fantasy could be rooted in that kind of reality,"[42] in " 'Errata' or, Unreliable Narration in *Midnight's Children*," he has conversely indicated that "one of the simplest truths about any set of memories is that many of them will be false."[43] These conflicting statements about "literal and remembered truth" and the ultimate disavowal of the act of faithfully remembering the past as a key to anagnorisis-as-truth may be read as a step forward from the Proustian project, which still reaches for the disclosure of an essential truth through the resurrecting work of involuntary memory, implictly exposing the latter's limitations for the postmodernist and/or postcolonial writer, who seeks the reappropriation of past history through a willful act of imagination and linguistic invention (compare, for example, with *MC*, 443).

Indeed, despite numerous structural and thematic parallels or recyclings, the uneasiness with "simple" anamnesic resurrection and with its opening on to the future is registered at both ends of *Midnight's Children* (which, like the ecstatic experiences of the *madeleine*, then of the badly adjusted cobbles in Guermantes in the first and last books of *A la recherche*, equally stake out the chronological bounds of Rushdie's novel)—from the earlier belief in the preservation of memory against the "corruption of the clocks" (*MC*, 36; quoted *supra*) or the green chutneys of fond remembrance which work as a cure against fever (*MC*, 209), through recurrent allusions to its immortalizing or pickling in words (for example, *MC*, 360), to "the impossible chutney of memory" (*MC*, 456) ironically manufactured by Mary Pereira, who confused family histories by swapping Saleem and Shiva at birth. Saleem's hesitancies between willful recollections, anamnesis (involuntary Proustian memory), but also, on one occasion, amnesia (in the dark rainforest of the Sundarbans (*MC*, 370), a parenthetical world of "the double-edged luxury of nostalgia" (*MC*, 363) which only faintly recalls the Proustian intermittences) and downright paramnesia (misrecollection) shaped by the novel's distorting and creative act of re(-)membering, reveal that the modernist Proustian solution will have worked only "partially" and its historically dated project must be supplanted. And it is to Rushdie's act of "promnesia" or remembering forward[44] in *Midnight's Children* that I would finally like to turn in order to illustrate this.

Whereas the individual hero of Proust's *A la recherche* only overcomes the strictures of linear time and history and resurrects the past in the present through the sporadic work of anamnesis which finally empowers him to "re(-)collect" through writing the narrative we have just read as one "novel" closes on the promise of another one to come, Rushdie's narrator, thanks to his transindividual fragmentation, encapsulates the "pickles" of history in order to open on to a prophetic utterance and offer a foretaste of the future of a nation: in the very act of the narrator's pointing forward to the empty jar of a future, after his final dissolution into six hundred million and more particles. In this fragmentation of the synecdochic individual who manipulates also collective history and memories, one must read the only possible acceptance of the double bind or, precisely, "pickles" in which the narrator finds himself.[45]

Chutneys are attempts at preservation in which the process of pickling dynamically changes the reality of the raw materials (compare with *MC*, 460) as it makes new, constantly changing commodities within the confined, "preserving" space of the sealed jar[46] (while baking merely effects a blending of components into a new homogenous result). The "chutnification" of history is then the ideal horizon of the narrator's pickling of chapters, each of which is "encapsulated" (*MC*, 75) in one pickle jar (and is different from the process of transubstantiation[47] or fabulous resurrection in Proust's writing, from the narrator's inkling of his essential plenitude in the *madeleine* episode [1:44] to the extratemporal enjoyment and "contemplation de l'essence des choses" [4:450, 454]). Thus we read towards the beginning of the twenty-seventh chapter of *Midnight's Children*:

> Twenty-six pickle-jars stand gravely on a shelf; twenty-six special blends, each with its identifying label, neatly inscribed with familiar phrases: [3 earlier chapter titles]. Twenty-six rattle eloquently when local trains go yellow-and- browning past; on my desk, five empty jars tickle urgently, reminding me of my uncompleted task. But now I cannot linger over empty pickle-jars; the night is for words, and green chutney must wait its turn. (*MC*, 384)

And in the thirtieth and last chapter, when Saleem Sinai is nearing his thirty-first birthday, which will also be the day of his death:

> Every pickle-jar [. . .] contains [. . .] the most exalted of possibilities: the feasibility of the chutnification of history; the grand hope of the pickling of time! I, however, have pickled chapters. Tonight, by screwing the lid firmly on to a jar bearing the legend *Special formula No 30: "Abracadabra,"* I reach the end of my long-winded autobiography; in words and pickles, I have immortalized my memories, although distortions are inevitable in both methods. We must live, I'm afraid, with the shadows of imperfection. (*MC*, 459)

> Thirty jars stand upon a shelf, waiting to be unleashed upon the amnesiac nation.
> (And beside them, one jar stands empty.) (*MC*, 460)

> In the spice bases, I reconcile myself to the inevitable distortions of the pickling process. To pickle is to give immortality [. . .] my thirty jars and a jar [. . .] One day, perhaps, the world may taste the pickles of history. [. . .] One empty jar . . . how to end? (*MC*, 461)

(The empty jar, we have known almost since the beginning ["While I sit like an empty pickle jar" (*MC*, 19)], is Saleem himself.)

But rather than bequeathing a text which fictitiously and deceptively prolongs itself into a new imaginary existence—*A la recherche*, but also Joyce's *A Portrait of the Artist as a Young Man*, which Stephen Dedalus, if he matures as an artist, will be capable of writing one day, thus achieving the same measure of ironic distancing that Joyce himself has—Rushdie's narrator-writer plunges into "[w]hat cannot be pickled, because it has not taken place" and gives us, on the threshold of the novel's solution, the thirtieth and last chapter, the substance of the thirty-first unwritten chapter of the narrator's dissolution:

> No, that won't do, I shall have to write the future as I have written the past, to set it down with the absolute certainty of a prophet. But the future cannot be preserved in a jar; one jar must remain empty ... What cannot be pickled, because it has not taken place, is that I shall reach my birthday, thirty-one today. (*MC*, 462, followed by a list of prospective, prophesied events)

Thus, though Proust's "real imaginary" oeuvre is not yet written and thus could be said to exist as an act of remembering forward (the typical modernist's retrospective glance over what will produce the work which will take the form we are reading), it is rather Rushdie's novel which captures the constructive spirit of promnesia by giving us as "physical text," beyond the point of convergence between experienced time and time of narration, the future not yet lived in the last pages, as if it were envisaged and remembered through narration-writing, willed into existence through the compelling (magical realistic) effect of food. Whereas "[t]he subject of the *Recherche* is indeed 'Marcel becomes a writer,' not 'Marcel the writer': the *Recherche* [...] is a novel of the future novelist," according to Rushdie himself, Saleem, towards the end of his life, directly "sets out to *write himself*."[48]

Rather than trying to break beyond the nightmarish trap of history in language like the modernist artist in Joyce's *Ulysses* or spiriting it away as social backdrop (Proust), Saleem, originally "handcuffed to history" like all his crossed generations of ascendants and descendants (just as, in the "sequel" of sorts, the Moor "tumbled towards history" [*Moor*, 5]), aims to encapsulate (hi)story, like djinns in a bottle, in as many chapters-in-a-book as there are names for pickle jars. But those "pickles" are precisely the impossible object of anamnesis, the *pharmakon* which is at once the restorative cure of self-preservation (in the sweetened form of the "green chutney of memory") and the destructive narrativized poison resulting in death, just as memory itself is "a clinical laboratory stocked with poison and remedy."[49] Rushdie's act of "remembering forward," also performed by the protagonist's three mothers in *Shame* who "were using the past, their only remaining capital, as a means of purchasing the future,"[50] may thus be seen as a way out of the modernist's angst towards (and occasional protective retreat from) history and political quandaries into the more visionary, "prophetic" fabric of the native/displaced East while yet facing its urgent national, political agendas. Whereas Proust converts food into spirit ("food for thought") in order to achieve the imaginary passage of book into work, and, within the larger economy of a semiotic dematerialization which Deleuze identified as Proust's Platonicism, the only (re)embodiment offered by Proust's oeuvre is the "temps incorporé" of the final pages of *Time Regained*,[51] Rushdie, through a process of narrative chutnification, gives us in a prophetic, magical, yet realist vision those future events which lie outside the scope of recollection-through-narration/writing, the repeated rituals of disincarnation/reincarnation, or (dis)embodiments, which confer on Indian food its irreducible materiality.

In deploying the full gamut of the emotional/culinary foretastes and aftertastes of (hi)story and memory (which also include the more "conventional" narrative uses of prolepsis and analepsis), *Midnight's Children* charts a tentative shift from the nostalgic Proustian modern(ist) anamnesis of involuntary memory (perhaps represented in Rushdie's text by the character Methwold, that is, "myth-world,"[52] through whom Eliot's "mythic method" can be aligned with a colonialist gesture), not only to a postmodern (Lyotardian) ana-mnesis as an analytic working through (according to the future perfect temporality of the unconscious), arguably already at work in the involuted temporality of *A la recherche*, but also to a more political and historical "remembering forward" or "promnesia" that would help to forge the amnesiac nation's "re-membrance of future things."[53] The sensualization of the narrative would thus "preserve" (in a dynamic sense) the possibility of a (trans-) individual/national "identity" through this "chutnification of history; the grand hope of the pickling of time!" so as to transcend "the impossible chutney of memory" (*MC*, 459). Proust's *madeleine*, dissolved in aunt

Léonie's *tilleul*, then in the mother's tea, is superseded by Rushdie's more vigorous, "historically aware"[54] (green) chutneys and spices, and the spiritual gourmet that consumes the physical into the metaphysical, the sensual into the "consensual" of synaesthesia (versus the "dissensus" of a "sensual politics"), has given way to gangs of picklers and spicers; exit essence, enter *sense*.

Notes

1. James Joyce, *Dubliners*, ed. Robert Scholes and A. Walton Litz (New York: Viking, 1969), 50.

2. Marcel Proust, *A la recherche du temps perdu*, édition publiée sous la direction de Jean-Yves Tadié, 4 vols. (Paris: Gallimard, 1987–89). All subsequent references to the most recent Pléiade édition of Proust's work—dismissed as "the portentous, over-annotated and illogically divided four-volume edition of 1987" by the crazed protagonist of John Lanchester's *The Debt to Pleasure* (London: Picador, 1996), 148—will appear parenthetically in the text, indicating the specific portion of the *Recherche* followed by Arabic numbers for volume and page identification. The translation immediately following the original quotation adopts the same convention for textual references, using C. K. Scott Moncrieff and Terence Kilmartin's six-volume *In Search of Lost Time*, rev. D. J. Enright (London: Chatto and Windus, 1992). For a comparative study of the two versions of the episode, see e.g. Richard Switzer, "The Madeleine and the Biscotte," *French Review* 30.4 (1957): 303–8, and especially Philippe Lejeune, "Écriture et sexualité," *Europe* 502–3: "Marcel Proust" (1971): 113–43. See also Jürg Bischoff's detailed genetic study, *La Genèse de l'épisode de la madeleine. Étude génétique d'un passage d'À la recherche du temps perdu de Marcel Proust* (Bern: Peter Lang, 1988). It is worth noting that the two earlier elements are recombined as "biscottes de pain grillé" in *Le Côté de Guermantes*, 1.2.327.

3. See also the osmosis of liquefaction and amorous feeling in the "orangeade scene" between Marcel and Albertine (*Sodome et Gomorrhe*, 3:156), briefly discussed by Julia Kristeva in "Orangeade and Ice Cream," in *Time and Sense: Proust and the Experience of Literature*, trans. Ross Guberman (New York: Columbia University Press, 1996), 207 [206–8].

4. (Paris: Seuil, 1974), especially 14ff. See also his earlier essay, "Proust et l'objet alimentaire," *Littérature* 6 (1972): 3–19.

5. Salman Rushdie, *Midnight's Children* (London: Picador, 1981); hereafter as *MC* with page references cited parenthetically in the text.

6. Salman Rushdie, *The Moor's Last Sigh* (London: Vintage, 1996); hereafter as *Moor* with page references given parenthetically in the text.

7. See e.g. the interview conducted by David Brooks in 1984 in "Adelaide," *Helix* 19 (1984): 57, and also Salman Rushdie, "*Midnight's Children* and *Shame*" (interview), *Kunapipi* 7.1 (1985): 8.

8. Cf. Salman Rushdie, " 'Errata': or, Unreliable Narration in *Midnight's Children*," in *Imaginary Homelands: Essays and Criticism 1981–1991* (London: Penguin, 1991), 23–24: "When I began the novel (as I've written else-

where) my purpose was somewhat Proustian. Time and migration had placed a double filter between me and my subject, and I hoped that if I could only imagine vividly enough it might be possible to see beyond those filters, to write as if the years had not passed, as if I had never left India for the West. But as I worked I found that what interested me was the process of filtration itself. So my subject changed, was no longer a search for lost time, had become the way in which we remake the past to suit our present purposes, using memory as our tool." In "Salman Rushdie's 'Use and Abuse of History' in *Midnight's Children*," *Ariel* 25.2 (1994), David W. Price reminds us of the project's inflection in the context of his own attempt to apply Nietzsche's three modes of history in the second of his *Untimely Meditations* to characters in Rushdie's novel: antiquarian history to Methwold, monumental history to the Widow, and critical history to the mixed hybrid Anglo-Indian Saleem, the latter struggling to present "a counter-narrative to the 'official' history of Indira Gandhi's government and the nostalgic histories of apologists for British imperialism" (93; see also 106). Nietzsche defines the goal of the critical mode in "On the Uses and Disadvantages of History for Life" as "an attempt to give oneself, as it were *a posteriori*, a past in which one would like to originate in opposition to that in which one did originate" (quoted in Price, 100).

9. Lanchester, *The Debt to Pleasure*, 123. Subsequent page references will be given parenthetically in the text. The trinity of French substantives is an apt allusion to Baudelaire's "L'invitation au voyage" for a novel which, in echo of, as much as unlike, Des Esseintes's fantasized trip across the Channel to England in Huysmans's *A Rebours*, also follows the course of the protagonist's real journey/quest of the senses from Portsmouth to Provence (see *infra*).

10. The unspeakable part or blood which the narrator refuses to spill is the shocking news that the aunt Mumtaz is still a virgin two years after her marriage to Nadir Khan.

11. Stuart Gilbert, "Prolegomena to *Work in Progress*," in Samuel Beckett et al., *Our Exagmination Round His Factification for Incamination of* Work in Progress (London: Faber, 1972), 61.

12. James Joyce, *Finnegans Wake* (London: Faber, 1975), 184.24. Subsequent page and line references will be given parenthetically in the text (all editions having the same pagination).

13. See also 171.13–18, and compare for example with Johns alias Shaun the butcher's self-advertisement in 172.05–10.

14. Donald Barthelme, "Conversations with Goethe," *Forty Stories* (London: Minerva, 1992), 67.

15. Beyond the tantalizing gratuity of the pun lies one of Rushdie's usual, politically motivated games with the geophysical shape of the subcontinent, perhaps suggestive here of a shrivelled yet fiery chilli pepper, an emblem for the explosiveness of family and state politics alike.

16. Laura Esquivel, *Like Water for Chocolate*, trans. Carol Christensen and Thomas Christensen (London: Black Swan, 1993), 45. Subsequent page references will be given parenthetically in the text.

17. Cf. also, soon after: "She felt her head about to burst, like a kernel of popcorn" (*ibid.*). An inviting parallel suggests itself here with Pound's modernist doctrine of the "true," "interpretative," as opposed to "ornamental," metaphor; see Ezra Pound's editorial comment in Ernest Fenollosa's *The Chinese Written Character as a Medium for Poetry* (London: Stanley Nott, 1936), 27.

18. Roland Barthes, *Mythologies*, sel. and trans. Annette Lavers (London: Cape, 1972), 78–80.

19. See Proust's letter to Jean de Gaigneron in *Correspondance*, texte établi, présenté et annoté par Philip Kolb, vol. 18: 1919 (Paris: Plon, 1990), 359, and e.g. *Le Temps retrouvé*, 4.610. In his excellent thematic dictionary *L'Œuvre cathédrale: Proust et l'architecture médiévale* (Paris: José Corti, 1990), s. v. "cathédrale" (77–119), Luc Fraisse concludes his discussion of the wide-ranging metaphorics of the architectural monument by saying that each of Proust's "phrases-cathédrales" ["cathedral-sentences"] "offre et tend au lecteur une miniature de l'immense cathédrale qui les abrite toutes" ["offers and gives to the reader a miniature version of the immense cathedral that encloses all of them"] (119). See also Richard Macksey, "The Architecture of Time: Dialectics and Structure," in *Proust: A Collection of Critical Essays*, ed. René Girard (Englewood Cliffs, N.J.: Prentice-Hall, 1962), 104–21, and Ellen Eve Frank, *Literary Architecture, Essays toward a Tradition: Walter Pater, Gerard Manley Hopkins, Marcel Proust, Henry James* (Berkeley: University of California Press, 1979), 113–65 (142–43 on food and architecture).

20. See n. 1, 1311 on the origin of the comparison, and Richard's remarkable analysis in "Proust et l'objet alimentaire," 18–19.

21. About the digestion and (literary) "assimilation" of aliments in Proust, cf. again Richard, "Proust et l'objet alimentaire," 6. The parallel between writing and the digestive function has also been noted by Serge Doubrovsky in *La Place de la Madeleine: Écriture et fantasme chez Proust* (Paris: Mercure de France, 1974).

22. Thomas Pynchon, *Gravity's Rainbow* (New York: Viking, 1973), 715; subsequent quotations on pages 716–17.

23. Cf., after describing Rabelais as "one of literature's great putter-inners"—which incidentally also applies to Winot's own all-inclusive, farraginous confessional "cook-novel": "My collaborator, pressed by me to provide a definition or distinction between Modernism and Post-modernism [. . .] said that 'Modernism is about finding how much you could get away with leaving out. Post-modernism is about how much you can get away with putting in'" (*The Debt to Pleasure*, 159). The reader will have already understood that the present essay resolutely purports to belong to the latter category.

24. This may also recall the ninth chapter, or "The Flaubert Apocrypha," in Julian Barnes's highly acclaimed *Flaubert's Parrot* (London: Pan Books, 1985), whose central question is: "Do the books that writers don't write matter?" (115), an important question since a parallel will be established between apocryphal texts never written and apocryphal lives never lived, the ousted possibilities and choices of life which fiction is free to explore serially: "With Flaubert, the apocrypha cast a second shadow. If the sweetest moment in life is a visit to the brothel which doesn't come off, perhaps the sweetest moment in writing is the arrival of that idea for a book which never has to be written, which is never sullied with a definite shape, which never needs be exposed to a less loving gaze than that of its author" (115–16—this may itself be a recall of the end of *L'Éducation sentimentale*, mentioned on p. 13, in which the hero's best memory from the past is of an unfulfilled event which thus saves intact the "pleasure of anticipation").

25. Despite noting the element of decadence in the use of flowers in cooking, Winot partakes of a similarly "degenerate" aesthetics as the one which characterized futurist cuisine, with its synaesthesia of cooking (food as art works; cf. *The Debt to Pleasure*, 99, about soups), politics, linguistics (its deforeignized glossary), nationalism, sexuality, art, and life. Antirealist, colonialist, and pa-

triotic, its "simultaneous style," notwithstanding its ideological program of harnessing the effects of "gastronomic chemistry" on thinking and action explored otherwise in Rushdie's and Esquivel's fiction, ultimately retained politics only as one among many ingredients in a generalized aesthetics. See [F.] [T.] Marinetti, *The Futurist Cookbook*, trans. Suzanne Brill, ed. Lesley Chamberlain (San Francisco: Bedford Arts, 1989).

26. Cf. Richard, *Proust et le monde sensible*, 31–32, n. 3.

27. Gilles Deleuze, *Proust and Signs*, trans. Richard Howard (New York: Braziller, 1972), 4. See also Jean-Yves Tadié, *Proust et le roman. Essai sur les formes et techniques du roman dans* A la recherche du temps perdu (Paris: Gallimard, 1971), 310: "le futur n'est nulle part aussi présent que dans ce roman du passé" (293–365 on time; quotes Deleuze on p. 312). In *Proust's Binoculars: A Study of Memory, Time, and Recognition in* A la recherche du temps perdu (Princeton: Princeton University Press, 1983), Roger Shattuck equally sees these provisional *moments bienheureux* brought about by involuntary memory's recreation of the past in the present as only transitorily essential, but ultimately devoid of the true (self-)recognition of the timelessness of art unfolded in *Time Regained* (31–39). (For the view of the transformation of linear time [of the "innumerable flashbacks, condensations, plots and digressions that make up the earlier volumes of *A la recherche*"] into the "timelessness of literature" in *Time Regained*, see also Julia Kristeva, *Proust and the Sense of Time*, trans. Stephen Bann [London: Faber, 1993], 23 [also in *Time and Sense*, 189].) Such reversals of the early "traditional" position, notably espoused by Samuel Beckett in his 1931 essay (republished in *Proust, and Three Dialogues: Samuel Beckett and Georges Duthuit* [London: Calder, 1965]), for whom Proust's entire book is "a monument to involuntary memory" (34), also imply a novel reinterpretation of what lost (and found) time ultimately stands for (cf. Deleuze, 17). Hence, for Gérard Genette in "Proust Palimpsest" (in *Figures of Literary Discourse*, trans. by Alan Sheridan [Oxford: Blackwell, 1982]), "For Proust, lost time is not, as is widely but mistakenly believed, 'past' time, but *time in its pure state*, which is really to say, through the fusion of a present moment and a past moment, the contrary of passing time: *the extra-temporal, eternity*" (226, n. 7). The same passage in *Time Regained* is also implicitly behind his later similar view, in *Figures 3*, of the Proustian hero as devoted to the search for the "extra-temporal" and "time in its pure state," and "want[ing] himself, and with him his future work, to be both together 'outside time' and 'in Time' " (Gérard Genette, *Narrative Discourse*, trans. Jane E. Lewin [Oxford: Blackwell, 1980], 160).

28. Deleuze, *Proust and Signs*, 19.

29. Maurice Blanchot, "Proust," *The Sirens' Song: Selected Essays*, ed. Gabriel Josipovici, trans. Sacha Rabinovitch (Bloomington: Indiana University Press, 1982), 71. The original essay, titled "L'Expérience de Proust" (in *Le Livre à venir* [Paris: Gallimard, coll. «idées nrf», 1959], 20–40), will be referred to whenever it is felt that the translation, even if modified, fails to render adequately Blanchot's thought. For another view of Proustian time as a metamorphosis, see e.g. Kristeva, *Proust and the Sense of Time*, 5ff.

30. Georges Poulet, "Marcel Proust," in *Études sur le temps humain 4: Mesure de l'instant* (Paris: Plon, 1968), 301. Subsequent page references will be given parenthetically in the text.

31. Witness also Proust's letter to Benjamin Crémieux—quoted in translation by Macksey (195), who notes (n. 2) several other instances in the overall

correspondance: "There will be no denying [that *A la recherche* is a construction] when the last page of *Le Temps retrouvé* (written before the rest of the book) closes precisely on the first page of *Swann*." This, and the more specific letter to Paul Souday in which Proust states that the last chapter of the last volume was written immediately after the first chapter of the first volume, are quoted by Jean Rousset and used as the basis for his argument about the circular structure of the *Recherche*; see his *Forme et signification. Essai sur les structures littéraires de Corneille à Claudel* (Paris: José Corti, 1964), 138ff.

The more complex view of a future perfect temporal structure is also expressed by Duncan Large in the fourth chapter of his *Nietzsche and Proust: A Comparative Study*, Unpublished Ph.D. diss., University of Oxford, 1995, 203–37 ("Logics of the Future Perfect"). For Large "*A la recherche* [. . .] emerges as a celebration of the superior point of view from 'after the event' which allows an appropriation of the past [. . .] through retrospective ('nachträglich' or 'après-coup') reinterpretation. [. . .] Since his narrator looks forward to the future as a redemption of the past, Proust actually inscribes the looped temporality of the eternal return in the conclusion to *A la recherche* itself, as a future perfect movement" (203). See also 220, 233 (about the future perfect as "a tense of wistful pre-emptive nostalgia"), 236–37, and 235, citing Gérard Cogez, *Marcel Proust,* A la recherche du temps perdu, Études littéraires 24 (Paris: Presses Universitaires de France, 1990), 60, for whom "l'écriture du roman va transformer [l'existence du Narrateur] progressivement en ce qu'elle aura été en fait, une longue gestation (signfication conférée après coup, au futur antérieur)." Poulet had already commented on Proust's frequent recourse, in *Jean Santeuil*, to the repeated interruption of the narrtion through a series of incursions into the future followed by returns to anterior time, i.e. a leap forward, then a withdrawal backward, whose effect was to turn the future into a future perfect ("Marcel Proust," 330–31).

32. Jacques Lacan, *Écrits: A Selection*, trans. Alan Sheridan (London: Tavistock, 1977), 86.

33. Blanchot, "Proust," 66; compare with "L'Expérience de Proust," 21. Genette expands on Blanchot's suspensive reading of the (in)complete Proustean work in "Proust Palimpsest."

34. Blanchot, "L'Expérience de Proust," 27.

35. Blanchot, "L'Expérience de Proust," 40. Josipovici opts for "indolence" but, in the light of earlier considerations about the movement from book to work (oeuvre) seen above, Blanchot's choice of word does more than merely recall the passage from indolence (*paresse*) to patience to tireless labor which he has just evoked (cf. also *infra*).

36. This is what, in an inverse movement, Proust described, as early as 1909 in a letter to Alfred Vallette referring to the prefatory project of *Contre Sainte-Beuve*, as an "en-working": "quand on aura fini le livre, on verra (je le voudrais) que tout le roman n'est que la *mise en oeuvre* des principes d'art émis dans cette dernière partie, sorte de préface si vous voulez mise à la fin" [when one has finished the book, one will see (I hope) that the entire novel is nothing other than the implementation ("en-working") of the artistic principles formulated in that final part, which would be a sort of preface placed at the end, so to speak] (*Correspondance*, vol. 9: 1909 [Paris: Plon, 1982], 156; my emphasis).

37. See e.g. Jean-François Lyotard, *The Postmodern Explained to Children. Correspondence 1982–1985*, trans. ed. by Julian Pefanis and Morgan Thomas (London: Turnaround, 1992), 9–25 ("Answer to the question: what is the Post-

modern?")—in which, however, Proust is seen as a modern, rather than a postmodern, artist as even the temporal deferments in his odyssey of consciousness nostalgically cling to the identity of writing with itself (23)—and 87–93 ("Note on the meaning of 'post-' "). Thus, for Large, "the temporal structures of *A la recherche* are already pointing towards a 'postmodern' grammatology," according to such strictly Lyotardian procedures (220). One could reread in this Lyotardian light, and therefore against Lyotard's judgment, Genette's identification, in the condensation of spaced-out moments, of the *ana*logy of a communal essence ("Proust Palimpsest," 204; cf. 207–8 about the passage from the ontological to the analogical), and Poulet's remark on the *ana*chronistic twinning of two such instants, joined together contiguously through an ellipsis of the distancing interval ("Marcel Proust," 328).

38. It is the doubling aspect of the experience of involuntary memory which confers on it its truly anamnesic quality, and this explains why the earlier episode of the *pain grillé*, which gave a more instant access to the childhood equivalent of the *biscotte*, was rewritten into the *madeleine* scene, with its dilatory recognition more capable of crystallizing powerful attendant feelings of happiness, love's power over death, etc., and of being prolonged again later (see Lejeune, "Écriture et sexualité").

39. Cf. Rushdie, "Imaginary Homelands," *Imaginary Homelands*, 19. The now well-accredited label "magic realism" (originally *magischer Realismus*), which designates both the sociopoliticization of the fictional and the fictionalization of the sociopolitical in a historically entrenched narration, owes its conceptual origin to a 1925 article by Franz Roh on German postexpressionnist art which was translated two years later by Ortega y Gasset in the influential journal *Revista de Occidente*, then imported into the South American literary context thanks to a famous essay, from 1949, by Alejo Carpentier on *lo real maravilloso americano*. These landmark contributions are both reprinted in translation in *Magic Realism: Theory, History, Community*, ed. Lois Parkinson Zamora and Wendy B. Faris (Durham and London: Duke University Press, 1995), 15–31, 75–88. For a more specific association between magic realism and postcolonial literature, see e.g. Stephen Slemon, "Magic Realism as Postcolonial Discourse," in the same volume (407–26), which offers the following conclusion: "By embedding the binary oppositions of past and present social relations into the 'speaking mirror' of their literary language, these [postcolonial] texts implicitly suggest that enabling strategies for the future require revisioning the seemingly tyrannical units of the past in a complex and imaginative double-think of 'remembering the future' " (422).

40. Rushdie, *Imaginary Homelands*, 13.

41. *Ibid.*

42. Quoted in Chandrabhanu Pattanayak, "Interview with Salman Rushdie," *The Literary Criterion* 18.3 (1983): 20.

43. Rushdie, *Imaginary Homelands*, 24. More recent neuroscientific theories stress that memory is never fixed but works differentially, and is more akin to the inventiveness of an incessantly revised fiction; see Margaret E. Gray, *Postmodern Proust* (Philadelphia: University of Pennsylvania Press, 1992), 67, who adds that "[t]he *Recherche* narration, now no longer credible as the masterly account of a knowledgeable, remembering narrator, might nonetheless be shown to be 'remembrance'—but through its very forgetfulness, invention, and repetition" (67), a critical correction which the project of *Midnight's Children* purposefully emphasizes. For a view of forgetting as the

prerequisite in Proust's "general law of memory" and recognition, see also e.g. Shattuck, *Proust's Binoculars*, 63ff. Thus the very first sentence of *A la recherche* ("Longtemps, je me suis couché de bonne heure" [For a long time I used to go to bed early]), with its conjunction of past action and present effect in the French *passé composé*, "begins a self-forgetfulness that will last until a coming-to, a novel and a lifetime later" (Shattuck, 81, 83).

44. I am using this phrase in a different sense from the one to which it has been set to work by Aruna Srivastava in " 'The Empire Writes Back': Language and History in *Shame* and *Midnight's Children*," *Ariel: A Review of International English Literature* 20.4 (1989): 63. (The phrase is mistakenly attributed to Barthes, rather than Nietzsche, as the wording in Hayden White's source article would seem to suggest).

45. This fragmentation is also that of the more fully individualized, autonomous senses in *Midnight's Children*, each (especially smell, hearing, and taste) being foregrounded in turn as a source of idiosyncratic experience and identity, whereas *A la recherche* works towards the synaesthesia of tastes and emotions needed for the epiphanic manifestation of a replenished essential subject (e.g. 3:636, where the vital metamorphosis of food reconciles all senses into a unifying aesthetic experience, from the crying of food to its palatability and the evocation of its [visual] architecture). The summing up of the itinerary or program of *A la recherche* as stretching from artistic self-contemplation to creative self-fecundation (cf. Doubrovsky, *La Place de la Madeleine*, 126) neatly captures the overall modern attempt at finally piecing back together or "re-membering" an essential fullness alien from Rushdie's (postmodern/postcolonial) eventually dis-membered "intersubject."

46. See also David Birch, "Postmodernist Chutneys," *Textual Practice* 5.1 (1991): 3.

47. For this view of Proustian writing, see e.g. Kristeva, *Time and Sense*, especially 22: "Proustian heroes and visions will eventually leave us with a singular and bizarre taste that is pungent and invigorating. It is the taste of the sense of time, of writing as transubstantiation."

48. See Genette, *Narrative Discourse*, 227 (translation slightly modified), and Rushdie, *Imaginary Homelands*, 24. The former adds: "The narrator's last sentence is when [. . .] the hero finally reaches his first. The interval between the end of the story and the moment of the narrating is therefore the time it takes the hero to write this book, which is and which is not the book the narrator, in his turn, reveals to us in a moment brief as a flash of lightning." It is this necessarily asymptotic conjunction which Rousset's more orthodox view of the *Recherche*'s circularity erases: "[hero and narrator] coincide with one another in the *dénouement*, which is the moment when the hero will become the narrator, that is, the author of his own story. The narrator is the hero revealed to himself [. . .]. The novel is conceived such that its ending leads to its beginning. (*Forme et signification*, 144).

49. Beckett, *Proust*, 35.

50. Salman Rushdie, *Shame* (London: Picador, 1983), 19.

51. For Genette, this *incorporation* designates the spatial sedimentation in Proust's aesthetic palimpsest of the effects of metamorphosis (of characters, places, etc.) through time; see "Proust Palimpsest," 212–13. See also Kristeva, *Proust and the Sense of Time*, 1–26: "Proust and Time Embodied."

52. This reading of the name of Saleem's real biological father was first suggested by Uma Parameswaran in "Handcuffed to History: Salman Rushdie's Art," *Ariel: A Review of International English Literature* 14.4 (1983): 45.

53. When I started working on this comparative project, *The Moor's Last Sigh*, as yet unpublished but no doubt already in the making, was that unknown/unknowable development—albeit in a different direction—of the "future" of *Midnight's Children*: a significant, though somewhat perfunctorily exploited, link between Rushdie's two novels is the reappearance of Saleem's offspring, Adam Sinai, now alias Braganza, in honor of the name of the pickle factory which he inherited from the two Pereira sisters after their deaths (*Moor*, 341–42; cf. also 199). Foregrounding the "pepperpot" and spice base of the earlier text, Rushdie's latest novel to date also extends the experiment with fictional time warping; whereas, in *Midnight's Children*, Rushdie allows the present of narration to catch up with fiction at the point of the narrator's dissolution (cf. *MC*, 457) and then proceeds to leap beyond death into the yet untold future, we realize retrospectively at the "end" of *The Moor's Last Sigh* (the fragment in italics, outside the "story" proper of the Moor, in which he is waiting for his imminent death) that the novel-as-retelling had started beyond the point of the story's/protagonist's demise, that, like him, it had already, from the start, gone through time faster than it should have (cf. *Moor*, 143).

54. I have borrowed this apt phrase from Günter Grass's *The Flounder*, trans. Ralph Manheim (London: Minerva, 1997), 340. Originally published in 1977 as *Der Butt* and first brought out in its English translation the year after, Grass's intricate fantasy reworking of sociopolitical history through spices, food, gastronomy, and cooking is an even likelier candidate for *Midnight's Children*'s literary ascendance than the earlier *Tin Drum*, to which Rushdie's novel has often been compared.

WORKS CITED

Barnes, Julian. *Flaubert's Parrot*. London: Pan Books, 1985.

Barthelme, Donald. *Forty Stories*. London: Minerva, 1992.

Barthes, Roland. *Mythologies*. Selected and translated by Annette Lavers. London: Cape, 1972.

Beckett, Samuel. *Proust, and Three Dialogues: Samuel Beckett and Georges Duthuit*. London: Calder, 1965.

Birch, David. "Postmodernist Chutneys." *Textual Practice* 5.1 (1991): 1–7.

Bischoff, Jürg. *La genèse de l'épisode de la madeleine. Étude génétique d'un passage d'A la recherche du temps perdu de Marcel Proust*. Bern: Peter Lang, 1988.

Blanchot, Maurice. "L'Expérience de Proust." In *Le Livre à venir*. Paris: Gallimard, coll. «idées nrf», 1959, 20–40.

———. "Proust." In *The Sirens' Song: Selected Essays*. Edited and introduced by Gabriel Josipovici. Translated by Sacha Rabinovitch. Bloomington: Indiana University Press, 1982, 66–78.

Brooks, David. "Salman Rushdie: An Interview." *Helix* 19 (1984): 55–69.

Cogez, Gérard. *Marcel Proust, A la recherche du temps perdu*. Études littéraires 24. Paris: Presses Universitaires de France, 1990.

Deleuze, Gilles. *Proust and Signs*. Translated by Richard Howard. New York: Braziller, 1972.

Doubrovsky, Serge. *La Place de la Madeleine: Écriture et fantasme chez Proust*. Paris: Mercure de France, 1974.

Esquivel, Laura. *Like Water for Chocolate*. Translated by Carol Christensen and Thomas Christensen. London: Black Swan, 1993.

Fenollosa, Ernest. *The Chinese Written Character as a Medium for Poetry*. Foreword and Notes by Ezra Pound. London: Stanley Nott, 1936.

Fraisse, Luc. *L'Œuvre cathédrale: Proust et l'architecture médiévale*. Paris: José Corti, 1990.

Frank, Ellen Eve. *Literary Architecture, Essays Toward a Tradition: Walter Pater, Gerard Manley Hopkins, Marcel Proust, Henry James*. Berkeley: University of California Press, 1979.

Genette, Gérard. *Narrative Discourse*. Translated by Jane E. Lewin, Foreword by Jonathan Culler. Oxford: Blackwell, 1980.

———. "Proust Palimpseste." In *Figures of Literary Discourse*, translated by Alan Sheridan. Introduction by Marie-Rose Logan. Oxford: Blackwell, 1982, 203–28.

Gilbert, Stuart. "Prolegomena to *Work in Progress*." In Samuel Beckett et al., *Our Exagmination Round His Factification for Incamination of* Work in Progress. London: Faber, 1972, 47–75.

Grass, Günter. *The Flounder*. Translated by Ralph Manheim. London: Minerva, 1997.

Gray, Margaret E. *Postmodern Proust*. Philadelphia: University of Pennsylvania Press, 1992.

Joyce, James. *Dubliners*. Text, Criticism, and Notes edited by Robert Scholes and A. Walton Litz. New York: Viking, 1969.

———. *Finnegans Wake*. London: Faber, 1975.

Kristeva, Julia. *Proust and the Sense of Time*. Translated and with an Introduction by Stephen Bann. London: Faber, 1993.

———. *Time and Sense: Proust and the Experience of Literature*. Translated by Ross Guberman. New York: Columbia University Press, 1996.

Lacan, Jacques. *Écrits: A Selection*. Translated by Alan Sheridan. London: Tavistock, 1977.

Lanchester, John. *The Debt to Pleasure*. London: Picador, 1996.

Large, Duncan. *Nietzsche and Proust: A Comparative Study*. Unpublished Ph.D. diss., University of Oxford, 1995.

Lejeune, Philippe. "Écriture et sexualité." *Europe* 502–3: "Marcel Proust" (1971): 113–43.

Lyotard, Jean-François. *The Postmodern Explained to Children. Correspondence 1982–1985*. Translations edited by Julian Pefanis and Morgan Thomas. London: Turnaround, 1992.

Macksey, Richard. "The Architecture of Time: Dialectics and Structure." In *Proust: A Collection of Critical Essays*. Edited by René Girard. Englewood Cliffs, N.J.: Prentice-Hall, 1962, 104–21.

Marinetti, [F.] [T.]. *The Futurist Cookbook*. Translated by Suzanne Brill. Edited with an introduction by Lesley Chamberlain. San Francisco: Bedford Arts, 1989.

Parameswaran, Uma. "Handcuffed to History: Salman Rushdie's Art." *Ariel: A Review of International English Literature* 14.4 (1983): 34–45.

Pattanayak, Chandrabhanu. "Interview with Salman Rushdie." *The Literary Criterion* 18.3 (1983): 19–22.

Poulet, Georges. "Marcel Proust." In *Études sur le temps humain* 4: *Mesure de l'instant*. Paris: Plon, 1968, 299–335.

Price, David W. "Salman Rushdie"s 'Use and Abuse of History' in *Midnight's Children*." *Ariel: A Review of International English Literature* 25.2 (1994): 91–107.

Proust, Marcel. *A la recherche du temps perdu*. 4 vols. Édition publiée sous la direction de Jean-Yves Tadié. Paris: Gallimard, collection «Pléiade», 1987–89.

——. *Correspondance*. 20 vols. Texte établi, présenté et annoté par Philip Kolb. Paris: Plon, 1976–92.

——. *In Search of Lost Time*. Translated by C. K. Scott Moncrieff and Terence Kilmartin. Revised by D. J. Enright. London: Chatto and Windus, 1992.

Pynchon, Thomas. *Gravity's Rainbow*. New York: Viking, 1973.

Richard, Jean-Pierre. *Proust et le monde sensible*. Paris: Seuil, 1974.

——. "Proust et l'objet alimentaire." *Littérature* 6 (1972): 3–19.

Rousset, Jean. *Forme et signification. Essai sur les structures littéraires de Corneille à Claudel*. Paris: José Corti, 1964.

Rushdie, Salman. *Imaginary Homelands. Essays and Criticism 1981–1991*. London: Penguin, 1991.

——. *Midnight's Children*. London: Picador, 1981.

——. *Shame*. London: Picador, 1983.

——. "*Midnight's Children* and *Shame*" (interview). *Kunapipi* 7.1 (1985): 1–19.

——. *The Moor's Last Sigh*. London: Vintage, 1996.

Shattuck, Roger. *Proust's Binoculars: A Study of Memory, Time, and Recognition in* A la recherche du temps perdu. Princeton: Princeton University Press, 1983.

Srivastava, Aruna. " 'The Empire Writes Back': Language and History in *Shame* and *Midnight's Children*." *Ariel: A Review of International English Literature* 20.4 (1989): 62–78.

Switzer, Richard. "The Madeleine and the Biscotte." *French Review*, 30.4 (1957): 303–8.

Tadié, Jean-Yves. *Proust et le roman. Essai sur les formes et techniques du roman dans* A la recherche du temps perdu. Paris: Gallimard, 1971.

Zamora, Lois Parkinson, and Wendy B. Faris, eds. and intr. *Magic Realism: Theory, History, Community*. Durham, N.C. and London: Duke University Press, 1995.

"Go hang yourself, you who have never been comfortably seated and eating an olive": The Taste and Defiance of an Adolescent Body

JO CROFT

> Happy the youth who comes to full maturity unstunted by perversions, excess or defect, and with true, trustworthy appetite and regular eating habits. Probably no period and no condition of life suffers reduced vitality and efficiency in diet so much as brain working and sedentary youth, despite the fact that none can better sustain such events so far as life and tolerable health are concerned.[1]
>
> There is generally a new relation to food. Appetite is often freaky, irregular, capricious, seeking a new equilibrium and larger variety, and the relation among the staple foods finally settled on almost always changes.[2]

INTRODUCTION: NOT QUITE EATING

"WHAT IS THE DIFFERENCE BETWEEN TASTING AND EATING"? WHEN I began working on this essay I found myself getting caught up with this unnervingly obvious question; much of the material I was looking at seemed to collapse these terms into one another. At one level, all of the five senses serve to communicate our experience of the world from outside to inside, and to this extent could be said to take place at the boundaries of our bodies. Of all the senses, however, taste seems, most acutely, to hover at the edge of another process, that is, eating. One only has to think of occupations based on tasting, such as wine taster, "royal taster," and so on, to get some idea of the complex ways in which "tasting" is defined as a constituent of eating while also being defined over and against eating. One way of describing "taste," then, is as a liminal activity—a process which takes place before (or as) food is swallowed, and which mediates between the outside and inside of the body. A definition given of "taste" in the *Oxford En-*

glish Dictionary is: "The quality or property of a substance which is perceived when it is brought into contact with certain organs of the mouth, etc. esp. the tongue."

Because tasting is "not quite" eating, it also carries with it the possibility of a refusal or expulsion of what is being eaten. More than the other senses, perhaps, taste is delimited by pleasure and disgust. Its transitional or intermediate function therefore is marked less by compromise than by ambivalence, which in turn is structured through a grammar of extremes. There is a difference, after all, between "both wanting and not wanting something at the same time" and "half-wanting/half-liking something." It is interesting to note that within psychoanalysis the term "ambivalence" has particularly close associations with eating and orality. For instance Bleuler, who first introduced the term in 1910, identified a key form of ambivalence as "ambivalence of the will (Ambitendenz)," that is, "when the subject wants to eat and not to eat at the same time."[3] The link between eating and ambivalence is further emphasized in Karl Abraham's paper "A Short Study of the Development of the Libido, Viewed in the Light of Mental Disorders"(1924) where he argues that the oral phase may in turn be subdivided into a "pre-ambivalent" (sucking) stage and an "ambivalent" (biting) stage:

> In the biting stage of the oral phase the individual incorporates the object in himself and in so doing destroys it. One only has to look at children to see how intense the impulse to bite is—an impulse in which the eating instinct and the libido still co-operate. This is the stage in which cannibalistic impulses predominate. As soon as the child is attracted by an object, it is liable, indeed bound, to attempt its destruction. It is in this stage that the ambivalent attitude of the ego to its object begins to grow up. We may say, therefore, that in the child's libidinal development the second stage of the oral-sadistic phase marks the beginning of its ambivalence conflict.[4]

Here Karl Abraham explicitly links the "ambivalence" of this "oral-sadistic" phase with the idea of "incorporation." Laplanche and Pontalis define incorporation as a phantasizing process which, roughly speaking, contains three meanings:

> it means to obtain pleasure by making an object penetrate oneself; it means to destroy this object; and it means, by keeping it within oneself, to appropriate the object's qualities. It is this last aspect that makes incorporation into the matrix of introjection and identification.[5]

Incorporation is a critical psychoanalytic concept as far as this study is concerned because it draws together three registers of object relationship: pleasure, destruction, and identification.[6] In other words, incorporation is a psychic mechanism through which we negotiate both the excesses of love and hate and the basic constituencies of identity formation. This association between ambivalent desire and identification summoned up by incorporation is one which also—mythically—besieges the adolescent subject. My central aim in this essay is to consider what happens when the terms "taste" and "adolescence" coincide. Mary MacLane's book exemplifies certain themes central to adolescent subjectivity and to adolescent writing. Published in 1902, when MacLane was nineteen, *The Story of Mary MacLane ("By Herself")*[7] takes the form of a confessional adolescent journal. It is an odd, outrageous text which both offers up a protest against the dreary "Nothingness" of the narrator's life with her family in Butte, Montana, and sets out a litany of her intense desires and loathings. Perhaps most significantly, this *Story* seems to be underlined by a paradigm of sexuality replete with hesitations and reversals—in which the subject apparently moves back and forth between positions associated with auto-eroticism and object-love. What I want to draw out in my reading of *The Story of Mary MacLane* is the way in which the processes both of writing and tasting enter into that paradigm—as agencies of transformation and as points of resistance.

For MacLane, an artist who knows "the art of Good Eating"[8] is diametrically opposed to "persons who eat for the sake of eating" (*MacLane*, 80). Implicitly, therefore, MacLane's formulation of this "art" turns upon the sense of taste, or "eating for the sake of tasting." This is not to say that MacLane separates her "art" from necessity or hunger. Far from it—she stresses that "the art of Good Eating has only two essential points: one must eat only when one is hungry, and one must take small bites" (*MacLane*, 80). Crucially, she also declares, much earlier on in the book, that "Writing is a necessity—like eating" (*MacLane*, 80). In MacLane's text, therefore, the "necessity" of both writing and eating is premised upon hunger, and as such seems to be inflected with an anticipatory or prolonged desire.

The Story of Mary MacLane is a book written for the world's attention, for the world's gaze. In a sense MacLane offers it up to her readers in a calculated act of exposure, demanding in return that they ("the world") satisfy her "Wanting"—that the world touch her:

> Had I been born a man I would by now have made a deep impression of myself on the world—on some part of it. But I am a woman, and God, or the Devil, or Fate, or whosoever it was, has flayed me of the thick outer skin and thrown me into the midst of life—has left me a lonely, damned thing filled with the red, red blood of ambition of desire, but afraid to be touched, for there is no thick skin between my sensitive skin and the world's fingers.
>
> But I want to be touched. (*MacLane*, 13)

The difference between a man and a woman is what holds MacLane apart from the world. Nothing else does, it seems, and certainly not her skin. Her brand of loneliness—made up of the "red, red blood of ambition and desire" is traced back in these lines to the fact that she is a woman and, more emphatically, to the fact that she is a not a man.[9] Here the world accrues a penetrative status, potentially capable of meeting her longing to be touched socially and sexually. This is what she desires and what she fears: this is what assails the edges of her body.

MacLane's writing seems to represent a layer—an inner skin of words through which its author can make contact with the world.[10] Her narrative comes from a bodily, yet written edge—a vantage point from which she can proclaim, "I stand on the edge, and I suffer"(*MacLane*, 5). However, MacLane's writing also seems to attempt to hold her "insides," her "red, red blood of ambition and desire" (*MacLane*, 13) in place. Her act of exposure resonates ambivalently both as an invitation for the reader to "taste" the inside and outside of her body, and as an assertion of her own embodied autonomy (that is, that she has a sovereign claim to "tasting" herself).

Crucially, MacLane's representations of both eating and writing far exceed the pragmatic, utilitarian connotations of the term "necessity." Whether producing writing or eating food, MacLane seeks to reflect, self-consciously, upon the *processes* of consuming and being consumed. And, strikingly, this self-reflexivity calls upon both narrator and reader to move between the internal and external topographies of MacLane's body. Fairly early on in the text, for example, MacLane throws a challenge to her readers that they read both across and beneath her body's surface. She writes: "You may gaze at and admire the picture in the front of this book. It is the picture of a genius—a genius with a good strong young woman's body,—and inside the pictured body is a liver, a MacLane liver, of admirable perfectness" (*MacLane*,27–28). In these lines MacLane's writing and her body seem to have become utterly enmeshed: the feminine adolescent subject is represented as self-conscious and as a form whose physicality is inextricable from its capacity for literary production. In other words, MacLane says, "I am a feminine writer, look at my picture because this is the body that you are reading." It is as if, in appealing to the reader's gaze, MacLane seeks to imbue the narrating "I" with a "good strong young woman's body," so that the narrative signifies as not-empty and locates its constant referent in the feminine body of Mary MacLane. Most noticeably, though, this body is not only "pictured," it has an *inside* which is full up with liver (traditionally held to be the "seat of emotion"[11]). The "fullness" of MacLane's literary identity can, it seems, only be conjured up through this double image of what lies within and beyond the boundaries of her skin.

Strong Food

According to Stanley Hall, an American psychologist writing at the turn of the century, adolescence is marked by "a new relation to food."[12] He argues that adolescent appetite "is often freaky, irregular, capricious, seeking a new equilibrium and variety, and the relation among the staple foods finally settled on almost always changes" (Hall, 11). He also stresses that "there is a lickerish daintiness, and it would seem that this upsetting coincides with a new love of spices, condiments, or very strong stimuli" (Hall, 13–14). For MacLane, the pleasures of eating certainly seem to be bound up with "strong" or extreme-tasting food. More specifically, it is through representing strong-tasting food such as olives being processed by her digestive system that MacLane seeks to open up her insides as a repository for both her readers' and her own desires.

MacLane cites the making and eating of fudge as a central event within her daily routine: "Nearly every day I make me a plate of hot, rich fudge, with brown sugar (I should be an entirely different person if I made it with white sugar—and the fudge would not be nearly so good)" (*MacLane*, 244). Not only does MacLane make much of her fudge's brownness and richness (a gesture which in itself closely parallels Freud's example of the cocoa manufacturer fantasy[13]), she also draws attention to the "boon" of her fudge in such a way as to affirm her own subjective uniqueness. Her value as an individual is both reflected in and heightened by the extreme taste—the brown richness of her fudge. Indeed, MacLane implies that so special and so excessive is this fudge that only *her* insides can adequately process it: "A very little of my fudge has been known to give some people a most terrific stomach-ache—but my own digestive organs seem to like nothing better. It's so brown—so rich!" (*MacLane*, 246).

Perhaps most significantly, Mary MacLane links the pleasure of eating fudge with the pleasure she takes in a particularly ritualistic form of reading (notably associated with a specific genre, the periodical for young people, which was a precursor of the teen magazine). She describes how she takes the fudge "upstairs to (her) room with a book or newspaper":

> My mind then takes in a part of what is contained in the book or newspaper, and the stomach of the MacLane takes in all of what is contained in the plate. I sit by my window in a miserable, uncomfortable, stiff-backed chair, but I relieve the strain by resting my feet on the edge of the low bureau. Usually the book I read is an old dilapidated volume of that erstwhile periodical, "Our Young Folks." It is a thing that possesses a charm for me. I never grow tired of it. As I eat my nice brown squares of fudge I read about a boy whose name is Jack Hazard and who, J. T. Trowbridge informs the reader, is doing his best, and who seems to find it somewhat difficult. I believe I could repeat pages of J. T. Trowbridge from memory, and that ancient bound volume has become part of my life. (*MacLane*, 244–45)

Here, then, a compacted scenario is set out before us, whereby we witness Mary MacLane "relieving herself" in the privacy of her own room. MacLane stresses how she "relieve(s) the strain" *with her feet on the bureau*, in a physical pose which seems to be very much in defiance of both "feminine" and "literary" respectability. As well as depicting her physical position in the room as she eats her fudge, she also makes an association between those two registers of consumption (of "taking in") which she holds onto as indulgent pleasures: first, eating a rich brown substance (she has made by herself, for herself); and second, reading a familiar text (the "erstwhile" nature of which suggests its significance as a textual memory both retained and repeated).

"An Exquisite Symphony of Sensualism . . ."

As MacLane writes about eating an olive so her narrative becomes more and more explicitly indulgent and celebratory. The description, from which I think it is worth quoting at length, in fact lasts a full eight pages:

> I bite the olive again. Again the bitter salt crisp ravishes my tongue. "If this be vanity—vanity let it be." The golden moments flit by and I heed them not. For am I not comfortably seated and eating an olive? Go hang yourself, you who have never been comfortably seated and eating an olive! My character evolves farther in its change. I am now bent on reckless sensuality, let it happen what will. The fair earth seems to resolve itself into a thing crisp and good and green and deliciously salt. I experience a feeling of fervent gladness that I am a female thing living, and that I have a tongue and some teeth, and salivary glands. . . .
>
> Also this bit slips down my red gullet, and again the festive Stomach lifts up its silent voice in psalms and rejoicing. It is now an absolute monarchy with the green olive at its head. The kisses of the gastric juice become hot and sensual and convulsive and ecstatic. "Avaunt, pale, shadowy ghosts of dyspepsia!" says my Stomach. "I know you not. I am of a brilliant, shining world. I dwell in Elysian fields. . . .
>
> Once more I bite the olive. Once more my tongue is electrified. And the third stage in my temporary transformation is complete. I am now a gross but supremely contented sensualist. An exquisite symphony of sensualism and pleasure seems to play somewhere within me. My heart purrs. My brain folds its arms and lounges. I put my feet up on the seat of another chair. The entire world is surely one delicious green olive. Therefore the green olive is a perfect thing—absolutely a perfect thing. . . .
>
> Disgust and approval are excited only by imperfections. When a thing is perfect, no matter how hard one may look at it, one can see only itself, and nothing beyond. . . .
>
> And so I have made my olive and my art perfect. (*MacLane*, 83–85)

What is perhaps most striking about Mary MacLane's description of eating an olive is that the act of tasting seems to be enacted far beyond the space of the mouth. For MacLane, in other words, "the art of eating" turns upon the ability to extend the process of tasting, of savoring downwards into "the red gullet" and "the Stomach." As MacLane's narrative explores her internal organs, it tells a story which is by no means a steady linear "tracking" of the olive's progress *through* the body. Instead its sensual movement back and forth between the mouth and the stomach seems a far remove from any clear-cut aim, function or ending, and is closer, perhaps, to Freud's 1905 conception of perversion than to biological narratives of food consumption and digestion. In his "Three Essays on Sexuality," for example, Freud describes perversions as:

> sexual activities which either (a) *extend*, in an anatomical sense, beyond the regions of the body which are designed for sexual union, or (b) *linger* over the intermediate relations to the sexual object which should normally be traversed rapidly on the path towards the final sexual aim. [14]

For Freud, then, perversion is characterized by *lingering, extending* and, implicitly, by *intermediacy*. Perhaps most crucially, as far as this essay is concerned, these perverse tendencies are defined in relation to a "normal sexual aim" which—without such perverse lingering, extending, and intermediacy—would lead directly to "a satisfaction analogous to the sating of hunger" (*Three Essays*, 61). The direct association here between hunger and sexuality makes it all the more tempting to read MacLane's representation of adolescent taste as perverse (a move which, almost too neatly, turns Freud's analogy back on itself).

In the second volume of *Adolescence*, Stanley Hall conceives the adolescent's sense of taste in a way which seems to be peculiarly appropriate as far as MacLane's adolescent tasting is concerned. As with *The Story of Mary MacLane*, what emerges from Hall's text is a version of the adolescent's sense of taste as "perverse." Tasting, in other words, has somehow strayed beyond the parameters of "normal" function and in doing so has distorted or arrested the linear logic of the bodily machine (compare with Hall's assertion that "the body is a machine for the conservation, distribution, and transmission of energy" [Hall, 9]). According to Hall, "every cell and tissue has its own hunger"(Hall, 9), and he is keen to stress that even the body's insides are subject to the evolutionary principle of "survival of the fittest": "There is a struggle for survival between the different organs of the same soma for the food supply which the blood contains, and sensation, and perhaps thought, are in one sense functions of nutrition" (Hall, 9).

As is the case with most of his work, Hall's formulation of adolescent taste seems to be riven by a tension between the functionalist schematizations of Darwinism and the far more crisis-bound speculations of early psychoanalysis.[15] The idea of individual organs competing for food conjures a paradoxical vision both of the activity of eating and of the body's inside: on the one hand, Hall represents the body as absolutely ordered and contained by notions of function, whereby there is a direct correspondence between the laws governing the body's internal and external worlds; on the other hand, though, this same image could be read as both chaotic and conflict-ridden, signaling the breakdown of corporal coherence.

Hall states that at adolescence: "It is as if taste now had a somewhat more independent value in itself, became more inward and more associated with the "Gemeingefühle" on the one hand, and more objectified on the other" (Hall, 9). This sentence seems rather hard to follow, both syntactically and conceptually. Perhaps most confusingly, Hall uses the German term *Gemeingefühle* here in a way that smacks of euphemism, almost as if he is alluding to something indecent (comparable perhaps with Freud's infamously ironic use of the phrase "J'appelle un chat un chat" [I call a cat a cat] in the Dora case history.[16] Judging by the surrounding sentence, the "Gemeingefühle" is implicitly linked to an "inward" (and introspective) realm of sensation, and yet the literal translation of this compound German noun is "common (or peer group) feeling." In other words, "Gemeingefühle" is a term that suggests an identification with a broader social group, the absolute obverse of inwardness. Hall therefore presents us with a highly equivocal model of adolescent taste in which the relationship between the inside and outside of the body seems "fluctuating" and "unsettled," mediated as it is through unstable identifications. As he says, "During or often before this transition stage there is a period of unsettlement, fluctuation, and freakiness"(Hall, 13). Far from fixing a secure demarcation between subject and object (consumer and consumed), here the act of *taking food in* seems to render the boundaries of adolescent identity less stable.

Narcissism and Unnamed Woe

Above all, perhaps, MacLane's description of eating an olive is an account of a sexualized relation between the subject and the inside of her body. Through a process of (magnified) introspection, MacLane erotically explores her own body—to the point where it begins to signify both as the perfection of all form and as a series of objects which relate separately and sensually to each other. The olive itself, when it enters the narrator's mouth, also becomes the narrative's point of entry into the narrator's body. As the olive "ravishes" her tongue so it seems to take on the status of another internal organ within MacLane's body. And just as MacLane's body tastes the olive, so the olive—or rather the language it carries—also somehow "tastes" her insides. Thus, the text frames its narcissism around the process of taking writing, as well as an olive, into the body.

MacLane identifies her acquisition of "the art of good eating" as a vital constituent of her genius (*MacLane*, 80). Her genius, in turn, is insistently associated with something inside her ("it is a hard thing to show" [*MacLane*, 119]): it is embodied by her "wondrous liver within" (*MacLane*, 64). Perhaps most significantly, though, MacLane states that genius "is prone equally to unreasoning joy and bitterest morbidness"(*MacLane*, 89). In other words, it is a sign that straddles two excessive states of feeling. The following passage illustrates how MacLane's genius comes to stand for the very opposite of a jubilatory narcissism. In doing so, it gives us some idea of what might be at stake—what might be being resisted—in MacLane's ecstatic narrativization of her body ingesting an olive:

> My genius is a sound, sure, earthly sense, with no suggestion of mystery or occultism. It is an inner sense that enables me to feel and know things that I could not possibly put into thought, much less words. It makes me know and analyze with deadly minuteness every keen, tiny damnation in my terrible lonely life. It is a mirror that shows me myself and something in myself in a merciless brilliant light, and the sight at once sickens and maddens me and fills me with an unnamed woe. It is something unspeakably dreadful. (*MacLane*, 191)

For MacLane, "the green olive is a perfect thing"(*MacLane*, 85), and in a way it has to be. After all, she writes: "Disgust and approval are excited only by imperfections. When a thing is perfect, no matter how hard one may look at it, one can see only itself, and nothing beyond" (*MacLane*, 85). To be more precise, then, internal perfection protects against the demand, or desire, to excite external "disgust and approval." Held, "perfect," within MacLane, the olive appears to guarantee that there is nothing beyond the walls of her body, that her body is full. This image presents us with an uncompromised and mythic version of narcissism. Crucially, though, this narcissistic position signifies here as "complete" only at the point of "temporary transformation." It is a very precarious kind of perfection.

> I set my teeth and my tongue upon the olive, and bite it. It is bitter, salt, delicious. The saliva rushes to meet it, and my tongue is a

happy tongue. As the morsel of olive rests in my mouth and is crunched and squeezed lusciously among my teeth, a quick, temporary change takes place in my character. I think of some adorable lines of the Persian poet: "Give thyself up to Joy, for thy Grief will be infinite. The stars shall again meet together at the same point in the firmament, but of thy body shall bricks be made for a palace wall." (*MacLane*, 82)

For MacLane, in these lines, poetry opens up the possibility of both loss and consuming joy. The pleasure of biting the olive is bound—through poetic discourse—to the body's most negative transformations, and the lusciousness of the object in MacLane's mouth is shadowed by the abjection of bodily waste (note the fecal image of "bricks"). In a sense, then, MacLane's text returns us here to the most ambivalent elements of orality[17], for as she bites the olive she ushers in not only pleasure but also destruction and (literary) identification.[18] Through writing, it seems, MacLane lays claim to her body as a locus of defiant autonomy. But as she takes words into her body, she also implicitly represents her "inside" as a site of transformations—of changes that she cannot quite secure. MacLane's written defiance hangs upon her capacity to hold her words within her body, both savoring and retaining the object (feces/money/gift) as part of the subject.[19] Paradoxically, though, the auto-erotic act of "tasting your own insides" seems to be transformed—through writing—into an act of reproducing the narrator's inner body as an object for the reader's desire.

Notes

1. Stanley Hall, *Adolescence: Its Psychology and Its Relation to Physiology, Anthropology, Sex, Crime, and Education*. vol. 2 (New York: Appleton, 1920).
2. Ibid.,11.
3. See entry under "Ambivalence," in J. Laplanche and J-B Pontalis, *The Language of Psychoanalysis* (London: Hogarth, 1985), 26–28.
4. Karl Abraham, *Selected Papers on Psychoanalysis* (London: Karnac Books, 1927), 451.
5. Laplanche and Pontalis, 211.
6. Ibid.
7. Note the use of the expression "By Herself"; in other words, MacLane is not explicitly named as the author. This convention was fairly commonly used for slave narratives, for example the authorship of Harriet A. Jacobs's *Incidents in the Life of a Slave Girl* is acknowledged with the phrase "Written by Herself."
8. Mary MacLane, *The Story of Mary MacLane* (London: Jonathan Cape,

1981), 80. Subsequent references to MacLane's journal will be given directly following the quotation in the text, abbreviated as *MacLane*.

9. In *Powers of Horror* (New York: Columbia University Press, 1982), 71, Kristeva argues that menstrual blood "stands for the danger issuing from within the identity (social or sexual)."

10. Note that Mary MacLane described one of her books (*I, Mary MacLane: A Diary of Human Days*) as an "examination of herself just beneath the skin." See Michael Yocum's introduction to the 1981 edition (x).

11. See entry under "liver" in the *Oxford English Dictionary*.

12. Stanley Hall is probably most famous for two things: for organizing the Clarke Conference of 1909, when Freud visited America for the first time, and as a pioneer in the field of child and adolescent psychology.

13. In an extensive footnote to his 1908 paper on "Character and Anal Erotism," Freud cites the example of a man's childhood phantasy of being a "cocoa manufacturer," which Freud interprets as a "screen phantasy": "from the back of the body to the front, excreting food became taking food in, and something that was shameful and had to be concealed became a secret that was a boon to humanity." *Pelican Freud Library*, vol. 7 (Harmondsworth: Penguin, 1977), 212.

14. Freud, "Three Essays on Sexuality," 1905, *Pelican Freud Library*, vol. 7, 62.

15. For further discussions of the tensions betweens these two epistemes see Nathan Hale's *Freud and the Americans* (Oxford and New York: Oxford University Press, 1971), and Dorothy Ross's *G. Stanley Hall: Psychologist as Prophet* (Chicago and London, 1972).

16. Freud, "Fragment of an Analysis of a Case of Hysteria ('Dora')," 1905 (1901), *Pelican Freud Library*, vol. 8.

17. Cf. Abraham's concept of the "ambivalent" biting stage.

18. Cf. Laplanche and Pontalis's definition of "incorporation."

19. See Freud's formulation of anal erotism in "Character and Anal Erotism," 1908, and "On Transformations of the Instinct as Exemplified in Anal Erotism," 1917, *Pelican Freud Library* vol. 7, 205–17 and 293–303.

Works Cited

Abraham, Karl. *Selected Papers on Psychoanalysis*. Translated by D. Bryan and A. Strachey London: Karnac Books, 1988 (1927).

Freud, Sigmund. *The Pelican Freud Library*, vols. 7 and 8. Harmondsworth, Penguin, 1977.

Hale, Nathan Jr. *Freud and the Americans: The Beginnings of Psychoanalysis in the United States, 1876–1917*. Oxford and New York: Oxford University Press, 1971.

Hall, G. Stanley. *Adolescence: Its Psychology and Its Relation to Physiology, Anthropology, Sex, Crime, and Education*. New York: Appleton, 1920 (1904).

Jacobs, Harriet A. *Incidents in the Life of a Slave Girl*. Massachusetts: Harvard University Press, 1987(1861).

Kristeva, Julia. *Powers of Horror: An Essay on Abjection*. Translation by Leon S. Roudiez. New York: Columbia University Press, 1982.

Laplanche, J., and J. B. Pontalis. *The Language of Psychoanalysis*. London: Hogarth, 1985.

MacLane, Mary. *The Story of Mary MacLane (By Herself)*. London: Jonathan Cape, 1981.

Ross, Dorothy. *G. Stanley Hall: The Psychologist as Prophet*. Chicago and London: University of Chicago Press, 1972.

V
SYNAESTHETICS/ ANAESTHETICS

Sight, Sound, and Synaesthesia: Reading the Senses in Victor Segalen

CHARLES FORSDICK

> It is perhaps just dawning on five or six minds that natural philosophy is only a world-exposition and world-arrangement (according to us, if I may say so!) and *not* a world-explanation; but in so far as it is based on belief in the senses, it is regarded as more, and for a long time to come must be regarded as more—namely, as an explanation. It has eyes and fingers of its own, it has ocular evidence and palpableness of its own: this operates fascinatingly, persuasively, and *convincingly* upon an age with fundamental plebeian tastes—in fact, it follows instinctively the canon of truth of eternal popular sensualism. What is clear, what is "explained"? Only that which can be seen and felt.[1]

FOR THE YOUNG DOCTOR VICTOR SEGALEN, MEDICINE WAS A ROUTE to literature, followed only grudgingly. Tension between career and vocation can be seen in two early, transdisciplinary works: the study of clinical observation in naturalist novelists, *Les Cliniciens ès lettres*, and the *Mercure de France* article on *dérèglement des sens*, "Les synesthésies et l'école symboliste," both of which avoid the Whiggish risks of the medico-literary movement to which they were allied—that is, retrospective diagnosis and reduction of literary text to author's case history—to propose a more advanced model of literature and medicine concerned with the mediation of bodily experience into language. It is this factor, linked specifically to an understanding of the senses within modern medicine, to which Segalen is drawn and which remained a central concern throughout the genesis and articulation of his own understanding of exoticism.

The principal contemporary French medico-literary critic, Augustin Cabanès, with whom Segalen had short-lived contact at the start of his career, devoted the second volume of his series *Les Curiosités de la médecine* to the senses.[2] Published in 1926, seven years after Segalen's death, this fragmented, exotico-ethnographic study of perception, is concerned more with the organs of sense than with the senses themselves.³ When Cabanès describes the sense ratios of other cultures, it is always unconsciously in terms of the Western sensorium and the hegemony which that implied. He cites, for example, contemporary ethnographic evidence from Guyana which suggests that visual deprivation causes heightened sensitivity of touch:

> Ceux qui ont pratiqué la jungle profonde de la Guyane, là où les rayons de soleil ne pénètrent pas et où règne sans cesse l'obscurité profonde, savent que les yeux des Indiens, déshabitués de la lumière, perdent peu à peu leur acuité visuelle et s'éteignent. Mais les habitants de la forêt continuent à percevoir sans hésitation la forme et la couleur des objets, en approchant simplement d'eux des mains.
> [People who have experience of the depths of the Guyanese jungle—where the rays of the sun never reach and extreme darkness constantly prevails—know the effect this has on the Amerindians. Their eyes become so unused to the light that the sharpness of their vision is gradually dulled and then fades away. But the people who dwell in the forest continue to perceive the shape and colour of objects, without hesitation, simply by using their hands.]⁴

This anecdotal evidence exemplifies contemporary ethnographic attitudes to "primitive" perception, the imagery of light and darkness supporting a degenerative shift from the visual to the tactile, from the traditionally "higher," intellectual senses to the "lower," animal ones. A commonplace of observations of sensory development (that is, that deprivation leads to compensation) is recast as an abnormality, allied in the text with aberrations viewed at home—such as "vision par la peau" [seeing with the skin] and the "nez oculifère" [ocular nose].⁵ Cabanès is drawn to instances of sensory exotica which he employs uncritically to awaken his reader to the "wonders of the senses." What he ignores—and what Segalen perceived—is that particular cultural codes of perception and sensory specializations occur in whole societies and are linked to ongoing processes of cultural conditioning. Moreover, as Walter J. Ong subsequently suggested, these varying processes of evolution are equally perceptible among Western cultures where literacy and printing have underpinned a transformation for hearing-domination to sight-domination. Before shifting his recent concern to this more narrow consideration of the oral-visual binary, Ong had gone some way to articulating an "anthropology of the senses" three decades before current attempts to do the same:

Man's sensory perceptions are abundant and overwhelming. [. . .] In great part a given culture teaches him one or another way of productive specialization. It brings him to organize his sensorium by attending to some types of perception more than others, by making an issue of certain ones while relatively neglecting other ones. The sensorium is a fascinating focus for cultural studies. Given sufficient knowledge of the sensorium exploited within a specific culture, one could probably define the culture as a whole in virtually all its aspects.[6]

Exoticism and the Senses

On the return journey from Tahiti in October 1904, Segalen wrote the first of a series of notes which he would collect over the next fifteen years as the unfinished, unfinishable *Essai sur l'Exotisme*:

Ecrire un livre sur l'exotisme. [. . .] Etudier chacun des sens dans ses rapports avec l'exotisme: la vue, les ciels. L'ouïe: musiques exotiques. L'odorat surtout. Le goût et le toucher nuls.
[Write a book on exoticism. [. . .] Study each of the senses in light of its relation to exoticism: sight and skies. Hearing: exotic music. Concentrate on smell. Nothing on taste and touch.][7]

This embryonic fragment clearly reveals not only an interest in the sensorium, but also a largely uncritical acceptance of the perceived dependence of exoticism on a matrix of sight, hearing, and—above all—smell. The location of writing—just off the coast of Java—is, however, significant.[8] On the one hand, Segalen had just passed through the Torres Straits, where five years previously Alfred Cort Haddon had led the Cambridge Anthropological Expedition—part of whose remit was measurement of "the senses and sensibilities of the natives"; on the other, it marks the midpoint of the return home from what Segalen describes as his sensory awakening in Tahiti.[9] Segalen had nearly died of typhoid while traveling to Tahiti: like the narrator and protagonist of Gide's *L'Immoraliste*, convalescence was accompanied by heightened, even excessive sensuality and a liberation from previous restrictions on sensation. This biographical detail is neither a gratuitous echo nor evidence of repetition of the exoticist trope of sensual release, for it points to the centrality of an understanding of sensation in Segalen's exoticism: "Commencer par la *sensation* d'exotisme. Terrain solide et fuyant"

[Begin with the *sensation* of exoticism which is a solid yet fleeting territory].[10]

Tension between solidity and ephemerality is evident and points to one of the central problematics of Segalen's attempted general theorization of the exotic: the question of individuality and subjectivity. Like the "uncanny," so closely linked to the intensity of experience that analysis is deranged, exoticism ultimately defies theorization. Segalen's paradigmatic traveler, the *exote*, in journeying to radically different cultures and resisting any assimilative impulse in order to perceive the irreducibility of their otherness, *feels*. The "fuyant" in the above quotation implies, however, not only the fleeting but also the vanishing. The entropic spread of tourism and mechanized travel implies for Segalen a spread of sameness and a diminution of the "choc" of meeting with otherness, a lessening of its assault on the senses. The *exote* is a sensuist, one of a minority of individuals with the ability to sense diversity who will have access to what Segalen calls sensory riches or "richesses sensorielles."[11] One implication of this search for extremes is the existence of the "para-sensory Exoticism" central to the short story "Dans un monde sonore," for Segalen describes in the *Essai*: "la construction d'un monde différent du nôtre par le choix de la sensation dominante (Monde sonore, monde olfactif, etc.) ou même par des propriétés différentes de l'Espace: Espace à quatre dimensions" [the construction of a world different from ours by the choice of the dominant sense (world of sound, of smell) or even as a result of different spatial properties: for example, four-dimensional space].[12]

Beyond the Sensorium:
"Les synesthésies et l'école symboliste"

Investigation of sensory ratios and awareness of the potential valency within the Western sensorium had marked Segalen's earlier article on synaesthesia, published before his departure for Polynesia. In the present article, there is not so much an interest in Segalen's use of synaesthetic imagery in his work—which has been studied elsewhere—but in the role of such breakdown of perceptual hermeticism and development of new matrices of the senses in his thought.[13] "Les synesthésies et l'école symboliste" is based on a discarded section of his doctoral thesis, shorn of academic niceties and presented to a nonscientific public as pro-Symbolist statement and antidegenerationist polemic. Synaesthesia had become a common literary device in the Romantic period, when rigid distinction between the senses proved insufficient for the explanation and description of sensual impressions.[14] There was a development of the earlier notion of the "concert" or "union" of the senses, since now sensations from different fields of perception were described as qualitatively identical and hence transferable. Its literary use as metaphor was countered, however, by a series of protoneurological analyses carried out by nineteenth-century French scientists seeking to discredit theological positions about the soul and to translate spiritual mysteries into entirely psychological ones. Symbolist adherence to the phenomenon reveals continuing resistance to such reduction.

Describing the phenomenon as organic development and metaphor, both medico and literary, Segalen's article seems inevitably and paradoxically split between these two poles.[15] Claiming to offer a scientific analysis of synaesthesia, it finally cast the phenomenon as unassimilable by science and the would-be impersonal, objective, positivist gaze. What strikes Segalen is the creative potential of such interpenetrative patterns of perception, a potential restricted by the individual nature of "des phénomènes dont la subjectivité même est la règle" [phenomena governed by their very subjectivity].[16] Like sense-based exoticism, synaesthesia is exclusive to the perceiver, its implicit associations untransferable. Attempts at public association—*le père* Castel's "clavecin oculaire" (1759) and more recent experiments with perceptual linking of sight, sound, and smell in the theater (for example, an experimental piece called *Cantique des cantiques* in which a series of sprays were placed in the prompt box)—are dismissed as excessively reductive and Segalen is drawn to artists such as Verlaine who appear to use synaesthesia more subtly to suggest rather than to prescribe.[17]

The confusion in the article is ultimately in the tension between medicine and literature, between synaesthesia as pathological phenomenon and synaesthesia as rhetorical device. Such ambiguity is accentuated in the second half of the article in which Segalen counters pathological understandings and endeavors to normalize the synaesthetic experience. Medical evidence used for such claims is hazy, but Segalen's purpose is specifically refutation of degenerationist understanding of synaesthesia as atavistic decline. He follows a series of British and American critics—including George Bernard Shaw, in "The Sanity of Art"—in attacking Max Nordau's *Entartung* (1894), published in the French translation *Dégénérescence* the following year.[18] This text was an attempt to transfer the attention of degenerationist theory from the asylum and the underworld to the literary avant-garde whose own perceived decadence and hypersensitivity had led to physical regression. Degeneration is, however, a vague concept whose elusive morphology and ambiguous teleology were applied loosely as part of a dialectic with "progress," and Nordau is often accordingly misconstrued as a comically intense individual, devoted to "outing" degenerate authors and other tainted individuals.[19] In *Degeneration*, however, he acted as popularizer rather than originator of a series of late nineteenth-century parascientific theories and social fears. Seeking an aetiology of degeneration, Nordau cited sensory overload as a specific cause, particularly brought about, he claims, by the increase of the practice of reading:

> A cook receives and sends more letters than a university professor did formerly, and a petty tradesman travels more and sees more countries and people than did the reigning prince of other times. All these activities, however, even the simplest, involve an effort of the nervous system and a wearing of tissue. Every line we read or write, every human face we see, every conversation we carry on, every scene we perceive through the window of the flying express, sets in activity our sensory nerves and our brain centres. Even the little shocks of railway travelling, not perceived by consciousness, the perpetual noises, and the varying sights in the streets of a large town [. . .] cost our brains wear and tear.[20]

The extreme outcome of such perceived sensory excess is, for Nordau, regression to the state of a mollusc incapable of distinguishing between sense impressions and unable to rely on distinct sense organs. The intersensory nature of such perception was allied with what he saw as the physiological abnormality of synaesthesia, the analysis of which ignores the different human sense organs and the unity within diversity which the phenomenon implies:

> The lowest animals perceive of the outer world only this, that something in it changes, and possibly also, whether this change is marked or slight, sudden or slow, they receive sensations differing quantitatively, but not qualitatively. We know, for example, that the proboscis, or syphon, of the Pholas dactylus, which contracts more or less vigorously and quickly at every excitation, is sensitive to all external impressions—light, noise, touch, smell, etc. This mollusc sees, hears,

feels and smells, therefore, with this simple organ; his proboscis is to him at once eye, ear, nose, finger, etc.[21]

An apparently similar analogy has been drawn by modern students of the synaesthetic: Richard Cytowic, for instance, sees the synaesthete as a "cognitive fossil" teaching us something about perceptual experience which has been obscured by the Cartesian approach to perception, that is, by dividing the sensorium into parts.[22] He eschews, however, links with the atavistic and vestigial to claim that accounts of such experiences bring us "closer to the essence of what it is to perceive."[23] Segalen's counterattack on Nordau has similarly enlightening implications, but instead places such perception within an ongoing pattern of human evolution. Subsequent development suggests that his scientific analysis had no more weight than Nordau's speculation, but contrast between the two is illuminating. Both Segalen and Nordau privilege the optical and the acoustic, but whereas the latter operates within a traditional, essentially Aristotelian, hierarchy of the senses which demotes the "animal" senses (smell, taste, and touch), the former considered these elements of the sensorium merely to be those seen hitherto as the most advanced. While for Segalen, the olfactory senses were dulled but nevertheless remaining to be refined, Nordau had sensed in Zola a perverse preoccupation with smell which underlined the abnormality of the olfactory while establishing sight and hearing as the only acceptable media for the perception of others: "[M]en and things do not present themselves to him as to normal individuals, viz., in the first instance as optical and acoustic phenomena, but as olfactory perceptions."[24] In stating the potentials of "olfaction sonore" or hearing mediated via the sense of smell, Segalen not only countered Nordau but also presented involuntary union of the senses as a prescient violation of perceptual convention, a new stage in the evolution of the senses and part of the development of new mental functions.[25]

"Dans un monde sonore": Towards an Anthropology of the Senses

Nordau's propensity to adopt imagery from natural history led him to describe the "type" represented by Huysmans's des Esseintes as "human sacculus," a creature which "has lost all its differentiated organs, and essentially only amounts to a vesicule (hence its name: little bag), which fills itself with juices from its host."²⁶ Despite reference to À rebours in Segalen's "Les synesthésies," the foundation of Huysmans's text in aristocratic decadence is obscured as Segalen's attempts to demedicalize the synaesthetic by marginalizing the antirealist and even supernatural overtones it is granted by Huysmans.²⁷ This tendency is central to the short story "Dans un monde sonore" which, in several aspects, can be allied to Huysmans's novel: that is, a character leaves the city to live in the border zone of the suburbs where he intends to create an enclave of sensory difference. Moreover, Segalen's protagonist, André, withdraws into a darkened echo chamber where sound is distorted and associated with a variety of flames and lights. Diagnosing his wife's requirement for daylight as a yielding to carnal sensuality, he privileges his acoustic perception at the expense of his other senses: gauchely handling cutlery, for example, he injures himself but feels no pain—"Il ne sentait rien!"²⁸ Between Huysmans and Segalen, there are similarly echoes in specific details: for example, the use of carpets to muffle sound and experimentation with synaesthetic machinery.²⁹

Eventually, both protagonists are led to conclude that what Huysmans calls the advantages of confinement are illusory and to abandon their attempted hermeticism. However, whereas des Esseintes considers the medical practitioner as an intruder and is eventually hostile to the existence to which medical intervention condemns him, Segalen's protagonist's recovery from his primarily auditory universe is perceived by him as a return to health and domestic bliss from a temporary "amusette de malade" [the passing fancy of a sick man].³⁰ This latter-day Orpheus, initially fleeing "le grossier monde matériel, muet et sourd" [the vulgar material world, which remains deaf and dumb], accepts reversion to visualism as a welcomed homecoming.³¹ It is rather the narrator—largely unstudied in accounts of the text which cast the work as science-fictional diversion—who resists such reversion and elaborates the understanding of the comment in the Essai sur l'Exotisme about the creation of new worlds by focusing on the domination of senses other than the visual. The text begins with a statement of narratorial ignorance: "Je ne sais comment l'idée me vint de renouer connaissance" [I do not know how the idea came to me to renew acquaintance with him], from which the text shifts towards gradual, seemingly illusory enlightenment.³² The narrator discovers confirmation in Bordeaux of what he had concluded from his ethnographic expedition to Malaysia—that is, that there is potential fluidity within hierarchies and combinations of the senses. Noticing the intersensory nature of his colleague's new mode of privileged perception,

> André me regardait des yeux—non, pas avec ses yeux . . .—mais tout son visage, tendu vers moi, semblait, dans un geste d'aveugle, attendre mes paroles, bien qu'assez innocentes. Ses oreilles s'épanouissait plus qu'il n'est d'usage, vraiment, dans nos attitudes de primates éduqués.
> [André was looking at me—not, however, with his eyes . . .—but his whole face was stretched towards me like that of a blind person as if it were anticipating my words despite their relative banality. His ears were more alert than is really usual for primates which have reached our advanced stage of development.][33]

He is drawn into collusion with the experiment/psychosis and develops complicity with this new sensory matrix. The initial "choc" of entering a "monde sonore" gradually subsides as the narrator is incorporated into his colleague's splendid isolation and the sensory subtleties of his existence.

In charting the development of Segalen as a maverick epistemologist, Noël Cordonier has recently revealed the sustained study of contemporary scientific and para-scientific research which followed Segalen's first circumnavigation of the globe and coincided with the period in which "Dans un monde sonore" was written.[34] One of the studies which influenced him is cited explicitly in the text of the short story, Alfred Binet's metaphysical study of relations between mind and body, consciousness and brain, L'Ame et le Corps. For Binet, this text represented a shift from psychology to philosophy, and the author admits he is only seeking fragments of truth for the text contains lacunae, inconsistencies and a series of open-ended questions.[35] There is a marked shift from the pathological study of sensory disorders in, for example, his article on "Audition colorée."[36] His central thesis appears to echo Descartes in the claim that the mental is indistinguishable from the physical because the exterior world is knowable only through the sensations: "We know all objects through the sensations they produce in us and we can only know them in this way. A landscape is only a collection of sensations."[37] It is, however, the development of this idea which is relevant: since each sense serves as an intermediary between object and faculty of knowledge, none, for Binet, offers a privileged revelation of exterior reality. The hegemony of certain senses over others which has evolved, foregrounding for instance the notion of supposedly "objective" eye and hand, is accordingly undermined.[38] Like Segalen, Binet is struck by the epistemological implications of such an observation:

> It may be possible then that entirely and extraordinarily new fields of knowledge will develop privileging hearing, smell, taste and even other types of sensation which we cannot for the moment perceive or understand because we are not yet able to distinguish them in ourselves.[39]

It is a hazy synopsis of these ideas which Segalen's narrator recalls when, having left André, he understands the potentials of drifting into "un monde sonore" in which the train, perceived in terms of sound and the visual, merely serves to disgust him:

> Brusquement tout ce déballage se brocha sous une couverture rouge, et je vis s'aligner sur une planche imaginaire dix ou douze volumes de même couleur, en même temps que ma mémoire, dressée à localiser, me récitait: "Alfred Binet, *L'Ame et le Corps*, Flammarion, éditeur . . . Bibliothèque de Philosophie scientifique. . . ." Je n'en demandais pas tant. Je fus ébahi.
> [Suddenly all this outpouring of ideas found itself bound in a red cover and I saw ten or twelve volumes of the same colour lining an imaginary shelf. At the same time, my memory—trained to pinpoint this type of reference—reeled off: "Alfred Binet, *L'Ame et le Corps*, published by Flammarion in the *Philosophie scientifique* collection. . . ." I was not expecting that. I was dumbfounded.][40]

Such apparent reversion to vision highlights one of the permanent tensions within Segalen's story, which suggests that the "monde sonore" is constantly threatened by all-pervading visual senses. In the textual account of a primarily aural world, it is ironic that Leurais refuses to correspond with André to avoid disturbing its balance. This openness to new means of perception, an idea echoed in a number of almost identical statements in the *Essai sur l'Exotisme*, accordingly appears to remain largely theoretical.

A specific element of the conventional exoticism of geographical displacement addressed in the *Essai* underpins the narrative of "Dans un monde sonore" but remains largely implicit. The narrator is said to have recently returned from an ethnographic expedition in Malaysia whose purpose was anthropometric: "mesurer les données sensorielles des Papous" [recording data about the senses of the Papuans].⁴¹ A fleeting comment that the voyage was undertaken as a result of personal inclinations suggests that his investment in this research was more than scientific. As the account of Leurais's travels echoes in the acoustic space, there is then clear resonance between the ethnographic experiments and the discovery of André's self-confinement. It is as if the narrator is more concerned with himself than with the subject of his observation, for he concludes: "[I]l advenait que j'étais mis en contact—non! encore un faux emploi de ces mots tactiles . . .—en résonance, avec ce nouveau mode de concevoir le monde autour de nous" [I happened to have been put in contact with—no! yet another wrong use of these images of touch—to have started resonating with a new way of understanding the world around us].⁴²

Ethnographic speculation is echoed in metropolitan experience as the findings of the Torres Straits expedition are recorded:

> J'en arrivais, de mon exposé, à des conclusions nouvelles, je crois: que les sens des peuples non civilisés ne diffèrent pas, en acuité réelle, des sens des races affinées; que le sauvage ne doit sa vue perçante qu'à une interprétation plus habile des objets familiers qui l'entourent, et surtout à sa connaissance pratique des aspects lointains: récifs, taillis sur la montagne.
> [I think that I was reaching new conclusions as a result of this account of my research. The senses of non-civilized peoples do not differ from those of more sophisticated races in terms of actual precision. The savage merely owes his sharp vision to a more skilled understanding of the everyday objects around him and above all to a practical knowledge of distant features such as reefs and copses on mountainsides].⁴³

It is significant that this section of the text is based on another (previously unrecognized) contemporary scientific study. A brief marginal annotation in the second manuscript version of the short story refers to a Cambridge University expedition to Murray Island in the Torres Straits, and in the manuscript dossiers of Segalen's Tahitian novel *Les Immémoriaux* are notes on a short article in *La Nature*: the ethnographer Frantz de Zeltner's "Les Sens des sauvages."⁴⁴ This is a summary of the Cambridge Anthropological Expedition to the Torres Straits led by Alfred Haddon between 1898–1899. The identification of this source is not a minor footnote to a reading of this text but crucial to its understanding. Haddon's expedition has become central to current histories and studies of an anthropology of the senses.⁴⁵ It was a turning point in the shift within the past two centuries of anthropology from taxonomy and measurement as ends in themselves to a sustained attempt to decipher specific indigenous meaning.⁴⁶ In the witty and erudite travelogue which he drew from his expedition, Haddon described this attempt to shift from anthropometry and craniometry to measurement of the senses:

> Although we have a fair amount of information about the external appearance, the shape of the head, and such-like data of most of the races of mankind, very little indeed is known about the keenness of their senses and those other matters that constitute the subject commonly known as experimental psychology. My colleagues were the first thoroughly to investigate primitive people in their own country, and it was the first time that a well-equipped psychological laboratory had been established among a people scarcely a generation removed from complete savagery.⁴⁷

The results are not, however, part of an analytical study exclusively of the senses, for Haddon's research on the expedition still involved the obsessive physical measurement of craniometry and attempts to discover racial distribution through consideration of cranial index which marked purely physical anthropology.⁴⁸ In *The Body Social*, Anthony Synnott comments accordingly on Haddon's work:

> This scientific perspective on sensory reactions does not constitute an anthropology of the senses as such; but it was a step forward in that this was the first systematic recognition of the senses in anthropology. The measurement of sensory reactions was a long way from the clarification of sensory meanings and lives in different societies, however; this was still physical rather than social anthropology.⁴⁹

The Torres Straits expedition marked then a gradual end to measuring in anthropology and a beginning of watching and listening in order to consider the role of the body in society.⁵⁰ Despite the lack of sustained analysis of the results collected,⁵¹ even the review of these which Segalen had read in *La Nature* revealed that the Islanders of the Torres Straits were not, as travelers' tales claimed, "doués de sens extraordinairement développés" [gifted with highly acute senses].⁵² Instead, cultural factors were responsible for the range and acuity of the senses: distinction of colors was hindered by paucity of nomenclature; in tests of taste, there was no word for bitterness; hearing in general seemed affected—undoubtedly by the widespread practice of pearl fishing; most subjects examined had highly accurate long sight. Haddon's comment that the Torres Straits islanders were "scarcely a generation removed from complete savagery" appeared to be corroborated by William Rivers's analysis of perceived visual acuity which continues to deny coevality while at the same time describes the ability to sense minute distinctions as a "hindrance to intellectual development."[53] His reasoning is surprisingly close to that of Nordau in *Degeneration*:

> If too much energy is expended on the sensory foundations, it is natural that the intellectual superstructure should suffer. It seems possible also that the overdevelopment of the sensory side of mental life may help to account for another characteristic of the savage mind. There is, I think, little doubt that the uncivilized man does not take the same aesthetic pleasure in nature which is found among civilized peoples.[54]

Denying such distinction, however, Segalen's notes on Zeltner's account stress the essential similarity: "Les Sens des Sauvages. Très analogues à ceux des civ(ilisés)" [Savages' senses. Very similar to those of civilized peoples].[55] His use of this material in "Dans un monde sonore" is an attempt to subvert the nascent ethnographic notion of differing sensorium as further marker of inferiority and to use it instead to develop the epistemological implications for the Western sensory matrix of the conclusions of the previous study, "Les synesthésies." With a touch of delicious irony, the narrator of the short story seems to accept André's description of his wife as an Australasian "sauvagesse" as a result of her privileging of touch and sight, the very senses which, according to Binet's critique, had been elevated in the Western sensorium. In an auditory space, reliance on sight is seen as a marker of insanity.

A fragment of the *Essai* states Segalen's passing fear that synaesthesia ignores the differences between the senses, that it is an entropic phenomenon with antiexotic implications: "Palinodie de mes synesthésies. [. . .] Oui ou Non? à méditer. Peut-être, attitude provisoire, prudente" [Palinode of my work on synesthesia. [. . .] Yes or No? think about this. Perhaps this is a sensible temporary approach].[56] His prevarication, however, reveals continued adherence to the implications of "dérèglement des sens" in its challenge of the assimilative, polarized, taxonomic, often kaleidoscopic visualism inherent in many contemporary accounts of otherness. In reviewing the received hegemony of the senses and suggesting the possibility of other configurations, Segalen reveals a vigorous awareness of the role of visual/textual bias within the construction of Western knowledge and suggests that consciousness of this is a new way not only of sensing other worlds, but also, more fundamentally, of making *sense* of others.

Notes

1. "L'idée de la physique n'est, elle aussi, qu'une interprétation du monde, une adaptation du monde [. . .] mais dans la mesure où la physique se fie aux témoignages des sens, elle passe et passera longtemps encore pour quelque chose de mieux, c'est-à-dire pour une explication. Les yeux et les doigts plaident pour elle, le visible et le tangible sont de son côté, voilà qui fascine, persuade et *convainc* un siècle dont le goût est foncièrement plébéen, car il se conforme instinctivement aux normes éternellement populaires du sensualisme. Qu'est-ce qui est clair? qu'est-ce qui nous 'éclaire'? Uniquement ce qui se laisse voir et toucher." Friedrich Nietzsche, *Par-delà bien et mal* (Paris: Mercure de France; Leipzig: Naumann, 1898), 17. Friedrich Nietzsche, *Beyond Good and Evil*, ed. Oscar Levy, trans. Helen Zimmer (Edinburgh: Foulis, 1909), 21. This quotation (from aphorism fourteenth, chapter 1, of the French translation of Nietzsche) was copied by Segalen into the manuscript of "Dans un monde sonore" to support the thesis which the short story explores. See Noël Cordonier, *Max-Anély et les Fantômes* (Paris: Kimé, 1995), 153.

2. On Cabanès, see Jane Govaerts-Régis, *Un Médecin au service de l'histoire. Augustin Cabanès* (Paris: Jouve, 1941). For details of Segalen's meeting with him in 1901, see "Lettres inédites de Victor Segalen," ed. Annie Joly-Segalen and Gabriel Germain, *Annales de Bretagne* 71 (1964): 429–43.

3. As an anecdotal and essentially nonanalytical work which fails to address the way in which the senses are not only ordered by culture but can also be indicative of cultural values, it could be allied with Diane Ackerman, *A Natural History of the Senses* (New York: Random House, 1990). For recent studies which attempt to begin to address these issues, see Constance Classen, *Worlds of Sense: Exploring the Senses in History and across Cultures* (London: Routledge, 1993), and David Howes, ed., *The Varieties of Sensory Experience. A Sourcebook in the Anthropology of the Senses* (Toronto: University of Toronto Press, 1991).

4. Augustin Cabanès, *Les Curiosités de la médecine II: les cinq sens* (Paris: Le François, 1926), 123.

5. Cabanès refers to sight impressions mediated via touch or smell. See ibid., 133 and 186.

6. Walter J. Ong, "The Shifting Sensorium," in *The Varieties of Sensory Experience. A Sourcebook in the Anthropology of the Senses*, ed. David Howes (Toronto: University of Toronto Press, 1991), 25–30 (28). Initially included in Ong's *The Presence of the Word* (New Haven: Yale University Press, 1967).

7. Victor Segalen, *Essai sur l'Exotisme*, in *Œuvres complètes*, ed. Henry Bouillier, 2 vols. (Paris: Laffont, 1995), 1: 745–81 (745).

8. Although Segalen was not necesarily aware of this, it is interesting to note that the understanding of the sensory matrix in Java—seeing, hearing, *talking*, smelling, and feeling—reveals that various cultures do not necessarily perceive the sensorium in the same terms. See David Howes and Constance Classen, "Sounding Sensory Profiles," in *The Varieties of Sensory Experience*, 257–88.

9. See Alfred C. Haddon, "The Cambridge Expedition to Torres Straits and Borneo," *Nature* 57 (1898): 276. This was a preliminary note published before departure and a request for "suggestions as to lines of investigation or methods of study." On the sensory aspects of his experience in Tahiti, see Segalen's letter to Henry Manceron (23 September 1911) in Victor Segalen and Henry Manceron, *Trahison fidèle. Correspondance 1907–1918*, ed. Gilles Manceron (Paris: Seuil, 1985), 106.

10. Victor Segalen, *Essai sur l'Exotisme*, 747.

11. Ibid., 749.

12. Ibid., 753.

13. See Ioanna Constandulaki-Chantzou, "La synesthésie dans le texte de Victor Segalen," in *Victor Segalen. Actes du Colloque de Brest* (Brest: Centre de Recherches Bretonne et Celtique, 1995), 273–84.

14. The first modern clinical case study seems, however, to have been attested in 1710 by the English ophthalmologist Thomas Woolhouse, who describes a blind man perceiving sound-induced colored visions. See Richard Cytowic, *Synesthesia: A Union of the Senses* (New York: Springer, 1989), ix, and Louise Vinge, *The Five Senses: Studies in a Literary Tradition* (Lund: CWK Gleerup, 1975), 166.

15. For a consideration of these issues of status, see June E. Downey, "Literary Synaesthesia," *The Journal of Philosophy, Psychology, and Scientific Methods* 9 (1912): 490–98; Cynthia Marsh, *M. A. Voloshin: Artist-Poet, a Study of the Synaesthetic Aspects of His Poetry* (Birmingham: University of Birmingham, 1984); and Richard Cytowic, op. cit, 238–83.

16. Victor Segalen, "Les Synesthésies et l'École Symboliste," in *Œuvres complètes* I, 61–81 (62).

17. In the same way, it is claimed that serious attempts to chart *correspondances* from Rimbaud's sonnet "Voyelles" fail, for Segalen comments that the work was "purement apocryphe d'intention et de sens" [of doubtful authenticity in terms of intention and meaning] (ibid., 65). A similar point is made in *Le Double Rimbaud* where Segalen cites Ernest Gaubert's "Une explication nouvelle du sonnet des voyelles d'Arthur Rimbaud" in which the author claims that the sonnet was inspired by the colors associated with letters in an alphabet primer. See Victor Segalen, *Le Double Rimbaud*, in *Œuvres complètes* 1: 486–502 (490).

18. For other critiques of Nordau, see George Bernard Shaw, "The Sanity of Art: An Exposure of the Current Nonsense about Artists being Degenerate," in *The Works of Bernard Shaw*, 20 vols. (London: Constable, 1930), 19: 293–346, and also [Alfred Hake], *Regeneration: A Reply to Max Nordau* (London: Constable, 1895).

19. For a general account, see *Degeneration: The Dark Side of Progress*, ed. J. Edward Chamberlin and Sander L. Gilman (New York: Columbia University Press, 1985). For a useful discussion of Nordau, see Hans-Peter Söder, "Disease and Health as Contexts of Modernity: Max Nordau as a Critic of Fin-de-Siècle Modernism," *German Studies Review* 14 (1991): 473–87; and Richard

Noll, "Max Nordau's *Degeneration*, C. J. Jung's Taint," *Spring* 55 (1994): 67–79.

20. Max Nordau, *Degeneration* (Lincoln: University of Nebraska Press, 1993), 39.

21. Ibid., 141.

22. Richard Cytowic, op. cit, 14

23. Ibid., 21.

24. Max Nordau, *Degeneration*, 502. See also *Aroma: The Cultural History of Smell*, ed. Constance Classen, David Howes, and Anthony Synnott (London: Routledge, 1994), 90. For a specific study of the anthropology of smell in eighteenth- and nineteenth-century France, see Alain Corbin, *The Foul and the Fragrant: Odour and the French Social Imagination* (London: Picador, 1994); first published as *Le Miasme et la jonquille* (Paris: Aubier Montaigne, 1982). See also Louise Vinge, *The Five Senses*, 25, for a consideration of Philo's discussion of the traditionally bestial and servile nature of the senses of taste, smell, and touch.

25. Victor Segalen, op. cit., 72 and 81.

26. Max Nordau, op. cit., 309.

27. See J.-K. Huysmans, *A rebours* (Paris: Flammarion, 1978), 61.

28. Victor Segalen, "Dans un monde sonore," in *Œuvres complètes* 1: 551–67 (564).

29. For references to sound-proofing, see *À rebours*, 76, and "Dans un monde sonore," 553; for Huysmans's "orgue à bouche," see 99, and the aural-visual machine in Segalen's text, 558. Another of Segalen's protagonists, Max in *Les Fantômales*, intends to "se meubler en des Esseintes" [to furnish his home like des Esseintes's]. Unpublished manuscript note, 25 May 1906, cited by Noël Cordonier, op. cit., 183.

30. Victor Segalen, "Dans un monde sonore," 567.

31. Ibid., 560.

32. Ibid., 551.

33. Ibid., 556.

34. See Noël Cordonier, op. cit., 13.

35. For a discussion of Alfred Binet's "Flight into metaphysics," see Theta Wolf, *Alfred Binet* (Chicago: University of Chicago Press, 1973), 339–47.

36. Alfred Binet, "Le Problème de l'Audition colorée," *Revue des Deux Mondes* 62 (1892): 586–613.

37. Alfred Binet, *L'Ame et le Corps* (Paris: Flammarion, 1905), 12.

38. On the privileged "objectivity" of sight and touch, see ibid., 74.

39. Ibid., 42.

40. Victor Segalen, "Dans un monde sonore," 566.

41. Ibid., 553.

42. Ibid., 566.

43. Ibid., 566.

44. See manuscript of "Dans un monde sonore," Paris, Bibliothèque Nationale, nouvelles acquisitions françaises, microfilm 3830, f.39, and Francis de Zeltner, "Les Sens des sauvages," *La Nature* (19 December 1903): 42. Segalen's notes on this article are contained in the file: *Protestantisme à Tahiti = le Tahitianisme*, Paris, Bibliothèque Nationale, nouvelles acquisitions françaises, papiers non classés.

45. I have found nothing yet to suggest that Segalen had read more than Zeltner's article on Haddon's work. For a factual account of the expedition,

however, see A. Hingston Quiggin, *Haddon the Head Hunter* (Cambridge: Cambridge University Press, 1942). The six volumes of reports are also of interest: *Reports of the Cambridge Anthropological Expedition to the Torres Straits*, 6 vols. (Cambridge: Cambridge University Press, 1901–1935). For an instance of application of its findings to contemporary sensory investigations, see Richard Cytowic, op. cit., 259.

46. See Anthony Synnott and David Howes, "From Measurement to Meaning: Anthropologies of the Body," *Anthropos* 87 (1992): 147–66.

47. Alfred Cort Haddon, *Head-Hunters: Black, White, and Brown* (London: Watts and Co., 1932), 15.

48. See Alfred Cort Haddon, "The Physical Characters of the Races and Peoples of Borneo," in Charles Hose and William McDougall, *The Pagan Tribes of Borneo*, 2 vols. (London: Macmillan, 1912), 2: 311–41. For a description of the methodology and practice of search for racial affinities, see A. C. Haddon, "Why We Measure People," *Science Progress* 7 (1898): 1–22.

49. Anthony Synnott, *The Body Social: Symbolism, Self, and Society* (London: Routledge, 1993), 145.

50. Synnott notes that this shift was largely influenced by the development of the first intelligence tests by Alfred Binet, which offered the first quantitative, qualitative but nevertheless still positivistic assessments of intelligence and intellectual abilities. See ibid., 245.

51. Haddon's colleague Dr. William Hale Rivers noted in the first part of the second volume of the reports that data had been collected to provide "facts to be processed later in comparison to subsequently collected material" (*Reports of the Cambridge Anthropological Expedition to the Torres Straits*, vol. 2). Rivers was lecturing on the psychology of the senses at Cambridge when he was recruited by Haddon to join his expedition in 1898. Work in the Torres Straits led to his ongoing interest in ethnology. See A. C. Haddon, "Obituary: Dr. W. H. R. Rivers," *Nature* (17 June 1922), 786–87.

52. Francis de Zeltner, op. cit., 42

53. W. H. Rivers, op. cit., 44.

54. Ibid., 44–45

55. For source, see note 44 above.

56. Victor Segalen, *Essai sur l'Exotisme*, 44–45.

WORKS CITED

———. *Reports of the Cambridge Anthropological Expedition to the Torres Straits*. 6 vols. Cambridge: Cambridge University Press, 1901–35.

Ackerman, Diane. *A Natural History of the Senses*. New York: Random House, 1990.

Binet, Alfred. *L'Âme et le Corps*. Paris: Flammarion, 1905.

———. "Le Problème de l'Audition colorée." *Revue des Deux Mondes* 62 (1892): 586–613.

Cabanès, Augustin. *Les Curiosités de la médecine II: les cinq sens*. Paris: Le François, 1926.

Chamberlin, J. Edward, and Sander L. Gilman, eds. *Degeneration: The Dark Side of Progress*. New York: Columbia University Press, 1985.

Classen, Constance. *Worlds of Sense: Exploring the Senses in History and across Cultures*. London: Routledge, 1993.
Classen, Constance, and David Howes. "Sounding Sensory Profiles." In *The Varieties of Sensory Experience: A Sourcebook in the Anthropology of the Senses*. Edited by David Howes. Toronto: University of Toronto Press, 1991, 257–88.
Classen, Constance, David Howes, and Anthony Synnott, eds. *Aroma: The Cultural History of Smell*. London: Routledge, 1994.
Constandulaki-Chantzou, Ioanna. "La synesthésie dans le texte de Victor Segalen." In *Victor Segalen. Actes du Colloque de Brest*. Brest: Centre de Recherches Bretonne et Celtique, 1995, 273–84.
Corbin, Alain. *The Foul and the Fragrant: Odour and the French Social Imagination*. London: Picador, 1994.
Cordonier, Noël. *Max-Anély et les fantômes*. Paris: Kimé, 1995.
Cytowic, Richard. *Synesthesia: A Union of the Senses*. New York: Springer, 1989.
Downey, June E. "Literary Synaesthesia." *The Journal of Philosophy, Psychology, and Scientific Methods* 9 (1912): 490–98.
Gaubert, Ernest. "Une explication nouvelle du sonnet des voyelles d'Arthur Rimbaud." *Mercure de France* 52 (1904): 551–53.
Govaerts-Régis, Jane. *Un Médecin au service de l'histoire. Augustin Cabanès*. Paris: Jouve, 1941.
Haddon, Alfred C., "The Cambridge Expedition to Torres Straits and Borneo." *Nature* 57 (1898): 276.
———. *Head-Hunters, Black, White, and Brown*. London: Watts and Co., 1932.
———. "Obituary: Dr. W. H. R. Rivers." *Nature* (17 June 1922): 786–87.
———. "The Physical Characters of the Races and Peoples of Borneo." In Charles Hose and William McDougall, eds., *The Pagan Tribes of Borneo*. 2 vols. London: Macmillan, 1912, 2. 311–41.
———. "Why We Measure People." *Science Progress* 7 (1898): 1–22.
Hake, Alfred. *Regeneration: A Reply to Max Nordau*. London: Constable, 1895.
Howes, David, ed. *The Varieties of Sensory Experience: A Sourcebook in the Anthropology of the Senses*. Toronto: University of Toronto Press, 1991.
Huysmans, J.-K. *A rebours*. Paris: Flammarion, 1978.
Marsh, Cynthia. *M. A. Voloshin: Artist-Poet: A Study of the Synaesthetic Aspects of His Poetry*. Birmingham, Ala.: University of Birmingham, 1984.
Nietzsche, Friedrich, *Beyond Good and Evil*. Edited by Oscar Levy. Translated by Helen Zimmer. Edinburgh: Foulis, 1909.
———. *Par-delà bien et mal*. Paris: Mercure de France; Leipzig: Naumann, 1898.
Noll, Richard. "Max Nordau's *Degeneration*, C. J. Jung's Taint." *Spring* 55 (1994): 67–79.
Nordau, Max. *Degeneration*. Lincoln: University of Nebraska Press, 1993.
Ong, Walter J. "The Shifting Sensorium." In *The Varieties of Sensory Experience. A Sourcebook in the Anthropology of the Senses*. Edited by David Howes. Toronto: University of Toronto Press, 1991, 25–30.
Quiggin, A. Hingston. *Haddon the Head Hunter*. Cambridge: Cambridge University Press, 1942.

Segalen, Victor. "Lettres inédites de Victor Segalen." Edited by Annie Joly-Segalen and Gabriel Germain. *Annales de Bretagne* 71 (1964): 429–43.

———. *Œuvres complètes*, 2 vols. Ed. by Henry Bouillier. Paris: Laffont, 1995.

Segalen, Victor, and Henry Manceron. *Trahison fidèle. Correspondance 1907–1918*. Edited by Gilles Manceron. Paris: Seuil, 1985.

Shaw, George Bernard. "The Sanity of Art: An Exposure of the Current Nonsense about Artists being Degenerate." In *The Works of Bernard Shaw*, 20 vols. London: Constable, 1930, 19, 293–346.

Söder, Hans-Peter. "Disease and Health as Contexts of Modernity: Max Nordau as a Critic of Fin-de-Siècle Modernism." *German Studies Review* 14 (1991): 473–87.

Synnott, Anthony. *The Body Social: Symbolism, Self, and Society*. London: Routledge, 1993.

Synnott, Anthony, and David Howes. "From Measurement to Meaning: Anthropologies of the Body." *Anthropos* 87 (1992): 147–66.

Vinge, Louise. *The Five Senses*. Lund: CWK Gleerup, 1975.

Wolf, Theta. *Alfred Binet*. Chicago: University of Chicago Press, 1973.

Zeltner, Francis de. "Les Sens des sauvages." *La Nature* (19 December 1903): 42.

The Anaesthesia of Charles Baudelaire's "Le Goût du néant"
KNUT OVE ELIASSEN

"Le Goût du Néant"

Morne esprit, autrefois amoureux de la lutte,
L'Espoir, dont l'éperon attisait ton ardeur,
Ne veut plus t'enfourcher! Couche-toi sans pudeur,
Vieux cheval dont le pied à chaque obstacle bute.

Résigne-toi, mon coeur; dors ton sommeil de brute.

Esprit vaincu, fourbu! Pour toi, vieux maraudeur,
L'amour n'a plus de goût, non plus que la dispute;
Adieu donc, chants du cuivre et soupirs de la flûte!
Plaisirs, ne tentez plus un coeur sombre et boudeur!

Le Printemps adorable a perdu son odeur!

Et le Temps m'engloutit minute par minute,
Comme la neige immense un corps pris de roideur;
Je contemple d'en haut le globe en sa rondeur
Et je n'y cherche plus l'abri d'une cahute.

Avalanche, veux-tu m'emporter dans ta chute?

["The Taste for (of) Nothingness": Dismal soul, once in love with strife, / Hope, whose spur once made your fervour flare / No longer wants to mount you! Lie down without shame / Old horse whose foot stumbles at each obstacle. // Resign yourself, my heart; sleep your sleep of beasts. // Vanquished, weary soul! For you, old marauder, / Love has lost its taste, so has dispute; / Hence goodbye songs of brass, and sighs of the flute! / Pleasures, tempt no more a dark and gloomy heart! // Adorable Spring has lost its scent! // And Time devours me minute by minute, / As the vast snows do a frozen body; / I contemplate from on high the globe in its roundness / Where I no longer seek a cabin's shelter. // Avalanche, will you take me with you in your fall?)[1]

THE NATURE OF THE RELATIONSHIP BETWEEN POETRY AND SENSUAL experience has played an important part in discussions about literature, at least since the Romantic movement at the end of the eighteenth century. One of the conceptions of poetry that emerged from Romanticism holds that the paramount characteristic of *true* poetry is the successful creation of an experience where the boundaries that separate subject and object, the individual and the world, the poet and the reader, are felt to dissolve. This effect has been appropriately called *the poetic moment*. "Moment" must here be understood as a kind of metaphorical nexus that draws its semantic energy from its creation of a complex interplay of meanings where at least three different significations are in play: the temporal sense of the poetic *nunc stans*, the "mechanical" sense of momentum (the poem as aesthetic gesture), and moment as the unveiling of a new aspect. Due to the transgressive nature of the poetic experience, it is seen as a moment that unifies or reconciles, as the common ground linking world and individual as well as individual and community is confirmed, even celebrated. The significance of the poetic operation is not limited to its effects on the present, but it is also a kind of recollection in which what has passed is again made present through the transformative spells of the poem's vivid linguistic representations. The result is a kind of simultaneity, or rather a temporal stasis of sorts. The poetic moment marks a stretching out of time, making it an instant filled with significance and being, where the pure and empty, "senseless," time of *chronos* yields to the full time of *kairos*. These spatial and temporal qualities of the poetic experience were later given a succinct (and untranslatable) formula by Proust—"l'espace et le temps rendus sensibles au coeur" [space and time made into something that the heart is able to feel].

Summed up in a more philosophical vocabulary, Romantic poetry can be said to be aiming at the dissolution of the three dimensions of Kantian philosophy. What is at stake is nothing less than the extrasubjective relation to the world, the intersubjective relation between individuals and the intrasubjective relation of the self (the historical me and the I of the present). Accordingly, the instant of poetic fulfillment—very aptly called the moment of "das lyrisches Ineinander" ["lyrical intertwining"] by Emil Staiger[2]—is accomplished by the erasure of the division, fundamental to Kantian thought, of time and space.

What remains, however, is the problem of language. Even poetry must, so to speak, bow to the rule of the metaphor. Or in the words of Paul de Man from his essay "The Resistance to Theory": "Mimesis becomes one trope among others."[3] Consequently the kind of literary aesthetics outlined above (admittedly a rather rough sketch) will need to justify the view that the distinction between experience and the representation of that experience *can* be effaced or, perhaps more correctly, "transcended." Looking at the history of literary theory, the appearance of such an idea must undoubtedly be seen in the shift from a poetics of allegory to a poetics of symbol. It is generally accepted that this is a change that takes place at the turn of the nineteenth century, in other words with what is usually referred to as the beginning of the Romantic era.

To claim that symbolist poetics has been out of fashion lately is not to exaggerate. Not only has it become commonly accepted that symbolist poetics more often than not are marred by a certain blindness in rhetorical matters, but it is also widely held that it continues an ideological heritage that in many ways appears to run counter to its professed belief in the sovereignty of man. One can easily demonstrate how the Romantic notion of poetry draws heavily on themes and ideas inherited from Christian mystical traditions. The idea of a full or fulfilled time is at least as old as the New Testament and the mental representation of sensual impressions has at least one famous precursor in the *compositio loci* of the Jesuits. The blind spots of the rhetorical and ideological reflexivity of the Romantic movement have become obvious when confronted with "modernist poetry" (to employ the kind of broad generalizations whose only excuse is that they permit a systematic approach); in other words, with a kind of poetry whose aim is no longer the representation of moments of fullness, but rather—thanks to its fundamental scepticism towards the symbolizing powers of language—one that is inclined to stress the impossibility of any representation whatsoever.

This is, generally speaking, Theodor W. Adorno's position when he argues that the hallmark of the modernist tradition is the emphasis on the rupture or breaking (*Bruch*) of the bonds that link the subject to the world in which it belongs.[4] Rather than being the medium of reconciliation and redemption, modernist poetry is and must be, according to Adorno, the aesthetic confirmation of the abyss that has opened up between man and his world in the alienation of capitalist society. Instead of being the mediator of symbols, affirming and realizing in the form of the successful work of art—the true token of which is the harmonious forms of the beautiful (*das Schöne*)—the common destiny of man, as a being of nature, and the nature he is immersed in, poetry is conceived as a linguistic practice that is monistic, folded in on itself and withdrawn from the world. In this gesture there emerges a poetics of absence or of negativity whose final justification consists in the possible conversion of poetic experience into conceptual philosophy. In fact, this position may even be seen as the continuation of the tradition of a mimetic concept of art, as the kind of negative aesthetics professed by Adorno, and in a paradoxical way is the true mimetic representation of alienated existence in late capitalism.

Whilst romanticist poetry aimed at the communication of the beauty and sensual richness of moments of spiritual and emotional fulfillment, modernist poetics of negativity on the contrary implies the use of language in a noncommunicating, nonbeautiful way. The task of the poet is no longer the celebration of being, but to bear witness to the poverty of our experience of the world. As the figures and tropes of the established poetic tradition are inscribed within a rhetoric of the beautiful, and thus must be considered as aesthetic language, a poetry that commits itself to the true state of things must resort to a different kind of rhetoric. As such a poetics does not allow for an aesthetics of literature, I will suggest Jean-François Lyotard's concept of the anaesthetic as a more appropriate term.[5] An(a-)aesthetic is a fitting denomination insofar as the concept stresses that what we are dealing with is a poetic practice that aims to negate the categories of the aisthesis, thus liberating aesthetics from the category of the beautiful. In denying the ideal of a unification of form and content by negating the subsuming or transformative powers of the beautiful shape, it thereby undoes form not only as the medium through which the subject realizes itself, but also as the central agent in the idea of the beautiful (beauty always appears as beautiful forms). As form is the means by which a bond or a passageway is established between subject and world, mind and matter, the anaesthetic gesture becomes the *signum* of the impossibility of (and thus the negation of) the conceiving (and receiving) of the world in the word (the concept). This (f)act in itself draws our attention to the conditions of the impossibility of naming, thereby opening up what Lyotard has called the ana-mnesis of modernity (playing on Freud's as well as Plato's use of the term), as the recalling of an original loss.[6] And finally the term "anaesthetics" bears witness to the general anaesthesia, the sensorial numbness, that is the precondition for a poetics of negativity and of modernity as a locus of loss.

However, one is tempted to ask how satisfactorily this settles the debate concerning the relation between poetry and sensual experience. Is poetic language, in Adorno's radical and rather melancholy critique of modernity, essentially a language of pure absence, of negativity, or does even modernist poetry have a sensual component? If so, what is the nature of poetry's sensual qualities? It is obvious that, to the degree that literature, or more precisely, poetry, can be seen as an aesthetic practice, it must somehow involve the five senses and thereby relate to sensual experience. With the theories currently in vogue stressing the negativity of literary language (from Blanchot and Derrida to Benjamin and Adorno), the aesthetic qualities of poetry are not self-evident. But how should the paradoxical, even oxymoronic, idea of an aesthetics of negativity, an anaesthetics, be understood? And furthermore, can the notion of an anaesthetics of literature be sustained without having recourse to the kind of artistic practice it negates? Does that entail that the prefix *ana-*, like the post-, the re-, the para-, and all the other prefixes circulating in current theory, can in fact, as Lyotard seems to be claiming, be seen as a reminder of a dependency that not only exists on a theoretical level—in the sense that negativity as a dialectical concept always subsists on positivity—but also on a more concrete level that is embedded in the poetic practice itself, be it either in its reliance on sensual metaphors or in the sensual qualities of the words themselves.

The following analysis of "Le Goût du néant" is an attempt to show how Baudelaire as a poet reflected upon this issue. I have chosen this poem from *Les Fleurs du Mal* for several reasons—primarily because it is generally held that one of the salient features of Baudelaire's poetry is an abundance of sensual metaphors that includes an unusually high frequency of nonvisual and nonaural sensations. Secondly, there are several good reasons for describing Baudelaire as the first post-Romantic poet in the sense that even though he clearly identifies himself with the ideas of the generations before him, he strongly signals that these ideas belong to a different time. The *modernité* that was his daily experience no longer allowed for beauty in the Romantic sense. Consequently, Baudelaire inferred, the moment of poetry was, if not forfeited, at least *dépassé*, a theme worked out allegorically in the opening poem of the collection *Les Epaves* from 1866, "Le Coucher du soleil romantique" [The Setting of the

Romantic Sun]. His explicit articulation of the dilemma of being split between, on the one hand, an identification with tradition and, on the other, the acknowledgement that the present has broken its bonds with the past, has made Baudelaire an emblematic figure for theories of modernity. This is not because this cleavage is articulated as an opposition or conflict between ideality and reality, but because it is formulated temporally and tragically, as a loss for which there is no amendment. Accordingly, Baudelaire's point of departure is quite the opposite of the Romantic movement, the acknowledgement of the fact that the conditions for a positive reception of poetry no longer existed. As Walter Benjamin has pointed out, he wrote for a reading public that had become indifferent to poetry. Due to "a change in the structure of experience," experience itself had fallen in value: "die Erfahrung ist im Kurse gefallen."[7] What is at stake in this claim is obviously the possibility of community itself, the rationale of the beautiful being, as Kant argues in the third Critique, the very foundation for intersubjectivity (the *sensus communis* manifesting itself through the judgement of taste, in other words in the aesthetics of the beautiful). But even though he took his audience's interest at best as a feigned one, Baudelaire nevertheless saw this lack of interest in the poetic medium as a common ground that made them his equals—"Hypocrite lecteur, mon semblable, mon frère!" [Hypocrite reader, my double, my brother!]

Written during the winter of 1858–59, "Le Goût du Néant" was published for the first time in 1859 in the January issue of *La Revue française*. It then appeared in a slightly different version as poem 80 in the second edition of *Les Fleurs du Mal*, where it is one of the last poems in the section called "Spleen et Idéal." The poem is interesting in the present context as it focuses thematically upon the problematic sensual relation between the lyrical I and the world, and gives an account of what might be described as a "sensorial collapse." It might be said thereby to corroborate Adorno's idea that modern poetry bears witness to the impossibility of any "true" aesthetic relation to the world. I will argue, however, that this does not necessarily preclude any relation whatsoever between poetry and sensual experience, a point Adorno himself stresses in *Ästhetische Theorie* (for instance in his two allusions to "Le Goût du Néant").[8] In my view, Baudelaire's poem contains a dimension that can be fruitfully discussed in the perspective opened up by Lyotard's idea of the "anaesthetic," and that in a wider scope can be seen as a corrective to Adorno's stern and pessimistic judgment.

It is well known that one of the central antagonisms in Baudelaire's anthology is the relation between spleen and ideality. This is an opposition between the low and the high, the pathological and the transcendent, and is also articulated by Baudelaire as a conflict between the corporeal and the spiritual. Significantly placed as the first and the largest of the six parts of *Les Fleurs du Mal*, the title "Spleen et Idéal" indicates the central elements in Baudelaire's vision of the human condition, the tragic incongruity between the corporeal world of reality and the spiritual world of ideals. We are, he puts it, forever fettered to the grave of the Ideal. Georg Lukács's tersely sums up this position in *Die Theorie des Romans* as a "Romanticism of disillusionment"; in other words a form of Romanticism that takes the defeat of the ideals of the spiritual world as an accomplished fact.[9] What sets this disillusioned Romanticism apart, is the experience (*Erfahrung*) that the soul (*die Seele*)—to employ Lukács's vocabulary—believes itself to be larger and grander than any destiny life has to offer. This incongruity leads to a protective reaction of withdrawal and isolation of the self. At the same time this is accompanied by an elevation of the self based on the certitude that by the very defeat of its ideals, the subject that professes them is raised above the profanity of the existing world. This double figure of defeat and victory sketched out by Lukács (a figure with a high degree of affinity with the Freudian conception of melancholy) is analogous to Baudelaire's double figure of spleen and ideal. It is, however, also reflected in a less conspicuous way, namely by the *correspondance* the title "Le Goût du Néant" establishes with another text written the same year, the first chapter of *Le Poème du Haschich*, "Le Goût de l'infini."

In itself "Le Goût du Néant" is an ambiguous formula, or more precisely, a polysemic one. Literally, it translates as "The Taste *for* Nothingness." "Taste" can obviously be read in many ways, as another word for "appetite" or "craving," "desire," and so on. However, bearing in mind Kant's words that "taste" is an eminently social concept, as well as the aristocratic ethos that permeates the Baudelairean universe, "predilection," with its connotations of evaluation, standard, and acquired faculty is probably a more appropriate translation of "Goût." This does not mean however that the one sense excludes the other, as the physical dimension of taste—taste as craving or *appetitus*—is maintained throughout the poem as an important part of the title's semantic backdrop. The title's prepositional *du* can also be rendered as a genitive, as in "The Taste *of* Nothingness." This phrase is equivocal in itself, in that "taste" contains both a subjective and an objective meaning. On the one hand, it designates the subjective perception of an object, the way something tastes for me (which is something unique that cannot be shared). On the other hand, it refers to a certain quality inherent in the object that can be sensed by anyone with his or her sensorial perception in normal working order. In addition, the titular *Goût* can be read as a genitive so that "Taste" is subordinated to Nothingness (Nothingness's taste). Finally this allows for two different understandings of "taste": it can be taken either in a metaphorical sense (which turns the title into a kind of catachresis), or *literally* as an actual gustatory impression.

When the titular *du* is read as a genitive, the title appears paradoxical, as it seems quite difficult to assign specific qualities, such as a certain taste, to that which is nothing, *le néant*. This would seem to confirm that both *goût* and *néant* should be understood metaphorically for instance in the way one of the English renderings of the poem translates the title as "The Craving for Oblivion." This is an interpretation that could be corroborated by considering one of the early working titles of *Les Fleurs du Mal*, namely *Les Limbes* (Limbo), a title that echoes the collection's many allusions to Catholic theology as well as to Dante.[10] I would, however, like to explore the opposite interpretation, that the titular "taste" should be read not only as a trope for the sensual experience of absence or nothingness (*néant*) but should be taken in the literal sense (to the degree it is meaningful to talk about nonmetaphorical language), and I suggest that this sensual experience of nothingness lies at the semantic core of the poem; or to put it more bluntly, that the poem deals with the experience of the absence of any sensual impressions at all. Its central theme is what one might call a "sensorial breakdown," or in Walter Benjamin's terms from "On some motifs in Baudelaire," the shock effect brought about by the collapse of the "aesthetic sensorium."[11] This does not exclude the notion of limbo as a key to the collection's allegorical imagery. It is neither pain nor suffering that characterizes the souls of Dante's Limbo (in the fourth canto of the *Inferno*) but rather a melancholic, indifferent, and terrible apathy, indeed a feeling not too distant from Baudelaire's *spleen*.

A few words about the formal features of "Le Goût du Néant" are in order before entering into the analysis. The layout is rather unusual in that the poem consists of three quatrains separated by three single, typographically isolated lines. It is a format that is unique in Baudelaire's oeuvre and has, according to several treatises on French versification, no precursors in French poetry.[12] The effect is a curious kind of "stop-go" rhythm that puts additional stress on the single lines (lines 5, 10, and 15). Another striking formal feature is that the poem contains only two rhymes, producing a sound effect that in its monotony contributes to the rather bleak and dreary images of the text. The particular status of the single lines becomes even more manifest given that not only their particular position vis-à-vis the chiastic rhyming pattern (*rimes embrassées*), but also their ending, echo the final line of the previous stanza (ABBA/A/BAAB/B/ABBA/A). It should be mentioned that the employment of chiastic rhymes is consistent with the traditional rules of French poetry insofar as paired rhymes were considered heroic, while the so-called *rimes embrassées* were seen as elegiac. The solemn mode is further emphasized by the use of the alexandrine, conventionally considered the most noble of French meters.

"Le Goût du Néant" takes the form of soliloquy as the lyrical I is apostrophizing his own soul. Apparently because of its dumb animal nature (at least this seems to be indicated by the central allegory of stanzas 1 and 2), the soul does not reply but remains silent throughout. The opening word of the first stanza establishes the poem's fundamental mood: *morne*—"sullen and weary." Here the poet appears to be reflecting upon his proper destiny as he sees himself in the light of what his soul once was but is no longer. The rather morose mood is emphasized through the prosodic likeness of *morne* to *mort* as well as their contrast with the assonant *amoureux*. The line's retrospective spirit is doubly underscored as *autrefois* is not only preceded by the comma, but also placed in front of the position of the conventional caesura, thus rhythmically bracketing its temporal aspect.

The second line introduces what is to be the central motif of the two first stanzas. The soul or the mind—*l'esprit*—is allegorically presented as an old and decrepit warhorse. The comparison hints at a conception of the human soul not as a spiritual center, but rather as something that by nature is bestial (characterized by its love for strife—*la lutte*—and its ardor). This impression is reinforced by line 5, in which the heart is solicited to sleep its "sleep of beasts." The image of the *esprit* having been mounted by the allegorical "Hope" (*L'Espoir*, with a capital E) is not only striking for its plastic qualities, as an allegory it subverts the traditional idea of the *esprit*. Baudelaire's allegory does not depict the soul as an independent or active entity, as the center of man's sovereignty or will, as it is commonly conceived, but rather as a subaltern (the *esprit* had at one time submitted itself to "Hope" and was explicitly *spurred on* by its master). The subversive character of the image is emphasized by the sexual connotations of *enfourcher*. The allegory's disparagement of the spiritual goes even further in that the image of Hope as the soul's master is a rather melancholic memory of times long gone, and now Hope no longer desires to mount the soul, thereby conveying a rather disillusioned and bleak outlook on the question of sovereignty. The spirit of the lyrical I (or that of man in general) is not represented as his own master, but as the subject of, or more precisely as the object of, foreign masters (and desiring to be so), which in this case is the illusion of Hope.

It is important to note how the contrast between the opening words of the two first lines, *Morne* and *espoir*, creates a tension that accentuates the opposition between past and present, retrospection and anticipation. In a tone that is resigned but calm, verging on the soothing (compare, for instance, the *sans pudeur* of line 3), the first stanza seems to conclude that old age has led to a condition where the vigorous appetite for life of former days is gone: "Résigne-toi, mon coeur." The present appears to be pervaded by an overall feeling of weariness bordering on collapse, illustrated by the lack of vigor as well as the motif of the old horse that stumbles at each step. This motif comes to prefigure and prepare the final fall that seems to be imminent in the last line of the poem. Finally the use of the past tense underscores the overall feeling of *la vie antérieure*.

The change of mood in the second stanza is apparent from the start in the shift from the prosodic qualities of *morne* in line 1 to the *esprit* of line 6. This is further accentuated by the following exclamation mark that breaks the calm, elegiac mood of the first stanza. This change in tone and prosodic quality mirrors the redirection of the temporal *setting* of the theme. While the first stanza, as we have seen, was oriented towards what once was, the second stanza marks a gradual turning towards the present condition. The transition from past to present is reflected in the stanza's sensual metaphors (as well as in the inversion of the rhymes). It is, however, a change that is more a matter of mood and of significance than of imagery as the image of the horse is maintained, maybe most strikingly in the word *fourbu* (rhythmically underscored both with an exclamation mark and by being situated before the caesura). The original meaning of *fourbu* is related to beasts of burden and signifies limpness or lameness as a consequence of being overstrained (for example, *cheval fourbu*). In everyday language *fourbu* denotes "exhausted" or "stiff" and hence comes to point toward the *roideur* of the last stanza, indicating a relationship between the stiffening limbs of the beast and the rigor mortis of the corpse. Consequently, the word works on both the allegorical and the literal levels of the text. What follows from the change in tone and mood is the dissolution of the feeling of intimacy that prevailed throughout the first stanza, a shift that is confirmed in the final word of the line, *maraudeur*, a term whose moral connotations are markedly more negative than those previously employed. The term *maraudeur* inevitably brands the poetic I (or rather *me*) as an outcast, a marginalized existence sustaining himself as a parasite, a marauder being equivalent to the French *pillard* and *voleur* (a thief and a robber).

The seventh line introduces a motif that will come to the forefront as we proceed: sensuality. The connection it establishes between *amour* and *dispute* gains significance in that it echoes the first line's *amoureux de la lutte*. Literally it states that both love and strife have lost their taste, as they neither appeal nor satisfy. This is the only echo of the title in the text itself, and the word is given extra weight by being placed immediately in front of the caesura. Furthermore, the echoing of the titular *goût* is amplified not only by the comma that succeeds it (that was not there in the first version of the poem), but more strikingly by the line's pun on the old proverb: "Des goûts et des couleurs on ne dispute point" [There's no accounting for taste]. The allusion underscores the disillusionment of the present position taken by the lyrical I, as the proverb offers a nihilistic outlook on aesthetics that from Baudelaire's point of view is quite incompatible with his own. Aesthetic value is of course, from the dandy's point of view, the only thing worth arguing about.

In the eighth line, a final goodbye is said to the active aggressiveness of the past. Though war is present, represented by the synecdoche of the "chants du cuivre et soupirs de la flûte," the goodbye is in fact an adieu to the sensual qualities of the battle, the *plaisirs*, and not the battle itself. The motif echoes one of the poems immediately preceding it, "Spleen" (poem 78), where in the final stanza a procession of hearses passes through his exhausted soul "sans tambour ni musique" [with neither drum nor music]. But although force and vigor are waning, the poem still appears to insist that the sleep of oblivion has not yet set in, in the sense that the memories of a different time appear to be aching like so many wounds. With the two last lines there is a noticeable shift from the calm, elegiac mood of the first half of the poem to a more dramatic mood. This is partly brought about by the use of diacritical signs, as three consecutive lines end with an exclamation mark, but is also due to the absence of any enjambment, a technique that dominates the first half of the poem. The result is an effect that seems to run counter to the stanza's semantic content, as exclamation marks, caesuras, and other rhythmical devices have to be seen as "vitality effects" that through the stressing or the breaking of the meter add materiality, or maybe more fittingly, *body*, to the text. Thus the first stanza's mixture of consolation and dejection has in the second stanza turned into something akin to desperation as the tension between content and rhythm in lines 6 to 9 creates a feeling of growing despair. This is summed up in the apostrophizing of sensual pleasures in line 9 and in the rhythmical emphasis on the *nevermore*, the "ne tentez plus."

The accumulated tension—both semantic and prosodic—of the second quatrain finds it relief in line 10. "Le printemps adorable a perdu son odeur" [Adorable Spring has lost its scent] is without doubt the best known line of the poem. This is its moment of peripety and disaster, the shock when it is acknowledged that the lyrical I's sensual relationship to the world has broken down, where it becomes clear that the despairing appeal to *les Plaisirs* in line 9 has been accepted. Or more precisely, what takes place is the acknowledgement that the present state is one in which the conditions of possibility of sensual experience no longer exist. The shock is intensified, as Walter Benjamin underlines in his essay on Baudelaire's lyrical motifs, by the fact that it is being articulated with "the utmost discretion" (*der äußersten Diskretion*).[13]

In referring to olfactory impression, line 10 continues the sensual theme of the previous lines—the "taste" of line 7, the aural metaphors of line 8, and the highlighting of the sensual pleasures of line 9. But line 10 also introduces a new motif, the seasons, the full importance of which we will return to later. The imagery seemingly continues the themes of the first two stanzas insofar as "spring" is a traditional metaphor for youth, that is, "the spring of life." This is all the more plausible given that an obvious interpretation of the following lines is that the snow and cold are synecdoches for wintertime, winter being a conventional image for old age and the absence of life. But it is not on the metaphorical level that the line has its strongest impact, but rather read in its literal sense. Literally, it states that the I of the poem experiences sensual isolation from the world; it thus relates the experience of aesthetic isolation *in strictu sensu*. What is presented as the brutal truth—prefigured by the "Adieu donc" of the previous stanza—is that sensuality is de facto a closed chapter: no more scents, no more taste, all that whets the appetite for life is history.

The literal reading of line 10 reveals the poem's central moment. This line also implies a break with the allegorical mood that has been predominant in the poem's first two stanzas. While the allegory of the warhorse is maintained and developed throughout lines 1 to 9, it is absent from the last stanza. This could be interpreted as the acknowledgement that there is no allegory that can aptly transform the experience of the loss of sensuality into meaningful metaphors of poetic language since the very condition for such an operation is the possibility of alluding to sensual experiences. Line 10 thus denotes both the breakdown of the aesthetic sensibility and the ability to render this particular experience in an allegorical form, that is, to *transport* lived experience into allegory. The *transport* itself has become unattainable.

If this line of argument is sustainable, I believe it would be fitting to call this the *sublime* moment of the poem, to use a term suggested by Auerbach in his important essay "On the aesthetic Dignity of the *Fleurs du Mal*."[14] In Kant's version from the "Analytic of the Sublime" in the *Critique of Judgement*, the sublime experience consists of two phases (which is a temporal differentiation within the sublime moment that sets him apart from Burke and other precursors). In the first phase, the faculty of understanding (*der Verstand*) is unable to muster categories or concepts that are adequate to the phenomena experienced; these therefore remain inconceivable, that which is outside the reach of intelligibility. This acknowledgement of the limits of human understanding brings forth, according to Kant, a feeling of despair, as it imposes upon us the idea that man is smaller than nature, or inversely, of matter's victory over mind. The most famous example of such a phenomenon is probably the infinity of the universe. As that which can be neither conceptualized nor represented, the immensity of the universe testifies to the shortcomings of our conceptual powers. The failure of our representative faculties is in the last instance a token of the human mind's intellectual deficit in relation to the material world. Within the framework of Kantian thought, this poses a major threat to his philosophy's central idea, namely the question of sovereignty, or more precisely the idea that man with the aid of his reason, can free himself from his embeddedness in nature, by being the founder of his own laws. This is where the second phase of the Kantian sublime comes in, marking the return of reason and the recovery of what has been lost. For that which cannot be conceived of with the categories of *der Verstand* and the powers of the imagination can be thought with the help of *die Vernunft* (the faculty of reason) as an idea—in this case, namely as the idea of infinity—and thereby confirms man's superiority to nature. "The sublime is that, the mere capacity of thinking which evidences a faculty of mind transcending every standard of sense."[15]

This leads us back into the bleak world of the last stanza, a stanza whose contents seem to confirm that what is taking place in the poem is an experience that can properly be called "sublime" (the sublime always being an experience and never an object). But it is a sublime that appears to be without the second phase in Kant's argument. To put it another way, it is sublime in the sense that it gives a description of an experience that cannot be transported into allegory; it cannot be translated into anything but itself, and only communicated literally. Thus, like the Kantian sublime, this is an experience that resists being subsumed by the existing categories of understanding, or stated differently, that cannot be translated into a metaphor. It is, nonetheless, negatively dependent on the faculty of understanding, as reason's recognition and acknowledgement of the lack of forms (that may well take the shape of allegories) through which the present phenomenon can be subsumed, is absolutely constitutive of the sublime experience. What is important in our context, however, is that Baudelaire's poem appears to contain a negative element alien to Kant's analysis of the sublime. The result is the creation of the kind of hopeless horror, characteristic of the Baudelairean sublime according to Auerbach, that offends against, as he puts it, "every traditional notion of the dignity of the sublime."[16] The poem does not explicitly thematize the element of negative pleasure which, for Kant, is something that follows from the faculty of reason, proving itself able to conceive of the sublime phenomenon as an idea. The question to be explored following the analyses of the last stanza is whether or not it makes sense to argue that the poetic representation itself can be seen as that second moment of the sublime experience, where the inconceivable is conceived as an idea. In other words, whether the poem's "regress" from an allegorical mode to a literal mode can be seen as a development that is analogous to the first part of the Kantian sublime, or whether the fact that the poem communicates the breakdown of the allegory parallels rather Kant's notion of "negative pleasure."

The breakdown of the senses in line 10 leads to a change of imagery. The contrast with the previous stanzas becomes even more apparent as the last five lines break with the pattern of interior monologue, of soliloquizing. As the allegory of the first half of the poem no longer seems sustainable, the allegorically presented theme of decrepitude and exhaustion is replaced by the acknowledgement of the passing of time. The lyrical I has turned away from its own past, the tense is no longer past but present, and the address is no longer directed to the self, to *l'esprit* (that is to the time of subjectivity), but to a nonpersonal, nonsubjective entity that exists outside and independent of the subject as *le Temps* (apostrophized as *Avalanche* in the last line). To understand the consequences of this shift, one must take into account the motif of the seasons. We have touched upon the notion of "spring" as a conventional metaphor for "virility" and "youth" and hence as an image of human time, but understood in a literal sense it designates a period within the natural cycle of the seasons and thus, metonymically, the time of nature. Natural time is a time outside of society, a time that is nonhuman; it is the time of natural history. This time is, properly speaking, "inhuman" and is thus, if not in opposition to—as it is not obvious that the character of the relation between natural time and human time is oppositional—at least foreign to and different from the experience of human time that was the dominant theme in the first nine lines of the poem. Thus the first and the second part of the poem juxtaposes and even confronts two different concepts of time; a human one, which, in principle at least, is meaningful, and a natural one, which from a human standpoint is devoid of meaning.

Seen from the perspective of human existence, the salient feature of natural history is its fatality as it is a time that can neither be stopped nor manipulated, but rather a time of eternal return. That we are dealing with a time that exists for itself, the pure time of the mechanical *tic-toc*, is indicated through the capital letter employed in *Temps* and the repetition of the word *minute*: "minute par minute" (further enhanced by the alliteration of "m'engloutit"). The alliterative rhyming of "m'engloutit minute par minute" makes the words resonate with a meaning that is stated *expressis verbis* by the poem itself, namely that time slowly but ceaselessly devours us: "le Temps m'engloutit minute par minute." This formula, with its allusions to the devouring Chronos, the merciless ancestor of the Greek pantheon, prominently placed in the final quartet, marks its central theme (echoed again in the last verse of line 15). It is an allusion that underlines that we are dealing with a form of time that is inhuman (the cannibalistic Chronos devouring his own children), and therefore offers no hope of redemption.

The idea of being devoured by time is curiously present in a double manner in the last line, since "avalanche" is not only prosodically but also etymologically related to "avaler," to "swallow." The poetic overdetermination of the slide and the act of swallowing is enhanced by the relation to "descendre" (meaning both to "descend" and to "swallow") common to both words. This is again echoed by the final word of the poem, "chute"—a word that in a Baudelairean context is limited to existentialist connotations but also takes on a religious and mythological meaning.

The season of the last stanza is winter, the season of death and absence of life, an image given further weight by the depiction of the dead body being covered by the falling and sublimely overwhelming ("immense") snow in line 12. The general feeling of its wintry scenery is one of "after the storm," an impression that can be supported by the absence of commas and exclamation marks, in short the vitality effects touched upon in our discussion of the second stanza. Furthermore, the sensual references from the earlier stanzas are absent. The poem seems to indicate that the dead body is that of the lyrical I as both lines 13 and 14 declare that the I no longer needs any shelter, as well as through the "roideur" that establishes a link to the earlier "fourbu" (while "roideur" is further emphasized by the neat prosodic contrast with the "rondeur" of the following line). The sensual death of line 10 seems to have turned into something bordering on actual death, a sort of existential *rigor mortis*, a numbed or anaesthetized phenomenological subject, emphasized prosodically not only through the assonance of "corps" and "roideur" but also with the "hardness" of the last five syllables, four of which contain the letter *r* (underlining the tactile associations linked to "roideur"). The feeling of distance and disconnectedness is further accentuated with the curious perspective of line 13. Here the nonterrestrial, out-of-this-world perspective views the earth from the outside, from the viewpoint of the "néant" so to speak; the lyrical I seems to have been catapulted out of this world and, no longer in need of any earthly dwelling ("l'abri d'une cahute"), looks back on the site of its previous life, in a manner that is characteristic of Baudelaire: "C'est là que j'ai vécu." Eventually this opens up the ambiguity of the final line, in which it is difficult to decide whether the plea should be understood as the expression of the wish to be taken away—as indicated by the title of the English translation we referred to earlier, "The Craving for Oblivion"—or rather the opposite, as a supplication to be allowed to stay.

Many commentators—Gaston Bachelard among others—have pointed to the importance played by smell in Baudelaire's poems and to a tendency to employ words related to olfactory perceptions in connection with experiences of oneness and wholeness. The most well-known example is probably the synaesthesias of "Correspondances" that relate to smell as the primary sense. I will argue that the sensual collapse of "Le Goût du Néant" can only be properly understood when seen in contrast to the rich synaesthetic impressions and sensual transports of "Correspondances." A striking feature of this poem is that all the other senses seem to be contained, or are at least containable, in the olfactory sensations. Smell is presented as the sense of oneness—the *sensus communis*, one is tempted to say—as when the poem describes smells ("parfums") "doux comme les hautbois, et verts comme les prairies" [soft and sweet like oboes, green like the meadows]; or in the last tercet, as "corrompus, riches et triomphants" that "chantent les transports de l'esprit et des sens" [corrupted, rich and triumphant, praising the raptures of the soul and the senses]. The sentence is ambiguous, as "transport" can be read as referring to sensual ecstasy and the loss of the self, as well as translation into metaphor. Thus the perfumes described become the causes of magical transformations, and the singing is not a praise, but rather a magical chant that seduces or even bewitches both the mind and the senses.

The olfactory experiences of "Correspondances" seem to confirm how smell in Baudelaire's poetic universe tends to be synonymous with the sense of being-in-the-world. The collapse of sensual perception in "Le Goût du Néant" leads to the recognition of the fact that the world is lost for the poetic I. The loss of the ability to sense the world, the breakdown of the aesthetic sensorium, seem to signify that the I is as if dead to this world. It is a loss that catapults the poem's perceiving agency out of this world to a position from which neither the sense of smell nor of taste, nor any other subjective and intimate sense, connects the individual to the world; from which one is left solely with the sense of vision, a sense that works only over distance—a sense that has distance as a condition of possibility. In the absence of smell and the other "low senses," the individual is only able to see and is thus no longer capable of a relationship based on intimacy and exchange with the world that surrounds it. Therefore the poem articulates the despair born of the recognition that the experienced world, the whole, total and sensually mitigated world, is closed off, no longer attainable even through the magical and sensual transportation of allegory—in the double sense of the German word for allegory, *Sinnbild*, meaning both an image with a meaning (*Sinn*), and a figure of speech using sensual imagery (*Sinn* in the sense of "sense"). But as Walter Benjamin puts it: "The word *perdu* acknowledges the present state of collapse of the experience he once shared (*das Insichzusammengesunkensein der Erfahrung*)."[17] Thus, even though the poem confirms the central idea of Adorno's modernist aesthetics, it also demonstrates that this shock can only appear against the background of aesthetic or sensual experience. Its deals with the sublime insofar as there is a memory, a reminiscence that is more than an idea. It is the memory of a world once sensed, once experienced as a whole, and given that smell is traditionally conceived of as a sense closely linked to memory, the loss of smell not only implies the loss of sensual impressions, it also seems to indicate the impossibility of remembering what once was. What seems to be remembered is the sole fact of forgetting, and the poem draws its poetic force from the memory of past experiences and of the sensual experience of the loss of sensual experience, of the experience of anaesthesia; in other words, nothing but "l'insensibilité du néant" spoken of in "Le Gouffre" (one of the poems added in the third version of *Les Fleurs du Mal* from 1868). It involves the experience in the present of that which can no longer be experienced, but which is experienced as a loss, its past tense marking that which is no longer present.

As Benjamin saw it, Baudelaire's poetry was formulated as a bulwark against the traumatic shocks of the modern urban life emerging in Paris in the 1840s and 1850s. Baudelaire's chief tool in erecting defences against the outside world was allegory. This, states Benjamin, is the meaning of the famous line from "Le Cygne": "pour moi, tout devient allégorie" [for me, everything turns into allegory]. But if Baudelaire saw the outer world devalued to a mere material already transformed by and subjected to conventional meanings and images, in itself devoid of any true differences whatsoever, the world is by the same token free to be disposed of by the artist at his will. What is gained is the absolute liberty of the artist that thereby confirms his own self-sufficiency. Seen from this angle, "Le Goût du Néant" comes across as a testimony of the fallibility of allegory as an aesthetic protective armor. At least this is one of the possible interpretations of the collapse of the central allegory of the poem or, more precisely, the collapse of the allegorical distance maintained throughout the two first stanzas, a distance that ceases to exist with the demand for a literal reading of line 10. The poem thus invites us to make the following two observations: first, that poetic language appears to be insufficient as a device for transforming the painful experiences of modern life into aesthetic imagery (that would procure the distance necessary to make the pain tolerable); second, that the translation of lived experience into aesthetic experience appears to be a thing of the past. In other words, the metaphorical operations of poetry, and more generally, of art, are no longer capable of mediating between man and world by providing the beautiful forms that confirm their common existence. These observations fit in well with the idea of an aesthetics of absence, or anaesthetics, discussed earlier. This aesthetics does not reflect any sensual experience, but is rather an affirmation of a condition of aesthetic numbness, of the historical decay of the conditions of possibility of aesthetic experience in the traditional sense (that is an aesthetics of beauty).

There is, however, one aspect that complicates such a reading: the question of the ambiguity of the titular *du*—both "the taste *for* nothingness," but also "the taste *of* nothingness." As the latter rendering indicates, the experience of anaesthesia is itself an experience, in the sense that the subject is somehow affected; something is obviously being perceived in the sensorial register. This could very well be the perception of the loss of perception, but it is nevertheless not possible to exclude the other meaning of the title, "The taste *for* nothingness," in other words, the desire for nothingness—or as Nietzsche would have put it: an active nihilism. But in what sense is it plausible to argue that the lyric I desires nothingness when, at the same time, it describes this experience as a disaster? Poetry is, of course, no stranger to such paradoxes. However with a poet like Baudelaire, whose level of self-consciousness in his poetry is extremely high, it seems reasonable to believe that these paradoxes are well calculated. I believe some light could be shed on this paradox if we reflect upon it at a metalevel, treating it as a paradox inherent to the aesthetic experience as such. In the article "Anima minima," Jean-François Lyotard proposes the following minimalist definition of the structure of philosophical aesthetics: it presupposes an object and a receptive entity, an experiencing agency that Lyotard calls anima (but which, to maintain Baudelaire's vocabulary in this poem, I will call *esprit*).[18] This receptive entity is that which is being affected, and thus is the locus where the aesthetic impression is born. This mind exists only insofar as it is being affected; without its ability to be affected, the mind would be soulless, it would remain sleeping—the sleep of beasts, to use the poem's own words. Aesthetic impressions are thus the marks of intrusions into what must by itself be considered as a nonexistence. What sensual excitement does to this nonexistence is to awaken the latent existence that lies more or less dormant within it. The kernel of Lyotard's argument is that what we call life emerges from the violence exerted from the outside on something that is in a condition of lethargy. The anima (*esprit*) exists only when forced to exist. Thus the *esprit* remains dependent on sensual impressions, that is, it has to be irritated or even be the object of violence in order to become aware of its own existence. Without this impetus from the outside, there is only numbness, anaesthesia. And the anima, the *esprit*, remains dumb without the possibility of this autonomy that rises out of self-awareness.

This could very appropriately be called a double-bind structure, and applied to Baudelaire's poem, it could give us a key to the ambiguity of the title. There is, on the one hand, a longing for annihilation, for anaesthesia, for the absence of any external stimuli that are possible temptations for a "morne esprit." On the other hand, there is the horror of nothingness, the fear of the void, of being devoured by time, and a longing for the life born out of the impacts of sensations. The very movement by which it once awoke holds the mind captive as it finds itself confronted by a hopeless choice: the alternative between extinction in imminent death or the dumb pain of a prolonged existence in sensorial limbo. This double structure also pertains to the aesthetics of Baudelaire's poem. Read on one level, it contains an implicit aesthetics of the allegory, where allegory is to be understood in the double sense of the German *Sinnbild* (amply demonstrated by the poem "Correspondances," in the double meaning of the word "transport"). On another level, the poem seems to be implying that there are certain experiences that cannot adequately be represented by allegory, experiences of a sublime character that cannot be communicated, or rendered by the traditional language of beauty or of poetic metaphor, but can only be signaled by a literal use of language (language thus functioning more deictically). I believe that this is the sense in which we can understand the literal use of language in poetry as sublime (the sublime being that which cannot be measured by anything other than itself). This indicates, finally, that at least in the case of Baudelaire, poetry exists neither as an aesthetic nor an anaesthetic use of language, but somewhere in between the two, existing or deriving its force from the simultaneous play of both registers.

Notes

1. The poem is taken from the 2d, 1861 edition of *Les Fleurs du Mal*. It is usually assumed that it was written during the winter of 1858–59. It was first published in *La Revue française* in January 1859. This English translation does not attempt to be anything other than a literal rendering of the poem. Unless otherwise indicated, all translations from the French and German are mine.
2. Emil Staiger, *Grundbegriffe der Poetik*, 7th ed. (Zürich: Atlantis, 1966).
3. Paul de Man, "The Resistance to Theory," in *The Resistance to Theory* (Minneapolis: University of Minnesota Press, 1986), 10.
4. Theodor W. Adorno, "Rede über Lyrik und Gesellschaft," in *Noten zur Literatur* (Frankfurt am Main: Suhrkamp, 1974 [1958]), 53.
5. The concept of an-aesthetics is developed by Lyotard in several articles. The one we will primarily be referring to in the following is "Anima minima," in *Moralités postmodernes* (Paris: Galilée, 1993).
6. "Ana-mnesis" is a term employed by Lyotard in much of his writing on the postmodern. See for example "Billett pour un nouveau décor," in *Le Postmoderne expliqué aux enfants* (Paris: Galilée, 1986).
7. Walter Benjamin, "Über einige Motive bei Baudelaire," in *Abhandlungen, Gesammelte Schriften* (Frankfurt am Main: Suhrkamp, 1991), vol. 1: 2, 608; see also "Der Erzähler," in *Gesammelte Schriften* vol. 2: 2, 439.
8. Theodor W. Adorno. *Ästhetische Theorie* (Frankfurt am Main: Suhrkamp, 1970), 40 and 66 (see also note 16).
9. Georg Lukács. *Die Theorie des Romans* (München, Hamburg: DTV, 1994), 98.
10. Per Buvik's *Poesiens skandale* (Oslo: Pax, 1996) focuses explicitly on ob-

vious Catholic aspects of Baudelaire's poetry that have been overlooked in the celebration of Baudelaire as the herald of modernism.

11. Walter Benjamin, "Über einige Motive bei Baudelaire," 641.
12. For example, Theodor Elwert, *Traité de versification française des origines à nos jours* (Paris: Klincksieck, 1965).
13. Benjamin, loc. cit.
14. "The Aesthetic Dignity of the *Fleurs du Mal*," in *Scenes from the Drama of European Literature* (Minneapolis: University of Minnesota Press, 1984 [1959]), 203.
15. Immanuel Kant, *The Critique of Judgement*, trans. James Creed Meredith (Oxford: Clarendon Press, 1952), 98.
16. Auerbach, loc. cit.
17. Benjamin, loc. cit.
18. See "Anima minima," in *Moralités postmodernes*.

Works Cited

Adorno, Theodor. *Ästhetische Theorie*. Frankfurt am Main: Suhrkamp, 1970.

Adorno, Theodor. "Rede über Lyrik und Gesellschaft." In *Noten zur Literatur*. Frankfurt am Main: Suhrkamp, 1974 [1958].

Auerbach, Erich. "The Aesthetic Dignity of the *Fleurs du Mal*." In *Scenes from the Drama of European Literature*. Minneapolis: University of Minnesota Press, 1984 [1959].

Baudelaire, Charles. *Œuvres complètes*, Bibliothèque de la Pléiade. Paris. Gallimard, 1975.

Benjamin, Walter. *Charles Baudelaire. Ein Lyriker im Zeitalter des Hochkapitalismus*. Frankfurt am Main: Suhrkamp, 1974. English translation: *Charles Baudelaire: A Lyric Poet in the Era of High Capitalism*. London: Verso, 1983.

Benjamin, Walter. "Der Erzähler." In *Aufsätze, Essays, Vorträge, Gesammelte Schriften* Band 2, 2. Frankfurt am Main: Suhrkamp, 1991.

Buvik, Per. *Poesiens skandale*. Oslo: Pax, 1996.

de Man, Paul. "The Rhetoric of Temporality." In *Essays in the Rhetoric of Contemporary Criticism*. London: Routledge, 1983.

———. "The Resistance to Theory." In *The Resistance to Theory*. Minneapolis: University of Minnesota Press, 1986.

Elwert, W. Theodor. *Traité de versification française des origines à nos jours*. Paris: Klincksieck, 1965.

Lukács, Georg. *Die Theorie des Romans*. München, Hamburg: DTV, 1994. English translation: *The Theory of the Novel*. London: Merlin Press, 1971.

Lyotard, Jean-François. "Billett pour un nouveau décor." In *Le Postmoderne expliqué aux enfants*. Paris: Galilée, 1986.

Lyotard, Jean-François. "Anima minima." In *Moralités postmodernes*. Paris: Galilée, 1993. English translation: *Postmodern fables*. Minneapolis: University of Minnesota Press, 1997.

Kant Immanuel. *Kritik der Urteilskraft*. Felix Meiner: Hamburg, 1974 [1790].

English translation: *The Critique of Judgement*. Translation by James Creed Meredith. Oxford: Clarendon Press, 1952.

Staiger, Emil. *Grundbegriffe der Poetik*, 7th ed. Zürich: Atlantis, 1966. English translation: *Basic Concepts of Poetics*. University Park: Pennsylvania State University Press, 1991.

Reading (in) Proust: With the Senses, beyond the Senses
JANE WALLING

IT HAS BECOME SOMETHING OF A COMMONPLACE IN PROUST STUDIES to talk about the centrality of reading in *A la recherche du temps perdu* both literally (the favorite books and authors of the hero/ narrator) and metaphorically in the sense of his attempts to decipher and understand experience, his interrogation of phenomena. The central figure is constantly engaged in the act of reading people, events, objects: his career is on one level what has been called "an apprenticeship in signs,"[1] where the most significant are those emitted by Jean-Pierre Richard's "hermeneutical objects,"[2] the madeleine, for example, and the spires of Martinville. One more recent critic has described the process of decoding as a major leitmotif in the novel and then goes on to say that the narrator's contact with the real world is constantly described as the reading of a text.[3]

What I propose to examine here is one particular type of reading, or sensual reading (I shall return to this shortly), namely "reading in the Book of Nature." It seems to me that Proust can fruitfully be considered as part of this long and honorable tradition which started with the idea that the whole of nature is like a book which the initiated is able to read as an expression of God's overall plan for creation. One of the earlier representatives of this tradition was Alain de Lille who died in 1203,[4] and since then there have been a considerable number of—often secular— variations on the theme which have received much critical attention.[5] However, if at the beginning of *A la recherche du temps perdu* there is nostalgia for a certain kind of nature spirituality, there is also during the course of the novel a gradual movement away from the natural world,[6] with the ascesis it requires being replaced by the increasingly cathected,[7] sensual reading of the human world. In this way, as in so many others, Proust is thus something of a Janus-figure: we have both "[a]n archaic Proust who still believes in old metaphysical systems,"[8] who, as I hope to show, is still greatly influenced by this tradition, and also a "Proust moderne" who denies nature any autonomy and uses it more and more for the illustration and explanation of human behavior.

I can obviously do no more here than say a few words about the largely literary tradition of reading in the Book of Nature. The central ideas of this tradition seem to be that nature constitutes a realm in which some kind of meaning or intention is manifested; it has its own language which can be read and interpreted by human beings; this act of reading puts the observer in touch with another transcendental realm; nature can thus mediate between the human and the spiritual worlds. These ideas are so widespread in French Romantic and pre-Romantic literature—especially poetry—that it is easy to forget to what extent they derive ultimately from quite esoteric sources.[9] Indeed, it is possible to trace an indirect influence on Proust here in that three nineteenth-century writers with whom he famously engaged—Sainte-Beuve, Balzac, and Baudelaire—were all, to varying degrees, writing in this tradition. Thus Sainte-Beuve includes in *Volupté* (1834) an account of the thought of the eighteenth-century philosopher and occultist Saint-Martin, with his hero coming to reject materialism and realizing that "all the visible things in the world and in nature" are signs to be interpreted, and finding himself able to "extract some syllables of this great word which, fixed here, wandering there, was trembling everywhere in nature."[10] Similarly, both Balzac in *Séraphita* and Baudelaire in *Les Fleurs du Mal* were writing under the influence of Swedenborg (1688–1772) and his principal idea that the spiritual world is more real than the material and is connected to it by correspondentia. Moreover, according to Swedenborg, everything in nature not only has some spiritual equivalent but also corresponds to something in man and, as Philip Knight points out, "this is no mere emblematic relation but one validated by visionary experience."[11]

In this tradition, German writers, such as Jean-Paul Richter and Novalis, have always played a central part, and it is perhaps characteristically to the German tradition that one has to turn in order to find a more systematic development of the idea of reading in the Book of Nature, where sensual reading of phenomena is combined with penetration beyond them. I use the term "characteristically" because one could argue that German thought and culture have been a great deal less influenced by

Descartes than is the case with French culture. In his book *Le Nouvel ordre écologique*, for example, the French philosopher Luc Ferry says of the French: "Nature is for us a dead letter. In the proper sense: it no longer speaks to us because long ago—at least since Descartes—we ceased to attribute a soul to it and to believe that it is inhabited by occult forces."[12] One might therefore suggest that German culture (and to a lesser extent English-speaking culture) is more able to conceive of the compatibility and continuity of the consciousness and the outside world, of nature and spirit, and less persuaded than many French writers of their total irreconcilability. For this reason it might be useful to consider sensual reading in Proust against the background of the German development of this tradition.

For a contemporary critic of Proust, Eliane Boucquey, writing from within the French Cartesian tradition, it thus goes without saying that, much as the narrator might like to try, he cannot be at once mystic and scientist, in other words, someone who both observes nature exactly and objectively and is also able to penetrate its secrets. "If this narrator is mad," she says, "it is because he wants to be at one and the same time a mystic and a scholar."[13] And yet it seems to me that there is one very obvious example of a writer who was both, who was, that is, able to combine the detailed and precise sensual reading of natural phenomena with an understanding of the forces behind them, who was able to see through *natura naturata*, nature as a series of created products or observable objects, to *natura naturans*, nature as a creative, dynamic force, an initiative center of activity.[14] The writer I am referring to here is Goethe. Goethe's method of reading the Book of Nature refused to recognize any gulf between the artistic and the scientific. Instead, he "strove to unite empirical observation and spiritual intuition" because "only by bringing observation and imaginative intuition into intimate interaction could man penetrate nature's appearances and discover its essence."[15] He was thus able to unite poet and scientist in an analysis and appreciation of nature that brought together sensuousness and spirituality. Although Proust was not directly influenced by Goethe, it seems to me that one can find striking echoes of what has become known as Goethean science in *A la recherche du temps perdu*, together with references to a very similar underlying epistemology. I hope therefore that a brief exposition of the Goethean approach will be a useful starting point for a discussion of the sensual reading of nature in Proust.

In his study of nature—particularly colors and plants—the first step for Goethe was the attentive, objective observation of the phenomenon, a detailed reading using all the senses and free of any preconceptions.[16] The second step was then to turn away from the object and attempt to produce an exact mental, sense-free equivalent, imaginatively conjuring it up in one's mind's eye. This process was known as "exakte sinnliche Phantasie,"[17] literally translated as "exact sensual imagination," which means that one is perceiving the object in imagination as if with the senses, although in reality this is an activity which transcends them. Sensual reading of the object thus makes way for a sense-free reproduction of it, where one is, as it were, thinking the object rather than thinking about it. This also means that the observer of nature (Goethe famously called himself a "Naturschauer" rather than a "Naturforscher," someone who observes nature rather than investigates it) is somehow imaginatively creating the flower, participating in the act of its creation or, as Goethe put it, "recreating in the wake of ever-creating."[18] In other words, he or she is internally reproducing the coming into being of the plant[19] rather than just visualizing a static mental equivalent of it. So development, movement, growth, the *gesture* of a plant (to use a key word in Goethean science) could be imaginatively intuited and this process would give one more insight into the particular individual essence of a plant than would be possible with conventional botany, where the organic realm is treated as if it were inorganic. By contrast, a Goethean reading of nature penetrates through to the life forces working and finding expression in natural phenomena, in other words, to *natura naturans*. Reading in the Book of Nature thus leads in Goethe to seeing in a higher sense.[20] This mental recreation of the growth patterns and gestures of living things could thus be said to lead to a knowledge of formative, organic processes which would complement a more analytical understanding of separate constituent parts or *natura naturata*. By imaginatively but precisely reproducing the gesture of a living thing, one is approaching an apprehension of its Gestalt, the complex wholeness which gives it its typical unique character.[21] This essence can, however, only be intuited when the senses have been given their due, when the total material reality of the object has been assimilated. This Goethean approach has been described as a hermeneutics of nature which avoids the false anthropomorphism of the pathetic fallacy in order to read the phenomenon in terms of itself, allowing it to speak for itself rather than imposing meaning on it.[22] A different kind of consciousness is operating here, one that is more intuitive, holistic, concerned with interrelationships rather than intellectual, linear, compartmentalizing.[23] Beyond the sensual experience it is the particular essence of a plant that is glimpsed, its interconnectedness, its necessity. As Saint-Martin says, "A flower represents the invisible reunion of all the properties which exist invisibly, from its root to the flower itself." The naturalist, he says, sees only the visible, whereas the occult philosopher (or Goethean scientist, one might add) sees "what we do not see there."[24]

The epistemology underlying the Goethean reading of nature is totally opposed to that of Cartesianism, in which the dualism between consciousness and the world has led to the so-called onlooker consciousness: the mind is detached from and observes the world outside itself. The other approach, however, sees the knowledge of a phenomenon as being intimately related to the phenomenon itself because for it the state of being known is understood as a further stage of the phenomenon, the stage it reaches in human consciousness. So the knower is not just an onlooker or reader but a participant in nature's processes and the state of being known can be seen as an evolutionary development of nature itself: it is the phenomenon itself which appears in consciousness when it is known. This means that the act of knowing is not a subjective human activity but the final stage in the development of the phenomenon.[25] In Richard Tarnas's description of "this participatory epistemology" we read: "from within its own depths the imagination directly contacts the creative process within nature, realizes that process within itself, and brings nature's reality to conscious expression."[26] Furthermore, one could say that the act of knowing par excellence takes place when the essence of a plant, for example, is articulated and captured in a work of art. Goethe himself said that beauty is the manifestation of secret laws of nature which would otherwise remain eternally hidden and, in a famous prose aphorism, that the person to whom nature begins to reveal her open secrets will feel an irresistible longing for its (nature's) worthiest interpreter or commentator, art.[27] In other words, the sensual reading of a natural object is followed by the production of an internal sense-free equivalent, and this in its turn is then translated, one might say reincarnated, in artistic form.

This more organic understanding of knowledge in fact preceded the modern period. It has been said, for example, that "the involvement of knowledge in being is the presupposition of all classical and medieval thought," where we see "knowledge as an element of being itself and not primarily as an attitude of the subject."[28] Goethe himself has been likened in this respect to Aristotle, who in *De Anima* talks of the reality (*eidos*) which only exists potentially (*dunamei*) until it is known and, when it is known, has its full existence actually (*energeia*). Goethe would have learned this too from German idealism and particularly Schelling, who said that in knowing nature the scientist was also producing it.[29] It should not be forgotten in this context that Proust was greatly influenced by Schelling and the whole *Naturphilosophie* movement. This means that both Proust and Goethe can in different ways be considered in the light of this tradition and its participatory, evolutionary epistemology. In her book *Marcel Proust: Théories pour une esthétique*, Anne Henry writes at length about Proust's debt to Schelling, particularly in the first half of his career, saying, for example: "*Jean Santeuil* is based on a happy confidence in the readability of nature. [. . .] There is not a single of its passages behind which one does not sense some page or other of Schelling or of his followers."[30] There is obviously a great deal more that could be said on the subject, but suffice it for the moment to suggest that the Goethean approach to nature, sensual reading followed by sense-free penetration, could be said to heal the so-called Cartesian split in that it transcends the division between the self and the world that we mentioned earlier.

There is in the central character in *A la recherche du temps perdu* a particularly marked sense of this division, of the gulf separating the *res cogitans* from the *res extensa* and, with it, a great longing to overcome it. In a celebrated early passage in the novel, the narrator is talking about his younger self reading in the garden at Combray. The points made seem equally applicable to other types of reading in the novel. He says: "Quand je voyais un objet extérieur, la conscience que je le voyais restait entre moi et lui, le bordait d'un mince liséré spirituel qui m'empêchait de jamais toucher directement sa matière" [When I saw an external object, my consciousness that I was seeing it would remain between me and it, surrounding it with a thin spiritual border that prevented me from ever touching its substance directly].[31] Here his consciousness, rather than engaging with the object, is perceived as standing between himself and it, preventing direct contact. In other words, a direct sensual reading is impossible; the narrator says much later that his imagination is the only organ with which he can appreciate beauty (3: 872). In order to be able fully to apprehend a phenomenon in the outside world, there needs to be some kind of internal response. The observer needs to complete the sensual experience, to produce "un équivalent spirituel" [a spiritual equivalent] (3: 879). The protagonist is therefore, as one critic puts it, constantly in search of "une extériorité convertible en intériorité" [an exteriority that can be converted into an interiority].³² As Proust himself says, in the discussion of literal reading mentioned above, the successful novelist is one who manages to replace "ces parties impénétrables à l'âme" by "une quantité égale de parties immatérielles, c'est-à-dire que notre âme peut s'assimiler" (1: 85) [Those parts which are impenetrable to the soul [. . .] with an equal quantity of immaterial parts, that is, which our soul can assimilate (1: 91)]. Real people are perceived by our senses, our physical organs, and are therefore opaque. Only via the intermediary of a sense-free, immaterial, internal, "disincarnated" equivalent can something come alive on the level of what Proust calls the soul.

In this famous early passage in the novel Proust is talking theoretically about successful reading. However, in order to find a practical example of sensual reading followed by sense-free assimilation, a prototypical example of what one might call Goethean reading in the Book of Nature, we must turn to the two seminal encounters with the hawthorns which also occur very early in the text. It is therefore these passages that I shall look at now in some detail. Here in fact we see particularly clearly the typical tension in the novel between a sense-free ascetic reading of nature and the cathected reading of people where sensual desire effectively prevents transcendence. These passages provide a striking illustration of different types of reading and both reflect and anticipate the movement in the novel away from the Goethean approach described above. It is as if the younger Proust's enthusiasm for Schelling is still vestigially present at the beginning of *A la recherche du temps perdu* but gradually fades during the writing of the novel.

It is interesting to note that the hawthorns make their first appearance in the text not in nature but in the church at Combray, the Book of Nature being thus immediately put into a religious context: "N'étant pas seulement dans l'église, si sainte, mais où nous avions le droit d'entrer, posées sur l'autel même, inséparables des mystères à la célébration desquels elles prenaient part" (1: 112) [Not only were they in the church, where, holy ground as it was, we had all of us a right of entry, but arranged upon the altar itself, inseparable from the mysteries in whose celebration they participated (1: 121)]. From the very beginning they are thus associated with the sacramental, with the visible pointing to and representing an invisible mystery, with the sensual reality standing for and leading to a spiritual truth. The language of flowers is here intimately connected to the symbolic language of cultic objects. Furthermore, there is a hint of a necessary relationship between nature, the mystery celebrated, and the time of year, the "mois de Marie." Nature is in fact personified here, as *natura naturans*. It is said to have actively shaped the leaves and added the ornaments of the flowers in order to render the hawthorns worthy of the occasion: "c'était la nature elle-même qui [. . .] avait rendu cette décoration digne de ce qui était à la fois une réjouissance populaire et une solennité mystique" (1: 112) [It was Nature herself who [. . .] had made the decorations worthy of what was at once a public rejoicing and a solemn mystery (1: 121)]. In other words, at this point the language used is suggestive of a meaning or intention behind or beyond the plant which is realized, visible, one might say legible in the plant.

Increasingly, however, it is the hawthorns themselves which are personified: "Plus haut s'ouvraient leurs corolles çà et là avec une grâce insouciante, retenant si négligemment le bouquet d'étamines" (1: 112) [Higher up on the altar, a flower had opened here and there with a careless grace, holding so unconcernedly [. . .] its bunch of stamens" (1: 121)]. And then we read the following striking phrase:

> en suivant, en essayant de mimer au fond de moi le geste de leur efflorescence, je l'imaginais comme si ç'avait été le mouvement de tête étourdi et rapide, au regard coquet, aux pupilles diminuées, d'une blanche jeune fille, distraite et vive. (1: 112)
> [In following, in trying to mimic to myself the action of their efflorescence, I imagined it as a swift and thoughtless movement of the head, with a provocative glance from her contracted pupils, by a young girl in white, insouciant and vivacious.] (1: 121)

This language is very reminiscent of the approach to nature that I attempted to characterize earlier, whereby the phenomenon is internally and imaginatively reproduced. Moreover, it is a process which is mentioned here—"efflorescence"—rather than a static image, and Proust uses the word "geste" to describe the particular movement, growth, the organic quality of the plants.

The internalized equivalent in this case is the image of a girl.

In other words, as with Goethe, we have the sensual reading of a natural object leading to its disembodied internal translation which in its turn then takes the form of something analogous in the outside world. It could be argued that this analogy is more of a metonymy than a metaphor, given that M. Vinteuil is described as sitting with his daughter next to Marcel and his family in the church. Indeed, the very next sentence begins "M. Vinteuil était venu avec sa fille" (1: 112) [M. Vinteuil had come in with his daughter" (1: 121)], so there is textual as well as spatial contiguity, and there follows a short digression on M. Vinteuil, to which I shall return later, which takes us right up to the moment when Marcel leaves the church and the hawthorns are mentioned again. Here the association between Mlle. Vinteuil and the hawthorn is made more explicit: "je remarquai alors sur les fleurs de petites places plus blondes sous lesquelles je me figurai que devait être cachée cette odeur, comme [. . .] sous leurs taches de rousseur, celui des joues de Mlle Vinteuil" (1: 113) [I then noticed on the flowers themselves little patches of a creamier colour, beneath which I imagined that this fragrance must lie concealed, as the taste of [. . .] Mlle Vinteuil's cheeks beneath their freckles" (1: 123)]. The notion of edibility is also introduced here and will be picked up again later. Finally we read of the flowers' "intermittente odeur" which "était comme le murmure de leur vie intense dont l'autel vibrait," and the reddish stamens are said to seem to have retained "la virulence printanière, le pouvoir irritant, d'insectes aujourd'hui metamorphosés en fleurs" (1: 114) [gusts of fragrance [. . .] like the murmuring of an intense organic life, with which the whole altar was quivering [. . .] the springtime virulence, the irritant power of stinging insects now transmuted into flowers (1: 123)]. We have therefore moved from the implied purity and chastity of bridal whiteness at the beginning to the more dangerous, libidinal qualities of pinkness and redness at the end of the passage. In this presentation of the plant there seems to be a necessary relationship between its being or essence and the color it takes on.

The next encounter with the hawthorns takes place shortly afterwards, this time in nature. The synaesthesia of smell and sound is immediately picked up again: the path is said to be "tout bourdonnant de l'odeur des aubépines" (1: 138) [throbbing with the fragrance of hawthorn-blossom (1: 150)]. Now, in an elaborate conceit ostensibly deriving from Marcel's first glimpse of the flowers in the church, the hedge is compared to a series of chapels; once again the hawthorns are closely, if more implicitly associated with a sacrament, the flowers being "amoncelées en reposoir" (1: 138) [heaped upon their altars (1:150)]. Here the stamens are said to be "fines et rayonnantes nervures du style flamboyant" (1: 138) [delicate radiating veins in the flamboyant style (1:150)]: the comparison between the patterns in the plant and the patterns of Gothic architecture (suggestive of order and intention) centers on the word "nervures" which is applicable to both (as well as to insects, incidentally) and is something Proust would have found in his reading of Ruskin. Personification of the hawthorns also continues: they are "parées" and holding "chacune d'un air distrait son étincelant bouquet d'étamines" (1: 138) [adorned [. . .] each its little bunch of glittering stamens with an absent-minded air" (1:150)].

Again Marcel feels called upon to go beyond a purely sensual reading of the hawthorns, "à m'unir au rythme qui jetait leurs fleurs" (1:139) [absorbing myself in the rhythm which disposed their flowers" (1: 151)], but this time he is unable to do so:

Mais j'avais beau rester devant les aubépines à respirer, à porter devant ma pensée qui ne savait ce qu'elle devait en faire [. . .] elles m'offraient indéfiniment le même charme avec une profusion inépuisable, mais sans me laisser approfondir davantage. (1: 139)
[But it was in vain that I lingered beside the hawthorns—inhaling, trying to fix in my mind (which did not know what to do with it) [. . .] they went on offering me the same charm in inexhaustible profusion, but without letting me delve any more deeply.] (1:151)

It is interesting to note that he speaks of the "rythme qui jetait leurs fleurs" and not "que jetaient leurs fleurs": the idea here seems to be that the rhythm—again movement, growth in time, and not a static image—comes before and is expressed in the flowers. This notion of an intention in nature is picked up again later when he mentions the "intention de festivité," translated by nature in the flowers and talks of "l'essence particulière, irrésistible de l'épine qui, partout où elle bourgeonnait, où elle allait fleurir, ne le pouvait qu'en rose"(1:140) [the special, irresistible quality of the thorn-bush which, wherever it budded, wherever it was about to blossom, could do so in pink alone (1: 153)], thereby also introducing the idea of necessity. It is as if pinkness is a quintessential attribute of the hawthorn.

One could obviously go into a great deal more detail here, but it might be useful to stop and summarize what we have seen so far: first, that the thinking subject can go beyond a purely sensual reading of an object and can internalize and imaginatively reproduce it; second, that each plant has a particular and unique gesture, essence, or language, an inner necessity, which is in this way apprehended by the participant in nature's processes (*natura naturans*); and third, that it is nature's own intentions, nature's meanings, which are articulated and thus legible in the plant. (The personification of the hawthorns holding out their stamens also to some extent reinforces this point.)

And yet these descriptions of the hawthorns, in many ways so reminiscent of Goethe's approach to nature and so rich in echoes of Schelling's world view, go hand in hand with a number of other features which subvert and relativize this reading in the Book of Nature, thereby anticipating the movement away from nature which we witness during the course of the novel. Indeed, this movement can be traced in microcosm in the differences between the two appearances of the hawthorns in that, with their second appearance, we are already beginning to move away from an appreciation of them in their autonomous essence into an increasingly human realm. The second time, as we have seen, Marcel does not succeed in internalizing them; he is unable to go beyond a sensual reading, although on both occasions he makes a similar effort: "sans oser les regarder qu'à la dérobée" [though I dared not look at it save through my fingers] the first time, and "je me détournais d'elles un moment" (1: 121) [I turned away from them for a moment (1: 151)] the second.

This is in fact a pattern which we find elsewhere in the novel. Descriptions frequently occur in pairs: a phenomenon appears, is described at length, only to reappear shortly afterwards in the text and form the basis of a second descriptive passage. This is also the case with, for example, the Martinville spires, where the narrator's retrospective account of their apparent movement is followed, this time immediately, by his younger self's first literary draft on the subject. Moreover, as one critic has noted: "Each of the two descriptions receives something like the reflection of the other, they illuminate each other like sun and moon; but it is always the first which is the source of light and movement, it is more humid, supple, united, an entity [. . .] While its reflection becomes fragmented, drier, darker" (Boucquey, 55). She goes on to suggest that the first passage is closer to the lost memory and is therefore fresher, less intellectual than the second. This is something of an imponderable and perhaps not immediately relevant here. What is important, however, is to note that the idea of *natura naturans* gradually recedes in order to make way for an increasingly human, domesticated realm. In this context one could mention the movement from the purer, more ascetic, and spiritual associations of white to the more erotic, cathected connotations of pink. Indeed, pinkness, as we have seen, is given explicitly childish and edible associations:

> Et justement ces fleurs avaient choisi une de ces teintes de chose mangeable ou de tendre embellissement à une toilette pour une grande fête, qui, parce qu'elles leur présentent la raison de leur supériorité, sont celles qui semblent belles avec le plus d'évidence aux yeux des enfants et, à cause de cela, gardent toujours pour eux quelque chose de plus vif et de plus naturel que les autres teintes, même lorsqu'ils ont compris qu'elles ne promettaient rien à leur gourmandise et n'avaient pas été choisies par la couturière. (1: 139–40)
> [And these flowers had chosen precisely one of those colours of some edible and delicious thing, or of some fond embellishment of a costume for a major feast, which, inasmuch as they make plain the reason for their superiority, are those whose beauty is most evident to the eyes of children, and for that reason must always seem more vivid and more natural than any other tints, even after the child's mind has realised that they offer no gratification to the appetite and have not been selected by the dressmaker.] (1: 152)]

This emphasis on the arbitrariness of the child's viewpoint seems to relativize and even slightly ironize the later reference to the essential pinkness of the flowers. The greater prestige of pinkness begins to seem to derive less from it being a necessary expression of an intention of nature and more from its associations with food the child enjoys eating. A sense of the autonomous working of *natura naturans* is eclipsed by this evocation of basic human needs and desires.

This association of aesthetic enjoyment with the pleasure of eating recalls another interesting passage in Combray where Marcel sees some buttercups which are as yellow as the yolk of an egg but which cannot satisfy the hunger they awake in him. They are described as "brillant d'autant plus [. . .] que ne pouvant dériver vers aucune velléité de dégustation le plaisir que leur vue me causait, je l'accumulais dans leur surface dorée, jusqu'à ce qu'il devînt assez puissant pour produire de l'inutile beauté" (1: 167–68) [glowing with an added lustre, [. . .], because, being powerless to consummate with my palate the pleasure which the sight of them never failed to give me, I would let it accumulate as my eyes ranged over their golden expanse, until it became potent enough to produce an effect of absolute, purposeless beauty" (1: 183)]. As Jean Pommier has said, this is a remarkable sentence: "Aesthetic pleasure would thus seem to result from the repetition that occurs near the surface of inedible things whose matter does not lend itself to a deeper assimilation. It too is thus derivative and second-best. Useless beauty indeed, if the disinterested joy of art replaces the animal pleasure of absorption, without entirely consoling the disappointed appetite."³³ As with the second appearance of the hawthorns, it is as if the sensual desires of the observer are interfering with and undermining the claims of a sense-free Goethean reading of the phenomenon. The physical appetite seems to take precedence over and thus implicitly to subvert or at least relativize the aesthetic sense as we are reminded to almost humorous effect of the child's perspective.

We move too from a comparison of nature to religious architecture, with its related implicit analogy between an intention in nature and artistic intention, to a comparison of nature to lesser, more decorative art forms. For example, the flowers are likened to "des pompons qui enguirlandent une houlette rococo" (1: 139) [the tassels wreathed about the crook of a rococo shepherdess" (1: 152)] and later to a "pompadour provincial" (1: 140) [this rustic "pompadour" (1: 153)]. There is a sense in which nature is increasingly denied its autonomy, becoming instead more and more humanized and domesticated. For example, Proust says: "ce n'était pas facticement, par un artifice de fabrication humaine, qu'était traduite l'intention de festivité dans les fleurs" but then continues: "c'était la nature qui, spontanément, l'avait exprimée avec la naïveté d'une commerçante de village travaillant pour un reposoir" (1: 140) [it was in no artificial manner, by no device of human fabrication that the festal intention of these flowers was revealed [. . .] it was Nature herself who had spontaneously expressed it, with the simplicity of a woman from a village shop labouring at the decoration of a street altar for some procession" (1: 152)]. In other words, we are told that nature is completely autonomous and nonhuman as it translates its intentions in the flowers only to see it personified in the very next phrase, and not as a great artist but rather as a simple "commerçante de village." This also seems to be a pattern that is repeated elsewhere in the novel. Marcel's desire to go to Balbec to witness "un moment dévoilé de la vie réelle de la nature [. . .] la force ou [. . .] la grâce de la nature telle qu'elle se manifeste, livrée à elle-même, sans l'intervention des hommes" (1: 384) [a momentary revelation of the true life of nature [. . .] the force or the grace of nature as it appeared when left entirely to itself, without human interference" (1: 417)] is ironically undercut a few sentences later by Legrandin's comment on the hotels which are now built there. Similarly, Tante Léonie's "tilleuls," to which a long descriptive passage is devoted very near the beginning of the novel (1: 51–52; 1: 55–56), are a dead, dried, cut-up version of the living trees outside, prepared for consumption by an aging hypochondriac.

Other factors also contribute towards this devaluing and relativizing of nature. Here, as so often in the novel, one could argue that the sheer quantity and complexity of the images sometimes has the effect of making us lose sight of the original phenomenon being described. The hawthorn passages are self-referential in this respect: nature, the "commerçante," is said to work "en surchargeant l'arbuste de ces rosettes d'un ton trop tendre et d'un pompadour provincial [. . .] de manière à ne laisser aucune place qui ne fût décorée" (1: 140) [by overloading the bush with these little rosettes, almost too ravishing in colour, this rustic "pompadour" [. . .] so thickly as to leave no part of the tree undecorated (1: 152–53)]. In other words, nature's art is here seen as precious, even gratuitous. There is indeed a rococo feel to much of the metaphorical writing in the novel (particularly about nature) where, as a number of critics have pointed out, the text no longer functions mimetically to describe an event or object but insistently refers to its own stylistic technique, thereby subverting representation.[34] Just as the virtuosity and ornamental inventiveness of nature make its creations begin, paradoxically, to seem unnatural, so does Proust's style increasingly draw attention to itself (and thereby to the human agent behind it) and away from any sense of the autonomous reality of the object being described.

Another important factor here is the role played by context. Following Paul de Man, it has now become quite common for critics to deconstruct Proust's metaphors as metonymies, in other words, to suggest that some images, far from being based on the necessary association of two disparate elements, derive instead from their chance contiguity.[35] In the case of the hawthorns, we have already seen that their first appearance is framed by references to M. Vinteuil and, particularly, his daughter, while their second appearance leads into a description of Marcel's first glimpse of another object of desire, Gilberte. Whether the contiguity operating here is the spatial contiguity of girl and flower on Marcel's experiential level or their textual contiguity on the narratorial level is perhaps less relevant than the fact that the juxtaposition of the two may make the comparison of hawthorns to girls seem less necessary, less essential. We have a sense that what one critic has called "seepage"[36] is going on here, and there seems to be some kind of blurring of the aesthetic and the erotic just as we have seen a blurring of the pleasures of observing nature and eating.

Context is important in other ways too, however. The first appearance of the hawthorns is framed by references to the Vinteuils, as we have seen, but in the middle of this passage there is also a long digression on the way in which Marcel through the window sees M. Vinteuil put a piece of music on the piano only to remove it a few minutes later with feigned embarrassment when his—Marcel's—parents arrive on a visit. This passage is crucial because of the way it anticipates and prepares for Marcel's later act of voyeurism through the same window when he witnesses a lesbian encounter between Mlle. Vinteuil and her friend. However, its position here in the text also seems to invite us to compare and contrast the two acts of seeing or reading, on the one hand the hawthorns, on the other hand M. Vinteuil. In the second tableau, we are presented with both the gesture and its hidden meaning, which is quickly and easily deciphered by Marcel. Human beings can emit deliberately deceptive signs[37] (Vinteuil puts on a show of modesty), but it is possible to see through these to the true intention (he wants to draw people's attention to his compositions). Nature, on the other hand, emits a different kind of sign, this being an expression of its true meaning or essence. In both cases the gesture is incomplete without human involvement and interpretation: for the first, Marcel can understand what M. Vinteuil really means; with the second, the observer of nature has to internalize the phenomenon in order to help it to realize its intention.

Something similar is happening with the second appearance of the hawthorns. This leads into a description of the sign emitted by Gilberte, a sign which also requires interpretation:

> sa main esquissait en même temps un geste indécent, auquel, quand il était adressé en public à une personne qu'on ne connaissait pas, le petit dictionnaire de civilité que je portais en moi ne donnait qu'un seul sens, celui d'une intention insolente. (1: 141)
> [her hand, at the same time, sketched in the air an indelicate gesture, for which, when it was addressed in public to a person whom one did not know, the little dictionary of manners which I carried in

my mind supplied only one meaning, namely, a deliberate insult.] (1: 154).

Note in the passage above the use of the word *geste* that translates Gilberte's intention.

This time, however, Marcel gets it wrong, just as he fails with the hawthorns: a couple of thousand pages later we learn that the gesture was not one of contempt but of desire. Human signs can therefore be misleading as well as deceptive. This whole passage seems to trace and prefigure Marcel's movement away from the more neutral, detached reading of nature to a reading of human gestures which is inextricably bound up with the senses and desire. The gestures of nature are gradually replaced by the human gestures of desire. Leo Bersani talks about the parallel between trying to understand the loved one's desires and trying to penetrate the hawthorns;[38] one might also add that the former activity gradually replaces the latter. In other words, girls become more important than flowers, as the title of the second volume, *A l'ombre des jeunes filles en fleurs,* also seems to suggest.

This second hawthorns passage is central because of the insight it gives into the tension between two different ways of reading experience. As such, it illuminates the future career of the central figure as well as of other characters in the novel. On the one hand, there is the involvement and yet inner detachment of the Goethean approach where one does not stop at the physical material reality of the phenomenon being observed but attempts to penetrate beyond it.[39] On the other hand, there is the reading which remains bound up with the senses and does not manage to transcend the physical. It will be apparent that it is the former approach, with its inner activity, ascesis and sublimation, which is necessary for the production of art, while the latter treats the object as an end in itself and is characteristic of the failed creativity of the would-be artists Swann and Charlus.

It seems therefore that, the more desire is present, the less clear and objective will be one's reading, the less able one will be to let the phenomenon speak for itself. The progression from ascetic reading to cathected reading can be clearly traced in the narrator's analysis of the different glances his younger self directs at Gilberte. He talks first of the sudden vision of the young girl appearing among the flowers, a vision which "ne s'adresse pas seulement à nos regards, mais requiert des perceptions plus profondes et dispose de notre être tout entier" (1: 140) [appeals not to our eyes only but requires a deeper kind of perception and takes possession of the whole of our being (1: 153)]. So far there seems to be little difference from the Goethean reading of nature which could also be said to demand more than just a sensual response and to require deeper involvement than is the case with the detached onlooker position implicit in the Cartesian world view.[40] Then, however, the narrator goes on to describe how his younger self looks at her "de ce regard qui n'est pas que le porte-parole des yeux, mais à la fenêtre duquel se penchent tous les sens, anxieux et pétrifiés, le regard qui voudrait toucher, capturer, emmener le corps qu'il regarde et l'âme avec lui" (1: 141) [with that gaze which is not merely the messenger of the eyes, but at whose window all the senses assemble and lean out, petrified and anxious, a gaze eager to reach, touch, capture, bear off in triumph the body at which it is aimed, and the soul with the body (1: 154)]. Here there is a reference to reading with all the senses but these are not in a state of alert but relaxed receptivity as is the case with Goethean reading: instead they are described as anxious and petrified, wanting to go beyond the sensual experience of touching in order to capture and possess. What is more, it will be apparent that the young Marcel wants to achieve an impossibility: he wants to penetrate and possess with his physical organs something which is immaterial, her soul, without this time going via the intermediary of an inner "spiritual equivalent." Finally, the third glance at Gilberte is even more cathected, being described as "inconsciemment supplicateur, qui tâchait de la forcer à faire attention à moi, à me connaître!" (1: 141) [an unconsciously imploring look, whose object was to force her to pay attention to me, to see, to know me (1:154)]. In other words, not only does he want to possess her, he also wants her to notice and acknowledge him. This can be seen as one stage further removed from the Goethean approach which considers the object without any prejudices or expectations but allows it total liberty to be itself and to speak for itself.

That a sense-free reading of nature is more difficult and demanding to achieve than a sensual reading of human beings seems to be implicit in the differences between the two passages we have considered which begin with the working of *natura naturans* and end with the boy's wistful interrogation of Gilberte. It also seems to be implied by a striking passage much later in the novel where the narrator says of his desire for Albertine that it was "une forme paresseuse, lâche et incomplète de posséder Balbec, comme si posséder matériellement une chose [...] équivalait à la posséder spirituellement" (2: 351) [a lazy, cowardly and incomplete form of possessing Balbec, as if to possess a thing materially [. . .] were tantamount to possessing it spiritually (2: 364)]. Physical possession may give the illusion of spiritual possession and thus distract from it. This is an illusion which Proust elsewhere describes as idolatry.[41] As we have seen, however, the only way in which a phenomenon can be spiritually possessed is through an act of inner creativity where the sensual reading of its physical materiality represents a necessary first step but is then transcended by the creation of a mental and, perhaps, artistic equivalent. This is what happens with the writing of *A la recherche du temps perdu*, whereas the story the novel tells is that of a man moving ever further away from his early epiphanic encounters with nature into an increasingly human, mental, even solipsistic world. Reading in the Book of Nature is gradually replaced by the sensual reading of other people.

Notes

1. This expression is used by Michel Raimond in *Proust romancier* (Paris: Société d'enseignement supérieur, 1984), chap. 6. See too Gilles Deleuze, *Marcel Proust et les signes* (Paris: P.U.F., 1964). Translations of all quotations, unless otherwise stated, are mine.

2. *Proust et le monde sensible* (Paris: Seuil, 1974), 133.

3. Edward Bizub, *La Venise intérieure: Proust et la poétique de la traduction* (Neuchâtel: A la Baconnière, 1991), 123.

4. Some lines he wrote neatly exemplify this tradition: "Omnis mundi creatura / quasi liber et pictura / nobis est in speculum. / Nostri status pingit rosa / nostri status decens glosa / nostrae vitae lectio." [As if it were a book and a picture Every plant and animal on earth holds up the mirror to us. The rose gives a picture of our condition, a fitting comment on our position and reading of our life] This verse is quoted in Philip Knight, *Flower Poetics in Nineteenth-Century France* (Oxford: Clarendon Press, 1986), 7.

5. See, for example, Ernst Robert Curtius, *Europäische Literatur und lateinisches Mittelalter* (Bern: A. Francke, 1948), and Hans Blumenberg, *Die Lesbarkeit der Welt* (Frankfurt: Suhrkamp, 1983).

6. Gilbert Gaston in *Proust, l'homme des mondes: Une lecture d' "A la recherche du temps perdu"* (Paris: Kimé, 1993), talks of "the shrinking of natural space as the novel unfolds. Nature is Proust's 'peau de chagrin,'" 273.

7. *Cathexis* is Freud's term for a charge of psychical energy concentrated upon an object, person, or idea. This is explained in his *Introductory Lectures on Psychoanalysis*, trans. James Strachey (Harmondsworth: Penguin, 1978), 380–82.

8. Eliane Boucquey, *Un Chasseur dans l'image: Proust et le temps caché* (Paris: Armand Colin, 1992), 60. See too Antoine Compagnon, *Proust entre deux siècles* (Paris: Seuil, 1989).

9. See particularly A. Viatte, *Les Sources occultes du romantisme*, 2 vols. (Paris: Champion, 1928).

10. Quoted in Knight, 43–44.
11. Ibid., 19.
12. Luc Ferry, *Le Nouvel ordre écologique* (Paris: Grasset, 1992), 20.
13. Boucquey, 147.
14. See, for example, Max Oelschlaeger, *The Idea of Wilderness: From Prehistory to the Age of Ecology* (New Haven: Yale University Press, 1991), 122–23.
15. Richard Tarnas, *The Passion of the Western Mind* (London: Pimlico, 1996), 378.
16. Goethe said, for example: "Ich [. . .] hatte die Maxime ergriffen, mich so viel als möglich zu verläugnen und das Objekt so rein, als nur zu tun wäre, in mich aufzunehmen" [I [. . .] had adopted the maxim of denying myself as much as possible and of assimilating the object as purely as was at all possible]. This is quoted in Peter Sachtleben, *Mit den Augen denken lernen: Einführung in die Naturstudien Goethes* (Schaffhausen: Novalis, 1994), 196.
17. This is explained in Charles Davy, *Towards a Third Culture* (Edinburgh: Floris, 1978), 69–70.
18. This is quoted in Henri Bortoft, *Goethe's Scientific Consciousness*, The Institute for Cultural Research Monograph Series, No. 22 (Nottingham: Russell Press, 1986), 14.
19. Goethe talks of observing the "Entstehung" [growth] of a phenomenon in order to achieve "das Anschauen eines Werdenden" [the observation of a process of development]. This is quoted in Sachtleben, 195.
20. Goethe said: "Wenn wir einen Gegenstand in allen seinen Teilen übersehen, recht fassen und ihn im Geiste wiederhervorbringen können, so dürfen wir sagen, daß wir ihn im eigentlichen und höheren Sinne anschauen" [When we can get an overview of an object in all its parts, really grasp it and can reproduce it in our mind, then we may say that we can—in the real and higher sense—observe it]. This is quoted in Sachtleben, 184.
21. Davy, 121.
22. Bortoft, 59.
23. Ibid., 29–34.
24. Quoted in Knight, 20.
25. This epistemology is very lucidly presented in Bortoft, 66–72, on which I have drawn here.
26. Op. cit., 434. Coleridge, for example, talked of the analogy and link between nature and the mind. He said, "If the artist copies the mere nature, the *natura naturata*, what idle rivalry! [. . .] Believe me, you must master the essence, the *natura naturans*, which presupposes a bond between nature in the higher sense and the soul of man." This is quoted in *The Theory of Criticism: From Plato to the Present*, ed. Raman Selden (London and New York: Longman, 1988), 26. Compare too with Joseph L. Esposito, *Schelling's Idealism and Philosophy of Nature* (Cranbury, N.J.: New Jersey, Associated University Presses, 1977), 112.
27. Both these quotations are to be found in *Readings in Goethean Science*, comp. Herbert H. Koepf and Linda S. Jolly (Spring Valley, N.Y.: Bio-Dynamic Literature, 1978), 24.
28. Gadamer quoted in Bortoft, 70.
29. See Bortoft, 70.
30. *Marcel Proust: Théories pour une esthétique* (Paris: Klincksieck, 1981), 140.
31. Proust, *A la recherche du temps perdu*, texte établi et présenté par

Pierre Clarac et André Ferré, 3 vols. (Paris: Gallimard, 1954), 1: 84. English translation: *Remembrance of Things Past*, trans. C. K. Scott Moncrieff and Terence Kilmartin (London: The Folio Society, 1981), 1: 90. All subsequent references to the French text and English translation will be made by volume and page number immediately following the quotation.

32. Gaëtan Picon, *Lecture de Proust* (Paris: Mercure de France, 1963), 108.

33. This is quoted in *Les Critiques de notre temps et Proust* (Paris: Garnier, 1971), 52.

34. See, for example, Margaret E. Gray, *Postmodern Proust* (Philadelphia: University of Pennsylvania Press, 1992), 118.

35. De Man talks of the "figural play in which contingent figures of chance masquerade deceptively as figures of necessity" in *Allegories of Reading: Figural Language in Rousseau, Nietzsche, Rilke, and Proust* (New Haven and London: Yale University Press, 1979), 67.

36. Gray, 86.

37. Compare much of Deleuze, *Marcel Proust et les signes*.

38. *Marcel Proust: The Fictions of Life and of Art* (Oxford: Oxford University Press, 1965), 61.

39. Davy, 120.

40. In her discussion of voyeuristic episodes in Proust, Gray talks of the narrator as a "dispassionate, withdrawn spectator" witnessing the homosexual encounter between Charlus and Jupien, 52. This sounds very much like the onlooker position and it is interesting to note that botanical analogies are used here in order to elucidate human behavior.

41. See, for example, the discussion in Walter Kasell, *Marcel Proust and the Strategy of Reading* (Amsterdam: John Benjamins B. V., 1980), 25.

Works Cited

Bersani, Jacques, ed. *Les Critiques de notre temps et Proust*. Paris: Garnier Frères, 1971.

Bersani, Leo. *Marcel Proust: The Fictions of Life and of Art*. Oxford: Oxford University Press, 1965.

Bizub, Edward. *La Venise intérieure: Proust et la poétique de la traduction*. Neuchâtel: A la Baconnière, 1991.

Blumenberg, Hans. *Die Lesbarkeit der Welt*. Frankfurt: Suhrkamp, 1983.

Bortoft, Henri. *Goethe's Scientific Consciousness*. Institute for Cultural Research Monograph Series, no. 22. Nottingham: Russell Press, 1986.

Boucquey, Eliane. *Un Chasseur dans l'image: Proust et le temps caché*. Paris: Armand Colin, 1992.

Compagnon, Antoine. *Proust entre deux siècles*. Paris: Seuil, 1989.

Curtius, Ernst Robert. *Europäische Literatur und lateinisches Mittelalter*. Bern: A. Francke, 1948.

Davy, Charles. *Towards a Third Culture*. Edinburgh: Floris, 1978.

Deleuze, Gilles. *Marcel Proust et les signes*. Paris: P. U. F., 1964.

de Man, Paul. *Allegories of Reading: Figural Language in Rousseau, Nietzsche, Rilke and Proust*. New Haven and London: Yale University Press, 1979.

Esposito, Joseph L. *Schelling's Idealism and Philosophy of Nature*. Cranbury, N.J.: Associated University Presses, 1977.

Ferry, Luc. *Le Nouvel ordre écologique*. Paris: Grasset, 1992.

Freud, Sigmund. *Introductory Lectures on Psychoanalysis*. Translated by James Strachey. Harmondsworth: Penguin, 1978.

Gaston, Gilbert. *Proust L'Homme des mondes: Une lecture d' "A la recherche du temps perdu*. Paris: Kimé, 1993.

Gray, Margaret E. *Postmodern Proust*. Philadelphia: University of Pennsylvania Press, 1992.

Henry, Anne. *Marcel Proust: Théories pour une esthétique*. Paris: Klincksieck, 1981.

Kasell, Walter. *Marcel Proust and the Strategy of Reading*. Amsterdam: John Benjamins B. V., 1980.

Knight, Philip. *Flower Poetics in Nineteenth-Century France*. Oxford: Clarendon, 1986.

Koepf, Herbert H., and Linda S. Jolly, *Readings in Goethean Science*. Spring Valley N. Y.: Bio-Dynamic Literature, 1978.

Oelschlaeger, Max. *The Idea of Wilderness: From prehistory to the Age of Ecology*. New Haven: Yale University Press, 1991.

Picon, Gaëtan. *Lecture de Proust*. Paris: Mercure de France, 1963.

Raimond, Michel. *Proust romancier*. Paris: Société d'enseignement supérieur, 1984.

Richard, Jean-Pierre. *Proust et le monde sensible*. Paris: Seuil, 1974.

Sachtleben, Peter. *Mit den Augen denken lernen: Einführung in die Naturstudien Goethes*. Schaffhausen: Novalis, 1984.

Selden, Raman, ed. *The Theory of Criticism: From Plato to the Present*. London and New York: Longman, 1988.

Tarnas, Richard. *The Passion of the Western Mind*. London: Pimlico, 1996.

Viatte, A. *Les Sources occultes du romantisme*, 2 vols. Paris: Champion, 1928.

VI
TELESENSUALITIES

Andy's Wedding: Reading Warhol
PETER KRAPP

omnibus auditur: sonus est, qui vivit in illa
—Ovid, *Metamorphoses*

FOR ANDY WARHOL, "NON-COMMUNICATION" WAS NOT A PROBLEM—"I think everyone understands everyone," he said; yet he remained detached, even remote: "I don't want to get involved in other people's lives. . . . I don't want to get too close. . . . I don't like to touch things . . . that's why my work is so distant from myself."[1] So how are we to read Andy Warhol—from afar? He tried, according to his own statements, to see and record everything, although he knew this to be impossible even with the help of all the technology he could get: " 'But it's impossible,' he said, 'it's impossible! I tried, but it is impossible. It's impossible to carry with you a movie camera, a tape recorder, and a still camera at the same time. I wish I could do it.' "[2] Thus reading Warhol in his obsession with witnessing might offer an experience of the impossible, something singularly volatile. On the other hand there is, again, a matter of repetition, a question of storage. While repetition is often considered tedious, infantile, and (especially in the tradition of the Frankfurt School[3]) unhappy, Andy Warhol's thoughts on these topics are seriously underrated: he was, after all, one of the foremost thinkers on such topics as repetition and aura, and perhaps the one who originally debunked originality. Warhol's use of modern media technology did not stop at works on paper or canvas or the screen; he also produced a novel in the Factory, a text which, taped and transcribed, returns to the question of writing anew. For writing, far from being reducible to mechanical repetition, nevertheless exhibits a certain "mechanical" resistance to presentation or analysis. Thus reading, in turn, can end up having to deal with tape-recorded speech, despite Hans Georg Gadamer's protestations to the contrary: a real text, he claims, would be written for the reader and not merely a fixation of voice, tone, and gesture by means of tape recording; consequently, the kind of text Warhol presents must remain impossible to understand for the Gadamerian reader. The ideality of the eminent text as an extension of the reach of communication, as that which "wants to be read," would have to remain linear and unchanged, untouched by reading.[4] Its sense would be prescribed, and only to be voiced by the reader. Arguably, to consider writing a mere addition to speech on the other hand would mean to admit that the sense of speech had from the beginning fallen short of itself. Navigating between the hermeneutic gesture which would exclude Warhol a priori and the journalistic amusement his written work was greeted with we will try to map out a way of reading Warhol.

Warhol's text requires the reader to decode the specific hiatus, the asymmetry of deferred communication: both voice and aura are considered inimitable and unrepeatable, and the task of teletechnology would be to capture their moment, preserve the voice, reproduce the aura. Warhol was so obsessed by this and so deeply in love with technology that eventually he considered himself married to it. Practically living by proxy, always on the phone, watching TV, he relentlessly recorded his Factory personnel on tape or on video. In his first book, *The Philosophy of Andy Warhol from a to b and back again*, he confessed:

> So in the 50s I started an affair with my television which has continued to the present, when I play around in my bedroom with as many as four at a time. But I didn't get married until 1964 when I got my first tape recorder. My wife. My tape recorder and I have been married for ten years now. When I say "we," I mean my tape recorder and me. A lot of people don't understand that.[5]

Therefore, when the *Andy Warhol Diaries* came out after his death, consisting of carefully edited transcriptions of tapes by Pat Hackett, it could be said that his wife had written his memoirs while he was still alive. When he started recording interviews for his book *POPism*, he would bring two tape recorders and run one while changing the tape in the other, so that nothing could escape.[6] And in the same manner, Warhol—who spent much of his time on the phone, while trying to take in everything that went on around him—produced the book published in 1968 as *a. a novel*, consisting of 451 pages of taped, transcribed Factory activities and telephone conversations.[7]

Warhol and his "wife" SONY had been following Robert Olivio, alias Ondine, one of the first Factory stars, and simply recorded him everywhere. As Olivio recalls three years later:

We tried to do 24 hours at one stop, and it became . . . it was just too much. I mean, Andy followed me into the toilet room when I was taking a shit. It was just impossible. It was literally impossible. It was literally like crawling up the walls. Have you ever had anyone do that to you? It's just . . . It's a fabulous book, isn't it? I mean, it is a totally fabulous book, but . . . but how can you say that to anybody?[8]

Warhol's intrusive witness protection program does not relieve the senses, nor does it heighten them; it offers love and attention, but only on condition of total control in repetition and recall. One day in the life of Ondine—the impossible Factory experience starts like this:

Rattle, gurgle, clink, tinkle.
Click, pause, click, ring.
Dial, dial.
ONDINE—You said (*dial*) that, that, if, if you pick, pick UP the Mayor's voice on the
other end (*dial, pause, dial-dial-dial*), the Mayor's sister would know us, be (*busy-busy-busy*).
DRELLA—We should start for the park, right? Okay. Hmm. *Coin drops. Money*
jingles as coins return. car noises in the background You're a clunk. Are there any way stations on the way that we have to (*honk, honk*) like uh, I, wha—(noise). If we go through, through the park, is there ANY place we can keep calling your uh, I mean right through the, uh, phone call. Is there any place where we can keep call him if we— Answering service . . . Are you (*cars honking, blasting*). Are there difFERent places—are there different places where we can call your ans—oh.

When *a* was sold for 10 dollars a copy in 1968, complete with carefully preserved typing mistakes, the reception was very reserved; it was read mostly as a frivolous portrait of sixties drug culture. The only good review it ever got was from *Playboy*, praising its "microcosm of words, mutilated sentences, grunts, giggles and blah blahs surrounding us."[9] We can safely infer, however, that Warhol was hardly bothered when confronted with the question as to whether or not there was any "realism" in it. Seven years after publishing *a*, Warhol explained: "Nothing was ever a problem again, because a problem just meant a good tape, and when a problem transforms itself into a good tape it's not a problem any more. An interesting problem was an interesting tape. Everybody knew that and performed for the tape. You couldn't tell which problems were real and which problems were exaggerated for the tape. Better yet, the people telling you the problems couldn't decide any more if they were really having the problems or if they were just performing."[10] At stake here is the very distinction between observer and observed: the other of interiority is not simply its opposite, it works the interior, from the interior, and yet is not itself inside. Suddenly, reading takes place within a much altered frame of reference. It seems as if today, one could not be outside the media. Can there be a detached vantage point of the observer, and what would this extra-mediatic position be? After Warhol, there is no such thing.

To figure out the conditions of possibility for reading and understanding a text produced not by an original, inspired author, but by the means of repetitive, automatic, apparently "senseless" technology—this is the challenge posed to us. "Mass-producing the moment,"[11] the technological innovations of the twentieth century have allowed mankind to break the limitations of space and time and to extend the means of understanding. Timing, efficiency, automated production rule; on the other hand, the spontaneous is in increasing demand. Fleeting images become recordable, food portable, experiences repeatable; it does not need a cunning technical apparatus to realize that reading also summons distant voices; "comme on ne peut pas téléphoner toujours, on lit. On ne lit qu'à la dernière extrémité. On téléphone d'abord beaucoup," [since we cannot always telephone, we read. We only read as a last resort. We prefer by far to telephone] as Proust put it.[12] The invention of the telephone arose from attempts to create a telegraph which would be able to send more than one message at once over a single line. And one of the earliest advertizements the Bell Company produced for the new technology was almost a user's manual: "Conversation can easily be carried on after slight practice and with occasional repetition of a word or sentence. On first listening to the Telephone, though the sound is perfectly audible, the articulation seems to be indistinct, but after a few trials the ear becomes accustomed to the peculiar sound."[13] The multiplicity of voices recorded and stored by Warhol are reminiscent of A. R. Luria's mnemonist S., whose memory seemed so inexhaustible that it took him decades to learn about forgetting. In his synaesthetic perception, even one person seemed to have many voices: "I got so interested in his voice," the patient recalls, "I couldn't follow what he was saying," and frequently experiencing trouble recognizing someone's voice over the phone, he found it was not because of a "bad connection," but "because the person happens to be someone whose voice changes twenty to thirty times in the course of a day." Without going into the potential import of "bad connections," suffice to say that eventually he succeeds: "he automatically screened off excess details by singling out key points of information," as his counselor reports proudly.[14]

Considering the enormous impact the telephone had, it is surprising that it took several decades before it was supplemented by the tape recorder to form a small surveillance unit: already in 1877, Thomas Alva Edison had considered the possibility of what he called a "telephone repeater." Afraid that the high cost of telephoning might deter people from using it widely, he hoped to profit from offering a device which people without a phone could use to record their voice and then have the message replayed over some central voicemail box to the prospective addressee.[15] But nothing came of his plans. Radio and television captured the attention, before the question of recording returned with a vengeance during World War II for the purposes of cryptology and propaganda. Although Alexander Graham Bell was the first to suggest the possibility of magnetic recording devices, it took until 1898 for Valdemar Poulsen to develop a "telegraphophone" in Denmark which could be used as a dictaphone, but was not loud enough for entertainment application. In the 1930s, magnetic recording on coated paper was developed in Germany and turned to commercial use, and soon, with the advent of magnetic recording, canned voices could withstand even the heat, cold, or vibration which disk recording could not have dealt with. Tape cassettes were introduced in the early 1960s, and outsold open-reel players for the first time in 1968.

Perhaps only the word "gadget"—derived from the French *gachette*, meaning a piece of machinery—comes close to describing Warhol's relationship with technology. Of course, the telephone was originally a gadget; and today's secondary gadgets attach themselves to it as fast as the whole Internet. Call waiting, call forwarding, beepers, quickdial, cordless extension phones, and conference calls became available in the late 1960s; recording devices have been in particular demand, as preferable to operators. In the mid-seventies, answering machines that replayed a prerecorded message, then took incoming messages and could be accessed remotely by the owner, became available for home use. In 1974 the Phone Mate, the Remote Mate, and the Automatic Electric Speaker Phone sold for several hundred dollars; and for considerably less money, the anxious user could not only monitor incoming calls without answering immediately, but also record every conversation that went over the phone line. At the time, such surveillance was legal as long as one party was informed of the call being recorded.[16]

If, as Freud has it, we ourselves are creating the gaps that we consequently have to bridge with the help of gadgets such as the telephone, this goes all the way back to the invention of writing as one of the first technologies, as a substitute for the voice of an absent person; furthermore, the telephone becomes an image of the transference, a projection of earliest contacts and connections. Then again, the telephone is also figured as something that is hooked up to the occult, or that which belongs to the past. Coming back home to seek repetition—which he considered happy, in sharp contrast to the Frankfurt School—Kierkegaard found that his servant had changed everything in his rooms and upon the unexpected return of his employer turned very white and shut the door in Kierkegaard's face, so that he felt "treated like a ghost." It would seem to me that there is a possible distinction between actively stalking repetition and an uncanny, uncalled-for, ghostly return. In both cases, as the work of Laurence Rickels demonstrates, Freudian psychoanalysis can serve us as a user's manual to mankind's ongoing technologization.[17] The desire to get in touch with the other side manifests itself in new technologies; one could cite spiritistic photography as a prime example, and radio was regarded, in its infancy, as a possible means of contacting the departed. Edison, the inventor of the phonograph, was also working on a device that was to enable him to communicate through a telepathic channel which he surmised between the long and the short wave frequencies, and Guglielmo Marconi believed he could capture Christ's last words on the cross by wireless transmission. All throughout the technology of telecommunication there is, as Nicholas Royle reminds us, a certain logic at work which puts us in touch with voices: "the question of the telephone cannot be dissociated from that of telepathy."[18] The voice is the other, more primal connection to mother, and it remains a direct connection to the one who is so close yet so far away. While the voice always comes life-size, video will always appear miniaturized and more abstract. The phone is very good at conveying unmixed messages, for we cannot see the conflicting nonverbal message that could accompany the voice; in this way, the phone gives rise to the fantasy of emotional directness. But at the same time, it is the same things that offer relief—anonymity, invisibility—that can just as well be uncanny, frightening, because the phone in effect always reanimates the earliest connections.

In Walter Rathenau's story, "Resurrection Co.," telephones are installed in each grave to ward off the fear of being buried alive on a graveyard in an American town. Soon enough, a lady who had been buried for several months calls up the switchboard, demanding to be put in touch with another grave. It turns out that it is precisely the technology that is supposed to offer the solace of salvation that can transform a whole society into a wired, technologized graveyard.[19] Electronic recording, as a logical consequence, must practically offer itself up to similar investigations. It was one of Warhol's contemporaries, the Swedish painter and filmmaker Friedrich Jürgenson, who made a "discovery" after taping birds in the forest in 1959: upon replaying the tapes, he heard his mother's voice address him from beyond the grave. He replayed the tape—his dead mother's voice was still there. By a series of subsequent experiments, he was convinced that one could capture multilingual voices of the dead on tape, usually just saying a word or two. Soon enough, others took up the recording of spirit voices, notably Konstantin Raudive. This use of electronic technology seemed to provide what parapsychological research had been waiting for: a medium people would consider credible. But Raudive admonished: "the experimenter must develop his hearing by constant listening to tapes. What at first seems like atmospheric buzzing is often many voices. They have to analyzed and amplified, of course."[20] Nothing else do we have before us in Andy Warhol's book. As a double of the living voice, the recorded one must appear uncanny, canned, straining to erase itself in order to shake off its technological constraints. In order to remain the live voice, it would rather die and disappear than be forced into repetition. At the same time, repetition can also mean cathexis of the same or narcissism in all its different forms.

Media theorists like Friedrich Kittler opine that the possibility for endless repetition on the basis of automatic recording was only one more reason to keep speaking: "to speak in particular about what writing is, and what it means psychoanalytically to be able to read one's own speech, even what is merely spoken off-the-cuff."[21] The odd scene is staged in Richard Matheson's short story, "Person to Person," where the protagonist has to deal with a phone ringing in his head. As he proceeds from one diagnosis to another, from stress to schizophrenia to telepathy to secret NSA operation experimenting with hypnosis to possession with an earthbound spirit, it transpires that every time he answers the ring, the voice gains more control over him, merely by making him lose himself. Whether the voice returns as that of his father, that of a spy, a Martian, or that of a lonely inventor trying to make contact, neither the protagonist's physician nor his analyst nor a psychic can figure out that it is in fact an acoustic mirror of the loser protagonist who kills himself a little, every time he answers, only to return within himself in the end as a more empowered, less frightened self, and it is only that new self that is strong enough to yank out the wire to that internal telephone.[22] Regardless of whether one calls it conscience, superego, or soul—in our teletechnological world, the pivotal repetition without which there would be no such thing as recognition will always have been deranged, as it were, by a mechanical double, an "internal telephone," as Derrida called it; to capture and replay is also to reply. Thus reading Andy Warhol will have to do with voice as much as with the mechanisms of repetition.

What is sensation, and what is the voice, when technological changes intrude into the realm of perception in such a way that the body is wedded to the machine? It is under these conditions, in response to this initial call that we must read. "We had to wait for the machine. It's just been delivered. It just got here."[23] Is the book an answering machine? In what sense can one claim that the reader must also be an answering machine? Memory and future become questionable when the last conversation can be recalled by means of a tape, and when the postmortem lies in the archive for decades. *a* confronts the reader with all the sounds of the Warhol Factory, but mainly with the half-recorded telephone conversation between people who call each other "Rotten Rita" or "The Duchess," "Billy Name" or "Tiger Morse"; there is an impressive amount of drug-taking and a depressing length of tape, the book being the result of almost complete technical surveillance. Everything happening in the Factory is stored on tape, video, and audio, and while some audio tapes are being transcribed, the next ones are being recorded with the clatter of typewriters in the background producing the book: "0—I had everything I wanted including *telephone rings typewriter writes telephone rings* 0-I'll get it; no I won't" (405). The book produced in this manner is utterly automatic in that it contains its own principle of movement; and while it does not erase but self-consciously foregrounds its own means of production, it would like to do away with forgetting. Nothing, technology seems to promise, can be lost anymore. However, all inscriptions presuppose a disappearance, a loss against which they must guard, and thus return to us as a cover-up for the inevitable, necessary forgetting which contaminates all commitment to memory. As Warhol, also a theorist of disappearance and aura, recalls:

> Some company recently was interested in buying my "aura." They didn't want my product. They kept saying, "we want your aura." I never figured out what they wanted. But they were willing to pay a lot for it. So then I thought that if somebody was willing to pay that much for it, I should try to figure out what it is. I think "aura" is something that only somebody else can see, and they only see as much of it as they want to. It's all in the other person's eyes. You can only see an aura on people you don't know very well or don't know at all. I was having dinner the other night with everybody from my office. The kids at the office treat me like dirt, because they know me and see me every day. But then there was this nice friend that somebody had brought along who had never met me, and this kid could hardly believe that he was having dinner with me! Everybody else was seeing me, but he was seeing my "aura." When you just see somebody on the street, they can really have an aura.[24]

An aura can only be sensed at a distance and by an other, and as soon as it is identified, it is lost: or as Walter Benjamin said, aura is always already being lost. Arguably, all technologies are there to serve as means of stalking and preserving such moments in order to repeat them, make them repeatable. Thus technology comes to reenforce the power of iterability. But we ought to ask ourselves, if repetition comes to constitute everything, what would the unrepeatable be? Perhaps the unrepeatable can be figured as nothing else than a peculiar singularity which cannot be subsumed, or rather which disappears when it is subsumed under generality. And singularity does precisely not consist in its being indivisible, not in a recollection or gathering, but rather in the sealed mark of division or doubling. Therefore it does not depend on a conceptual nature or an essence, but can only appear in its disappearance as that which is radically nonconceptual. This fury of disappearance depends on an obsession with repetition, and is thinkable only as a disappearance of repetition, as a negative function of repetition[25]—and thus Warhol's aura is so singular because it evaporates as soon as it is reproduced, which is to say, produced.

The intrusion of technology, then, can be figured as a means of stalking the unrepeatable. The moment of connection in *a* is cathected: "I'm sorry baby, listen, I'm sorry but I, I have been calling you since I've arrived and you've been busy; this is the first time you haven't been and there was nobody at the factory and there should have been someone here to receive the uh, the camera" (36). As the use of taperecorders, video equipment, and answering machines serves to capture the uncalculable moment, the impossible goal of total witnessing, total surveillance, total recall becomes contaminated by itself or by forgetting itself. Forgetting is difficult to circumscribe, since it is never just loss of memory, or the effacement of objective representation. "The curse of total recall," as it is put on the back flap of the 1968 translation of Luria's *The Mind of a Mnemonist*, is that memory is never exhausted by taking in more. In fact, keeping more mnesic representations inevitably entails the contamination of memory with forgetting: a pure remembrance would be nothing but forgetting, detail but no difference, images without categories. If forgetting and memory are not opposites, then we might say that Warhol tried to gain a hold in the moment through the forgetting of forgetting.[26]

Of course the apparatus of writing is already a technology. But talk of a "challenge" of the new, electronic media abounds, and many commentators share the surmise that "an entire epoch of so-called literature, if not all of it, cannot survive a certain technological regime of telecommunications."[27] It is taken as read that this inability to survive hinges on a supposed loss of the topological anchor, on an alleged dislocation or even loss of body, and of a sense of reality and perception that is bound to the body, and I find this conservative instinct touching.[28] However, it could well be the case, I think, that writing has always been touching on the body in this manner, namely on the body lost or estranged, and that writing and other technologies are instances of a certain excarnation. Unaccommodated, unappropriated, unassimilated, estranged, and contaminated, the body touches on the senses of reading; lost at the limits of language, it returns as a foreign body within. This sense of loss is restored again and again by dint of a reiteration of the Platonic argument that all new media appear as machines of forgetting from the perspective of the old mediascape.

Therefore it becomes a matter of selectivity, of inclusions and exclusions:

> No it's novel that it's being a novel as a matter of fact, we can read in the book, protesting novelty; "vut do you mean by a novel?" uhhh-hhh I know it just . . . there's no other brush stroke. 12 hours of On-

dine a novel? you're not going—are you going to put it in a book or what make it one whole book. (100)

This unity is of course forever postponed by means of the ongoing tape recording. The penultimate chapter is a soliloquy that begins like this: "This is a supposedly long m-o-n-o-logue about whatever it is that I talk about uh—I'm no brain—and I never have had a brain—and I don't want one; I dun know what else to say—this tape should be finished—I wish I were a brai-n" (405). In this parody of post-Joycean monologue, Warhol confounds not only the apparently so-easy distinctions between ear and mind, or between bodily senses and electronic technology; even the spiritual is no longer opposed to the mechanical, but the mechanical comes back to haunt the spiritual: "Hello may. I'm making love t o th e taperecord er. Hehh Hehh Hehh I don't know what to say to i t. Uhh—religiou s" (445). And this marriage with the mechanical bride, made in technological heaven, does not allow for a divorce, because writing and reading presuppose the technological to such an extent that they are inseparable.

To many commentators, the history of memory and of mnemonics seems divided into a rhetorical tradition that constantly invents technical models, and a psychological one that holds them to be mere metaphors unable to represent either incorporation or hypomnetic excarnation. However, if speech is communicated above our heads, we will have needed the ferro-heads of tape recorders to make speech "immortal."[29] As Mina realizes in Bram Stoker's *Dracula*, though, audio taping is less than ideal for later access, for the replay remains analogous, and the information recorded becomes manageable only when transcribed. In passing through circuits and terminals, the voice will have been terminated.[30] But it survives—the shortcircuiting of the voice results in a technologized text, a computerized telephone, that is to say, an answering machine. The question will have been how to respond to this kind of antihermeneutical teletext that automatically creates itself and has already swallowed the reader. An approach to Andy Warhol's book must take into account the way in which the phone is already off the hook; the receiver dangles in front of us, and we have to respond as we are sucked into the telephonic structure of the book, remembering and foiling all recall. When we speak of technology, we speak of repetition and of memory: but isn't this use of technology against forgetting precisely an attempt to forget about forgetting by means of technology? If there could be no literature without the technologies of writing, we also need an anamnesis of that which is erased and forgotten.

The last words of *a* are: "Out of the garbage, into The Book" (451). The recycling of the voice in writing is figured, here, as the return of remembrance in forgetting. As Kittler put it, "after all, tape recorders, television cameras and radio microphones were invented for the very purpose of recording gibberish (Blabla). Precisely because they 'understand nothing.' "[31] It is an attempt to use tape and paper against forgetting, while at the same time covertly trying to forget about forgetting. And yet, a memory of forgetting only turns the forgotten into something phenomenal and thus betrays forgetting in turn. It would seem that an "automatic forgetting" is redundant: how could forgetting be anything else? The materiality of the act of reading itself is all too easily forgotten, as on the tape of incoming messages on an answering machine, erasing older messages. The automatic keeps erasing itself automatically, and intervenes in order to facilitate a forgetting of forgetting. It automatically functions like a cover-up, and I have momentarily forgotten who told me that—it might have been left on my ansaphone, though. The case of Andy Warhol's *a* demonstrates that literature must be an answering machine. We are left with little alternative if we are not to embrace the pessimism of the *New York Review of Books*, concluding "that in its errant pages can be heard the death knell of American literature."[32]

Notes

1. Both citations from the interview with Gretchen Berg, *Cahiers du Cinema in English*, 10 (1967).

2. Jordan Mekas, "Notes after Reseeing the Movies of Andy Warhol," in *Andy Warhol*. Ed. J. Coplan. (New York: New York Graphic Society, 1970), 139–46; here: 146; compare also Warhol, "Why I Love to Live Fast," *High Times* 33 (May 1978).

3. E.g., Theodor W. Adorno, "Freudian Theory and the Pattern of Fascist Propaganda," in *The Essential Frankfurt School Reader*, ed. Andrew Arato and Eike Gebhardt (New York: Continuum 1982), 133, Max Horkheimer and Theodor W. Adorno, *Dialectic of Enlightenment* (New York: Continuum, 1972), 172. What his estate makes of Warhol's delight in repetition in conjunction with the voice is perhaps best illustrated by his 4 times 15 minutes of fame, consisting of nothing but "Uh yes. Uh no," ad infinitum, recorded on CD with an introduction by Ivan Karp (Sooj Records 1996).

4. Hans Georg Gadamer, "Der 'eminente' Text und seine Wahrheit," *Sprache und Literatur in Wissenschaft und Unterricht* 57 (1986): 4–10; here, 6.

5. Andy Warhol, *The Philosophy of Andy Warhol from a to b and back again* (London: Picador, 1975), 32.

6. Pat Hackett, ed. *The Andy Warhol Diaries* (New York: Warner Books, 1989); Andy Warhol and Pat Hackett, *POP-ism: The Warhol '60s* (London: Hutchinson, 1981).

7. Andy Warhol, *a. a novel* (New York: Grove Press, 1968). Interestingly enough, extracts from this book, this novel way of writing "a novel," were published in French as "How to become a professional homosexual": *Comment devenir un homosexuel professionnel. Extrait de A.* (Paris: Panoplie de l'Amateur, 1979).

8. R. Olivio, "Ondine, New York 16. December 1978," *Köln &* 1 (1995); in a variation on Ovid, "sony est, qui vivit in illa," see *Metamorphoses*, trans. Rolfe Humphries, (Bloomington: Indiana University Press, 1955), verses 400–401.

9. Paul Carroll, "What's a Warhol." *Playboy* 16.9 (1969).

10. Warhol, *The Philosophy of Andy Warhol from a to b and back again*, 26.

11. Daniel Boorstin, *The Americans: The Democratic Experience*. (New York: Vintage, 1974), 359ff.

12. Marcel Proust, "Journées de lecture 1907," *Journées de Lecture*. (Paris: 10/18 Editions, 1980), 59–66, giving rise to Jean Cocteau's play with the *voix humaine*; see also Walter Benjamin, "Telephon," *Berliner Kindheit um Neunzehnhundert*. (Frankfurt: Suhrkamp, 1950), 22–25.

13. Cited in Robert Lucky, *Silicon Dreams: Information, Man, and Machine* (New York: St. Martin's Press 1989), 202.

14. A. R. Luria, *The Mind of a Mnemonist*. (New York: Basic Book, 1968), 66ff. "The Art of Forgetting," developed here long before Umberto Eco, took Luria's patient deeply into the realm of screen memories, which we will have to take up elsewhere. It is perhaps sufficient to stress here that writing down and burning his notes of what he wanted to forget did not work, contrary to a widespread assumption about this text. (This method is used in Orwell's *1984*, though.)

15. *North American Review* (June 1878); see Boorstin, 379, and Robert Conot, *A Streak of Luck* (New York: Da Capo Press: 1980).

16. Tania Grossinger, *The Book of Gadgets*. (New York: McKay, 1974), 76–77.

17. E.g. Laurence Rickels, *Aberrations of Mourning: Writing on German Crypts*. (Detroit: Wayne State University Press, 1988), and *The Case of California* (Baltimore: Johns Hopkins University Press, 1991).

18. Nicholas Royle, *Telepathy and Literature*. (Oxford: Blackwell, 1991), 168.

19. Walter Rathenau, *Gesammelte Schriften* vol. 4 (Berlin 1918–1919), 345f.

20. Raudive's book on how "The Inaudible becomes Audible," published in German in 1968 (as "Das Unhörbare wird Hörbar"), appeared in English in 1971 with Taplinger in New York. See also the report by David Ellis in *Psychic* (February 1974) for an account of possible telekinetic and telepathic interference in the experimental setup used by Raudive.

21. Friedrich Kittler, "Draculas Vermächtnis," ed. Dieter Hombach *ZETA 02 Mit Lacan* (Berlin: Rotation Verlag, 1982), 103–36; translated into English as "Dracula's Legacy," *Literature, Media, Information Systems* (Amsterdam: G + B Arts, 1997), 50–84; here, 51.

22. Richard Matheson, "Person to Person," *I Am Legend*. (New York: Tom Doherty Asociates, 1995), 294–317.

23. *a*, 36; compare also Andy Warhol, "Sunday with Mister C: an audio-documentary by Andy Warhol starring Truman Capote," *Rolling Stone* 132 (April 12, 1973).

24. Andy Warhol, *The Philosophy of Andy Warhol from a to b and back again* (London: Picador, 1975), 75.

25. Karl Heinz Haag, "Das Unwiederholbare," ed. Max Horkheimer, *Zeugnisse*. Theodor W. Adorno zum sechzigsten Geburtstag (Europäische Verlagsanstalt, 1963), 152–61.

26. In the original version of this paper, the word "Gegenwart," German for "present," allowed me to pun on "gegen" [against] and "warten" [waiting, delaying].

27. Jacques Derrida, *The Post Card from Socrates to Freud and Beyond* (Chicago: University of Chicago Press, 1987), 197; as I finish the corrections on this text, I receive an uncanny postcard, with a picture of Andy Warhol on the telephone at Silver Factory 1965, photographed by Billy Name. The writing on this card, mentioning Friedrich Kittler as well as the publishing of a novel, was started, but then covered over with white sticky tape, and covered with new text. However, the US Postal Service had found it necessary to stick bar code labels on both sides of the card, obscuring the handwriting as well as the photograph once more.

28. Bernhard Waldenfels, "Hearing Oneself Speak: Derrida's Recording of the Phenomenological Voice," *Southern Journal of Philosophy* 32 (supplement) (1994).

29. As the *Scientific American* wrote when reporting about Edison a century ago: "A Wonderful Invention—Speech Capable of Indefinite Repetition" . . . cited in Oliver Read and Walter L. Welsh, *From Tin Foil to Stereo—Evolution of the Phonograph*. (Indianapolis and New York: H. W. Sams 1959), 12; all of Lacan's seminars were saved on tape and transcribed for the next session because, as he said himself, people were not listening, they were trying to understand. Jacques Lacan, "Radiophonie" *Scilicet* 2/3 (1970): 94ff.

30. See Jonathan Goldberg, *Voice Terminal Echo* (London: Methuen, 1986); Avital Ronell, *The Telephone Book* (Lincoln: University of Nebraska Press, 1989); Garrett Stewart, *Reading Voices* (Berkeley: University of California Press,1992); and Donald Wesling and Tadeusz Slawek, *Literary Voice. The Calling of Jonah* (New York: SUNY Press, 1995).

31. Friedrich Kittler, "Dracula's Legacy," *Literature, Media, Information Systems*. (Amsterdam: G+B Arts, 1997), 50–84; here, 53 (Warhol's nickname "Drella" is of course a conjuncture of Dracula and Cinderella. . .).

32. Robert Mazzocco, "aaaaaa . . . " *New York Review of Books* 12.8 (1969).

Works Cited

Adorno, Theodor W. "Freudian Theory and the Pattern of Fascist Propaganda," *The Essential Frankfurt School Reader*. Edited by Andrew Arato and Eike Gebhardt. New York: Continuum 1982.

Benjamin, Walter. "Telephon," *Berliner Kindheit um Neunzehnhundert*. Frankfurt: Suhr kamp, 1950.

Berg, Gretchen. *Cahiers du Cinema in English*, 10 (1967).

Boorstin, Daniel. *The Americans: The Democratic Experience*. New York: Vintage, 1974.

Carroll, Paul. "What's a Warhol." *Playboy* 16.9 (1969).

Derrida, Jacques. *The Post Card from Socrates to Freud and Beyond*. University of Chicago Press, 1987.

Goldberg, Jonathan.*Voice Terminal Echo*. London: Methuen, 1986.

Grossinger, Tania. *The Book of Gadgets*. New York: McKay, 1974.

Haag, Karl Heinz. "Das Unwiederholbare." *Zeugnisse. Theodor W. Adorno zum sechzigsten Geburtstag*. Edited by Max Horkheimer. Europäische Verlagsanstalt, 1963.

Hackett, Pat, ed. *The Andy Warhol Diaries*. New York: Warner Books, 1989.

Horkheimer, Max, and Theodor W. Adorno. *Dialectic of Enlightenment*. New York: Continuum, 1972.

Kittler, Friedrich. "Dracula's Legacy," *Literature, Media, Information Systems*. Amsterdam: G+B Arts, 1997.

Kittler, Friedrich. "Draculas Vermächtnis." *ZETA 02 Mit Lacan*. Edited by Dieter Hombach (Berlin: Rotation Verlag, 1982), 103–36; translated into English as "Dracula's Legacy," *Literature, Media, Information Systems*. Amsterdam: G+B Arts, 1997.

Lacan, Jacques. "Radiophonie." *Scilicet* 2/3 (1970).

Matheson, Richard. "Person to Person," *I Am Legend*. New York: Tom Doherty Associates, 1995.

Lucky, Robert. *Silicon Dreams: Information, Man, and Machine*. New York, 1989.

Luria, A. R. *The Mind of a Mnemonist*. New York: Basic Book, 1968.

Mazzocco, Robert. "aaaaaa . . ." *New York Review of Books* 12.8 (1969).

Ovid. *Metamorphoses*. Translated by Rolfe Humphries. Bloomington: Indiana University Press, 1955.

Proust, Marcel. "Journées de lecture 1907." *Journées de Lecture*. Paris: 10/18 Editions, 1980.

Rathenau, Walter. *Gesammelte Schriften*, vol. 4. Berlin 1918–1919.

Read, Oliver and Welsh, Walter L. *From Tin Foil to Stereo: Evolution of the Phonograph*. H. W. Sams: Indianapolis and New York, 1959.

Rickels, Laurence. *Aberrations of Mourning: Writing on German Crypts*. Detroit: Wayne State University Press, 1988.

———. *The Case of California*. Baltimore: Johns Hopkins University Press, 1991.

Ronell, Avital. *The Telephone Book*. Lincoln: University of Nebraska Press, 1989.

Stewart, Garrett. *Reading Voices*. Berkeley: University of California Press,1992.

Waldenfels, Bernhard. "Hearing Oneself Speak: Derrida's Recording of the Phenomenological Voice." *Southern Journal of Philosophy* 32 (supplement), 1994.

Warhol, Andy. *a. a novel*. New York: Grove Press, 1968.

———. "Sunday with Mister C: An Audio-Documentary by Andy Warhol Starring Truman Capote." *Rolling Stone* 132 (12 April 1973).

———. *The Philosophy of Andy Warhol from a to b and back again.* London: Picador, 1975.

———. "Why I Love to Live Fast." *High Times* 33 (May 1978).

Warhol, Andy, and Pat Hackett. *POP-ism: The Warhol '60s.* London: Hutchinson, 1981.

Wesling, Donald, and Tadeusz Slawek. *Literary Voice: The Calling of Jonah.* New York: SUNY Press, 1995.

Singular Sense, Second Hand
PEGGY KAMUF

"It has a second hand," she said.
"Oh, I don't care about that," was the reply.

THE WATCH HAD A SMALL FACE RINGED IN A GOLD-COLORED METAL that could be slid on and off a slim leather wristband. The novelty was its adaptability, the possibility of changing the color of the band. There were four of these: one of black suede, another white, a red one, and a fourth whose color I've forgotten (blue?). The whole set was presented in a long white jeweler's box that sprang smartly open and shut.

It was the first "grown-up" gift her parents had given her, its numbered face denoting a new responsibility and accountability. But from the first, this gift was confused with a verbal exchange. Many years later, she would learn a very precise word for the kind of confusion that had to remain unspoken in her own idiom. In the Babel of more than one language, it was what would be called a malentendu—mishearing as misunderstanding. For lack of such a term's precision, not hearing or knowing its range across the random senselessness between idioms, the misunderstood, misheard word left traces far more durable than the object that was their concrete occasion.

"It has a second hand," said her mother after the girl had had time to give the first signs of gratified pleasure. As these did not give any indication that she had noticed the special feature, her attention was being drawn to it.

"Oh, I don't care about that," she replied.

Shocked by her daughter's bald-faced ingratitude, the older woman's face decomposed. The dismay almost choked off her voice.

"What a thing to say!"

In a flash, the whole scene came crashing down around the girl's ears, the very ears that had somehow tricked her into reading lines from the wrong script.

"It's second-hand" said her mother.

"Oh, I don't care about that," was the girl's reply.

While her own ears were ringing with the utterly plausible interference of the two declarations, the effect of which ought to have been comic but which under the circumstances stung her with the sudden and, for the moment, useless awareness of the treachery of words, her mother heard only the one version of the exchange, which cast the girl in such an inexplicably disagreeable role. Fumbling to explain what she understood too late to have happened, the girl managed only to make matters worse since it had then to come out that she saw nothing incongruous in the idea that her parents, not rich but hardly poor, might buy a used watch for their only daughter. Besides, one had only to look at it in its crisply clean box to see that the watch and its assortment of wristbands were perfectly new.

The damage was irreparable and there was no retrieving her mother's generous humor. She looked at her daughter now with mistrust, making no attempt to dispel the sense of the latter's trespass. The girl protested but only in silence. The confounding homonymy of a language had asserted itself at the very juncture of her *entente* with the being who, more than any other, was supposed to know her meaning even before she put words to it. Was this misunderstanding proof to the contrary? What had happened? No doubt she never succeeded in convincing her mother of the innocence of the mistake, either because she rapidly gave up trying or because she herself grew to suspect that her mother's version had some truth in it. Already by then, the exchange of gifts was freighted with a certain anxiety (was she worthy of this?), but there is no telling how much this affect was a cause before becoming a result of the episode of the second(-)hand. A silence settled around the affair. Yet, there was anything but silence within where the girl kept up a running dialogue with a new, dangerous interlocutor, this mother tongue that had suddenly become the parent of monstrous offspring—the same words, plus or minus an inaudible hyphen, telling two incompatible tales. "Here, look, a second hand," in other words, an extra measure of my affection, in fact a third hand that will divide the minutes of your impatient young life so that you will see how, yes, time has not been arrested by the past but is propelling you toward whatever you wish, the gifts of the future. But also "Look, it's (only) second-hand," meaning I could do no better than an *objet trouvé* that comes with a past, tales it could tell of the times marked on some other young—or perhaps not-so-young—wrist, accompanying the movements of another hand, used, a hand-me-down of unknown provenance.

An elementary lesson in the vicissitudes of speech: saying and meaning could be dissociated quite ruthlessly without, apparently, the least intention on the speaker's part. My meaning is not mine so long as it depends on hearing and therefore on others. None of these potentially interesting vistas opened up at the time. On the contrary, the lights dimmed for awhile as if someone had just clumsily tripped over the Christmas tree light cord. The fault gaped too large and had to be accounted for; there was blame to be assigned.

In her internal dialogue, the girl fought off the notion that the blame should come to her: Why was Mother so unwilling to credit the reasonable explanation she had given as the disculpating truth? She awaited in vain a sign that her mother had done so—a laugh they could have shared over the absurdity of the bad joke, the lame pun. Instead, the dialogue pursued implacably; she must have been listening for some confirmation of the suspicion that hers was a thankless task of raising a heartless child. This might have been one of the first occasions the daughter heard her speak the words that would later become a relentless refrain, words that had the power to send her into a rage that, on the rare occasions it exploded on the outside, disturbed with disastrous effects the familial policy of silence. "You're just like your father," her mother would say. The words carried no perceptible tenderness for the personality of the man she'd married after giving up her plans to be a geneticist. Rather, that he had turned out to have the dominant genes, at least in the case of her daughter, was apparently a cause of considerable chagrin for her and no reason to cherish either that parent or his child. Decoded it meant: you are secretive, uncommunicative or, in its worst intonation, you are unfeeling, insensitive. The reproach invariably stung in its unreasonableness, as if the daughter should have chosen different genes instead of her mother a different husband. But even if it was not uttered on that occasion, like an answer to the riddle of the second(-)hand or some premature moral to the story of the child's barely begun life, the phrase began to resonate in an inner ear from that moment, striking a chord ever afterward on the notes of her father's hearing. The resonance was dim, but that was perhaps the way her father, who had lost the hearing in his right ear at about age twelve or thirteen, perceived only irregularly the muted sounds of his world. To be "just like her father" meant also therefore—but inadvertently, ironically—to turn a deaf ear to what others were saying. His infirmity, with its accidental etiology, had become a generation later the girl's willful disposition; his incapacity, her insensitivity. He was not to blame if he couldn't always hear. (But, to the ironic inner ear, was there not also a note of doubt even as regards that physical disability? After all, who could tell if he didn't hear or if he just pretended not to hear? The partial deafness might be a sort of reverse crutch that he relied on to blot out the world.) As for her, she had no such excuse.

This, then, was the obscure region of the fault to be avoided, if possible, in her ponderings over the curious impasse into which she had been led as if by some mischievous hand turning senselessly in its own little circumference. It was an impasse because the quickest exit inexorably turned out to lead right back over the gap where she was suspended again. The way out took the form of an alternative: "not my fault, therefore hers." Although this simple, two-step reasoning brought a certain satisfaction, it wasn't very long before the trap shut in a neat vice. The more she seized upon the disculpating hypothesis, the more it grabbed her back with the proof of her ingratitude, the very charge she charged her mother with bringing against her unjustly. Round and round, the two versions always came down to and back to just one as the rotating hand swept forward to its point of departure that was never a point of arrival or rest. "If I am right—she listened to me only to hear signs of my unworthy nature—then I am wrong and in the wrong." And vice versa, or almost. The strange logic of the equation never simply reversed, an asymmetry difficult to grasp seeming to veer it towards the, for her, more discomfiting side of the balance. The hand just touched the point of her possible innocence before setting off again to pull her into the gulf of another minute of certain guilt. The little measured intervals of grim satisfaction could have been enough to keep the whole thing turning indefinitely, despite the repeated pricks to the floated balloons of her good conscience. And, indeed, perhaps it did just that for many years.

But perhaps as well, less clearly and certainly less consciously, what remained always just out of reach was a way to admit the fault, to assume it but as a desire that had chosen to speak at the wrong moment and in a confused manner. To have heard "it's second-hand" she had to have wished to overlook the obvious—the brand newness of the thing that came wrapped in the absence of a past and that could change its appearance in order to efface whatever traces of wear it would inevitably accumulate. Had she wanted, then, a device that would tell a story as it told the time, a kind of book with hands and springs? A gift from the past, of the past, which is to say her mother's, her father's, some concrete link to the history of all those other hands that had left so few marks on the things she saw around her?

But that would have been unspeakable, unthinkable even, and she surely did not think it at the time.

Why tell you this story of a second hand? And why tell it in the third person as if it did not happen to me, but to another? And why, if I wanted you to think it was a fiction or a story reported second-hand, do I now assume it to the order of the first-hand and first person? In other words, if the genre is autobiography, then why not mark it in the conventional fashion, by grammatical person? Good questions. But here's the thing: the first-hand experience I related came to me only as experience of the second-hand, that is, as a repetition by another of what was not simply itself but first of all doubled, multiplied, of the order of the more-than-one. The story I wanted to tell is that of a singular articulation in this more-than-one, our so-called common language, and for that the first-person convention of autobiography seemed not only inadequate but a disavowal of the very interval or space by virtue of which the singular can be repeated. The story I've told would be about, in effect, the interval that holds apart the first-hand and the second-hand, but also the interval that alone can allow the first to be repeated in its difference from the other.

Reading is our subject, and reading with the senses, rather than with sense in general, in the sense of a conventional, single meaning: it is to this articulation of plural senses with single sense that I bring my not-autobiographical story. You will not have heard, perhaps, that the articulation happens there as what cannot be heard, as an unspoken mark of punctuation—or not. You may not have heard this because between "second hand" and "second-hand" (or "secondhand") not only is the difference inaudible, but there is disagreement among the orthographic conventions governing the spacing (or not) of this word. If the OED is still a reliable guide to British usage, then "second-hand" is the preferred spelling of the adjective, as in "second-hand automobile" or "second-hand watch." However, both the Webster's Unabridged and the Random House dictionaries recommend for their primarily American users "secondhand" with no space and no hyphen, forming what is called a solid or closed compound word. British and American conventions agree, on the other hand, that the open compound "second hand" is correct when referring to the hand on a watch or clock that counts off the seconds. According to Eric Partridge, "hyphen" is a Late Latin word that derives from the Greek *huphen*, which is itself a compound word formed by the joining of *hupo*, "under," and *hen*, "one"; literally, then hyphen means "under one," and hence "into one" or "together."[1] From its earliest use by manuscript scribes to signal the linked syllables or letters of a word that have become separated at the end of a line, its range of later print uses has been extended considerably: the linking of commonly associated words, the affixing of occasional prefixes, the indication of a specific syntactic combination, or even a typographical convention for the representation of an abnormal speech pattern, such as stuttering or unusual emphasis on separate syllables of a word.

This variety of conventional uses (and there are still others one could mention) already points to the hyphen's double sense of articulation, which both joins what it separates and separates what it joins.[2] Unlike other conventions of punctuation, moreover, hyphenation signals articulation not at the level of propositions, clauses, or phrases but at a more elementary level of the formation of units of sense. Perhaps hyphenation does not even belong to the category of punctuation, as commonly defined, but signals a discernibly different act, which could explain in part why, in English at least, we have both this noun, hyphenation, and a verb, to hyphenate, whereas no equivalents have been formed for the other common marks of punctuation ("periodization" and "to periodize" have ordinarily nothing to do with placing a period at the end of a sentence). Linguistic treatises one may consult on punctuation either exclude consideration of the hyphen or mention it only in passing.[3] Prescriptive manuals, such as Eric Partridge's *You Have a Point There*, classify hyphens among what it calls the "allies and accessories" of punctuation proper. The standard reference for American university presses, *The Chicago Manual of Style*, treats hyphens principally in its chapter on spelling and introduces the section with the remark that the cloudy distinctions among solid, hyphenated, and open compounds are responsible for probably "nine out of ten spelling questions that arise in writing or editing."[4] After setting out "general principles" that conform to the trend away from the use of hyphens and underscoring that this is a trend and not a rule, the same authority admits that there are "quite literally, scores of other rules for the spelling of compound words. Many of them are nearly useless because of the great numbers of exceptions" (164). This problem is itself compounded if one has to take account of differences between American and British usage, as already mentioned. According once again to the Englishman Partridge, ever since World War I, which "taught many people that superfluities should be treated as such and therefore discarded" (138), the tendency toward the formation of nonhyphenated compound words in English has accelerated and among Americans more so than Britons. American alacrity in discarding "superfluities" alarms many Britons, says Partridge, and results in some "ugly continuities (for example, *nonresistance*)." At the same time, however, he does not seem to doubt that such ugliness is our common future as speakers of the English language: "So why," he asks, "resist the inevitable?" (138). Why resist, in other words, the unhyphenated "nonresistance"?

It is a version of that question I want to take up briefly, not, however, to explore any further what the vicissitudes of hyphenation may indicate about different national characters, even though that is doubtless an interesting subject.[5] Rather, because it marks the space of a certain resistance to nonresistance, a minimal jot left as a reminder to hold apart the two (or more) terms that are all the same being pulled together "under one," hyphenation perhaps supplies an opening, albeit a tiny one, for remarking the insertion of singular differences within general structures of meaning. This opening can be described in one of the effects already noted, the largely non-rule-governed practice of hyphenation in different English idioms. What may be provisionally called the hypothesis of the hyphen, which, for structural reasons cannot be fully raised to or posed as a thesis, is this: hyphenation makes room for or gives place to a mark that arrests the disappearance of a singular sense at the limit of common sense, common language, the rule of the under- and into- one.

At this point, one should attempt to say something general about singularity if only to demonstrate the predictable failure of any such an attempt. Fortunately, we don't have to venture into this territory unassisted. I am going to rely on two seasoned guides and two recent works elaborated around a thinking of singular articulations within the general space of sense. They will also allow us to run a few preliminary tests on the hypothesis of the hyphen.

In the introduction to his collection of essays, *Inventions of*

Difference: On Jacques Derrida, a book described by its author as "about singularity," Rodolphe Gasché sharply disputes the idea, advanced by another commentator, that "the distinctive trait of Derrida's writing imparts its singularity to his texts in a way that renders their generic categorization impossible."[6] This assertion, which has all the appearance of a certain common sense, posits in effect an impermeable barrier between singular sense and, precisely, common sense. It renders singularity, as Gasché puts it, "opaque, silent, or immediate in a nondialectical sense" (14). Gasché, by contrast, wants to insist that if indeed singularity were simply inaccessible in this sense, then it would be "quite simply thoroughly unintelligible" (ibid.). That is, one could not possibly have any idea of it at all. The reasoning here might bring to mind a similar observation of Freud's concerning the unconscious drive, which "can never become an object of consciousness"; the drive has access to conscious thought only as and on condition of representation in an idea. This condition is the condition of knowing anything at all about the drive, for, as Freud puts it: "If the drive did not *attach itself* to an idea or manifest itself as an affective state, we would know nothing about it."[7] Likewise, Gasché underscores that the condition of singularity's intelligibility is its repetition "in an idealizing doubling." If one is to have any idea at all of singularity, then it "must translate itself, interpret itself as intelligible in its unintelligibility." As Freud put it, it must "*attach* itself to an idea." Or as we might now begin to be able to say with some understanding, it must hyphenate.

Gasché does not name the hyphen as such. Nevertheless, the language he selects from a passage in *Shibboleth*, Derrida's essay on the iteration of singular dates in Celan, and in particular the word "ligament" will allow us to translate, to hyphenate.

> Singularity . . . cannot be simply demarcated from the universal. As with the ciphers encountered in Celan's poetry, with the singular "chance and necessity cross and in crossing are both at once consigned. Within its strictures a ligament binds together, in a manner at once significant and insignificant, fatality and its opposite: chance and coming-due, coincidence in the event, what *falls*—well or ill-together." It is thus imperative to acknowledge this *togetherness* of the unique, the one-and-only-time, of the utter singular's refusal of all possible repetition *and* necessity, ideality, universality, in order to do justice to the singular itself. For the singular to be understood as what it is, that is, in its utter singularity, the ligament that within it holds together, each time in a singular manner, contingency and

necessity, sheer punctuality and universality, must, in one way or another, be acknowledged. (15–16)

I said that Gasché does not name the hyphen; nevertheless, the above passage, in addition to excising and then reattaching the term "ligament," practices hyphenation at two different levels. Whether this is an accidental or necessary gesture is not a question one should rush to decide, given what the passage has to say about the coming- or falling-due together of chance and necessity and despite the fact that an accident seems indeed to have been responsible for at least one of the hyphens that shows up here.

At a first level, then, the passage repeats a translation of Derrida's sentences from *Shibboleth* that have been rendered into English with the help of two hyphenated words—or so it appears. The compound "coming-due" hyphenates the translation of "échéance," which is the falling-due of the deadline (a word that perhaps used to be hyphenated). Derrida's text, which is working to retrieve and repeat Celan's singular idiom of the date, crosses into and crosses *with* the English idiom by means of this uncommon yet intelligible compound word. As for the second hyphenated word Gasché quotes, "ill-together," it turns out to have been formed by a typographical error in the quotation, both the translation and the original having used a dash here.[8] By chance, accident, or error an ill-formed word results, and it is one which says precisely, that is, badly, the ill-fitting joint of the singular's repetition in generality: "ill-together."

At a second level, Gasché's own language, as it continues after the quoted lines, picks up the hyphenating trait remarked there: he forges the four-part compound "one-and-only-time" and sets it in balance with "necessity, ideality, universality." This hyphenated general name of absolute singularity, of that which can only take up a name through universalizing repetition, has by the end of the passage, after a number of repetitions, been transformed into the common word "punctuality." "For the singular to be understood as what it is, that is, in its utter singularity, the ligament that within it holds together, each time in a singular manner, contingency and necessity, sheer punctuality and universality, *must*, in one way or another, be acknowledged." The ligament must be acknowledged. The force of Gasché's repeated imperative here carries over the force of a hyphenating punctuality or punctuation at the singular crossing of chance and necessity traced in his own text. The hyphenating imperative, in other words, dictates not just a duty to acknowledge what can and therefore must be acknowledged; it is that which is also imperatively punctuating the language of common understanding at its limits.[9]

To follow the inscriptions of this double imperative, we will turn to our second guide. Jean-Luc Nancy, no less although differently than Jacques Derrida, has set his thought within the space of articulated singularity. For his most recent collection of essays, Nancy announces this preoccupation clearly enough in the chosen title: *Être singulier pluriel [Plural Singular (or Singular Plural) Being]*. The reversibility of the two modifying adjectives, their co-priority and co-secondarity (with the shift in sense that is thereby allowed), supplies the syntactic and semantic matrix that is worked through most explicitly in the initial chapter of the book. I am not going to try to summarize the intricate movements of this essay. I merely want to remark on the considerable extent to which the hyphenating gesture imposes itself on these pages. This can be seen, once again, at two levels.

At a first level, there is the regular and constant occurrence of hyphenated compounds, formed either through the insertion of hyphens in normally unhyphenated words (for example, pre-position, dis-position, ex-position, co-appear, co-existence, co-incidence) or through the forging of hyphenated word-phrases. The latter practice is heavily relied on as a vehicle of the exposition of "singular-plural/plural-singular-being," which is indeed, at one point at least, explicitly hyphenated in this way (58). Other formations dictated by this thinking-in-hyphenation precipitate out of the Heideggerian elaboration of *Mitsein*, which both French and English translate with the help of a hyphen: *être-avec* and Being-with. Indeed, Nancy quite clearly positions what he is doing here as what would be called in French an "explication avec" *Being and Time*, that is, an "explanation with," a coming-to-terms, and in particular a coming-to-terms with the "with" of *Mitsein* or Being-with.

After asserting that the existential analytic of *Being and Time* is "the enterprise from which all subsequent thinking derives" inasmuch as this analytic registered "the seismic jolt of a decisive rupture in the constitution or the consideration of sense," Nancy then remarks:

> The analytic of *Mitsein*, however, remains only sketched [in *Being and Time*] and subordinated, even though the trait of *Mitsein* is said

to be co-essential to *Dasein*. In this way, no doubt, the entire existential analytic hides the principle of a closing down of its own opening. It is thus necessary to re-open and to force a passage through the obstruction that, without any doubt, determined the filling-in and the folding-back of Being-with by means of the "folk" and its "destiny." This does not mean that it is necessary to "finish off" an analysis that is merely sketched, or to give *Mitsein* a "principial" place that is rightly its due. Being-with no doubt escapes "on principle" from both finishing and the principial position. But it is necessary to go back over the trait of the sketch and bear down on it so as to bring out the fact that the co-essentiality of Being-with implies nothing less than a co-originarity of sense.[10]

The French word *trait* that I have twice translated above as "trait" means as well a line drawn, which is why it figures in the French term for hyphen: *trait d'union*, literally, "line or mark of union." But it is not this semantic coincidence alone that can lead one to hear the above passage and the imperatives it issues as announcing a necessary rehyphenation of what has been filled in, occluded, obstructed, or closed down. Nancy's language, at this point, adopts a specifically graphic description for what must be done: "go back over the trait of the sketch and bear down on it." This redrawing of the line, however, does not figure a setting down of some boundary or limit; rather, it is always the double gesture of an articulation in difference of the singular-plural/plural-singular, of "being-several-together" (61), of "being-the-ones-with-the-others" (108), of "being-each-time-with" (121).[11] These latter sort of hyphenated formations, then, which arise regularly and constantly here, carry out the graphic imperative that Nancy formulates above, the necessity of going back over the articulating trait that has been covered over or closed down.

At a second level, this graphic practice is thematized, so to speak, around the preposition "with" or "avec." Here, I will have to be even more cursory in the description of how this thematization remains a spacing practice of the sort I am calling hyphenation. What comes to be thematized in this way is a preposition, "with" or "avec," which is to say, a lexical unit that belongs to the class of syntactic or logical terms called syncategorems: words which do not have meaning by themselves but only when used in conjunction with another word or words. What I have called Nancy's thematization of "avec" is the movement that carries over this syncategoremic character of the pre-position into affirmations or propositions that bear out the non-categorical sense of the in-conjunction-with-another. I will take two examples and propose a minimal commentary on them:

> A unique subject could not even designate *itself* and refer or relate to *itself* as subject. A subject, in the most classical sense of the term, supposes not only its own distinction from [*d'avec*] the object of its representation or its mastery: it supposes at least equally its own distinction from [*d'avec*] other subjects whose ipseity (or even, if one prefers, aseity) it can distinguish from [*d'avec*] its own center of representation or mastery. The *avec* is thus the supposition of "self" in general. But it is precisely not an underlying supposition, in the mode of the infinite auto-presupposition of subjective sub-stance. As its syntactic function indicates, "avec" is the pre-position of position in general, and it thus makes for its dis-position. (60–61)

In addition to the introduced hyphens in the words "sub-stance," "pre-position," and "dis-position,"[12] what one may remark here is the idiomatic effect that shows up when one translates the three occurrences of "d'avec," a French preposition that in fact combines two prepositions and that one must normally render, as I did here, not as "with" but "from" (for example, the "distinction from other subjects"). Literally, "d'avec" stages a kind of tug-of-war in two directions, away from/with, and is itself an articulated formation, marked not by a hyphen but by an apostrophe. In any case, the last sentences of the passage thematize, substantialize, or categorize not the "d'avec" but the "avec," when they make of it the grammatical subject of three predicating propositions, beginning with "The *avec* is thus the supposition of 'self' in general." This movement, then, can also be described as taking the risk that such a predication or substantialization of the "avec" will once again occlude, close down, cover over, or simply drop the difference articulated in the idiomatic, untranslatable formation "d'avec."

To generalize very quickly, and without further corroboration, I would be tempted to say that Nancy's writing is quite precisely, graphically dictated by this sort of risky gesture, which then requires, as the first passage I quoted put it, a doubling back over the trait so as to bear down once again on the occluded articulation. This could explain perhaps two prevalent features of the Nancien idiom: on the one hand, the frequency of copulative propositions in the third person present singular of the verb "to be," propositions, therefore, that take the risk of categorization, and on the other hand, the frequent imperatives, some modality of the impersonal "it is necessary," "il faut." If we are correct in reading such a text according to the hypothesis or the pre-position of the hyphen, then the "it is necessary" each time re-inscribes, bears down on the imperative Nancy relays in the wake of Heidegger's "sketch" of *Mitsein*: "it is necessary to go back over the trait of the sketch and bear down on it." In other words, the imperatives regularly issued here would be given above all or first of all to the writing itself—or to thinking, as Nancy prefers to say, for example in this sentence that combines the two features I have just isolated, the copulative proposition and the order of the imperative: "That being, absolutely, is being-with, this is what we must think [Que l'être, absolument, soit être-avec, voilà ce qu'il nous faut penser]" (83–84). What we might call the syncategoremical imperative, given to thinking, to writing, is also given to reading and all the more clearly so, perhaps, when it is placed under the command of "sensual reading."

> I select the second example because it will bear down on the hyphen by name: The *with* is not "unpresentable" like a withdrawn presence or like an Other. If there is no subject except with other subjects, the "with" itself is not a subject. It is or it draws the hyphen, the mark of union/disunion that by itself appropriates neither the union nor the disunion as substances posed under the mark: the latter is not a sign for a reality, not even for an "intersubjective dimension." It is truly—"in truth"—a line drawn on the void that at the same time traverses and underscores this void, which makes for its tension and traction, the tension and traction—attraction/repulsion—of the "among"-us [*l' "entre"-nous*]. The "with" remains among or between us, and we remain among ourselves: nothing but us, but nothing but interval between us. (84)

These sentences thematize the hyphen or rather the *trait d'union*, that is, they are general propositions on the hyphenating effects of "between," "among," or "with." And yet, just as with the previous examples, these general propositions are inflected by an idiom and thereby limited in their generality, as may be verified by attempting to translate them. Thus, for example, Nancy takes the rather considerable risk of re-inscribing the French phrase "entre nous," which is first cited and hyphenated as "the 'entre'-nous" and then inserted twice without any further punctuation in the sentence: "L' 'avec' reste entre nous, et nous restons entre nous." What cannot be simply repeated in another idiom, English for example, are the several resonances of the phrase "entre nous," which range from the aside or the secrecy of "just between us" to the sense of a closed circle of intimacy, family, friends, or neighbors: in this latter sense "nous restons entre nous" could therefore also mean "we are alone among ourselves, no outsider is present." It is precisely such gestures of closure or ex-clusion, whereby "we" pose and appropriate a substantial subject of community, that Nancy's re-inscriptions of the pre-positions—with, between, among—are working to expose. But this ex-position is undertaken at the risk of a re-inscription of the idiom that is "entre nous," just between us, unrepeatable or imperceptible for outsiders.

What I have just described is a marking effect of the common idiom, the possibility of a repetition of sense that exercises its tractorlike pull on the hyphenating or pre-positioned instance of the singular. Having recourse to his idiom, Nancy consigns this effect to the co-originarity and co-secondarity of a "singulier-pluriel," singular plurality/plural singularity. It is not, then, conceptual or categorical generalization as such that risks effacing without trace the singular trait here, because "entre nous" defines and performs only a *limited* generality, collectivity, or community, that which can be assembled in the *entente* of a common idiom. For this common idiom repeats singularity's effacement and, in the same trait, re-marks the limit at which, *entre nous*, we will have been *overheard* by another, by a different idiom, no longer speaking therefore just among ourselves.

What does it mean to overhear a hyphen? To overhear that which, under one, stands at the limit of a common under-standing? Is it to hear more than one should and is meant to or, on the contrary, as we can also say in our idiom by appealing to another sense, to overlook an essential something at once under and over, before and beyond the sense of our common meanings? What sense, hyphenation? Inaudible, odorless, tasteless, untouchable, the hyphen is finally invisible as well, even when its conventional mark has not already been effaced by the tendencies of the common idiom. In the sensorial array, no organ or faculty is set to read the hyphenating pulse. And yet, precisely: a pulse, the repetition of a beat, seconds ticking off beyond counting, but not to infinity, finite, rather, and always approaching the end, the one-and-only-times of our watches never quite synchronized, on the second. A sense of the singular counts with the unaccountable repetition of what has no number, not even one. The sense, perhaps, of a vigil and a vigilance, the sense of being *on watch* for the passing of the singular other.

Notes

1. See Eric Partridge, *You Have a Point There: A Guide to Punctuation and Its Allies* (London: Hamish Hamilton, 1953),134.

2. For a more complete inventory and a very witty analysis of hyphenation, see John McDermott, *Punctuation for Now* (London: MacMillan, 1990), 113–28. McDermott cites the "conventional wisdom" that "dashes divide and hyphens join," but is then careful to observe that "the hyphen performs two apparently contradictory tasks. It holds together two (or more) word-elements that would not normally occur in combination (such as, well, *word-elements*, or *fish-hooks*), and keeps apart word-elements which, though linked, must be shown as separate (such as *word-elements or fish-hooks*)" (113–14). On the "conventional wisdom" regarding hyphens, see Harold Herd, *Everybody's Guide to Punctuation* (London: Allen and Unwin, 1925), who reduces the hyphen to a single function: "The hyphen is used to join two words together" (38). (My thanks to Peter Krapp for these references.)

3. See, for example, Charles F. Meyer, *A Descriptive Study of American Punctuation* (Ann Arbor, Mich.: University Microfilms International, 1983) and Geoffrey Nunberg, *The Linguistics of Punctuation* (Stanford, Calif.: Center for the Study of Language and Information, 1990).

4. *The Chicago Manual of Style*, 13th ed. (Chicago: University of Chicago Press, 1982), 162.

5. Studies of punctuation in English frequently accept to speculate rather freely, or all too predictably, on the sociopsychological determinants of the general differences between American and British usage in this domain. In the appendix to Partridge's book, "A Chapter on American Practice," John W. Clark comments on Partridge's repeated assertion that "American punctuation tends to be more rigid than British, and more uniform, more systematic," for which reason it is also, in Clark's estimation, "easier to teach and, once learnt, easier to use." Two "facts" are then adduced to explain this difference: the greater tolerance for "individualism and independence" in Britain than the U.S., and the greater reliance among "cultivated" Americans on written rather than oral/aural tradition. These facts are in turn attributed to various ambient conditions: greater "fluidity" of American social classes, greater frequency of successful social climbing among Americans, which also produces greater anxiety among Americans about "correctness" or idiosyncrasies. "In short," he concludes, "an American is likely to punctuate unconventionally only because he doesn't know any better; a Briton, at least the typical British writer, because he is jolly well sure he does" (211–12).

6. Rodolphe Gasché, *Inventions of Difference: On Jacques Derrida* (Cambridge: Harvard University Press, 1994), 13; Gasché is quoting from Mark C. Taylor, "Failing Reflection," in Taylor, *Tears* (Albany, N.Y.: SUNY Press, 1990), 101.

7. "The Unconscious," in *The Standard Edition of the Complete Psychological Works*, ed. and trans. James Strachey, vol. 14 (London: Hogarth Press), 177; my emphasis.

8. Gasché is quoting from the selections of Joshua Wilner's translation of *Shibboleth* included in *Acts of Literature*, ed. Derek Attridge (New York: Routledge, 1992), 398; for the original language, see *Schibboleth, pour Paul Celan* (Paris: Galilée, 1986), 43.

9. This punctuality, if not punctuation, could also be the point of articulation with Roland Barthes's distinction between the *punctum* and the *studium* as he elaborates it throughout *La Chambre claire: Note sur la photographie* (Paris: Gallimard, 1980).

10. Jean-Luc Nancy, *Etre singulier pluriel* (Paris: Galilée, 1996), 117–18; my trans.

11. In French: "l'être-à-plusieurs-ensemble," "être-les-uns-avec-les-autres," "l'être-à-chaque-fois-avec."

12. In fact, the last word falls at the end of a line and therefore the hyphenation following its first syllable appears dictated by typographic convention. However, Nancy elsewhere hyphenates the word "dis-position" in this way.

WORKS CITED

Attridge, Derek, ed. *Acts of Literature*. New York: Routledge, 1992.

Barthes, Roland. *La Chambre claire: Note sur la photographie*. Paris: Gallimard, 1980.

Derrida, Jacques. *Schibboleth, pour Paul Celan*. Paris: Galilée, 1986.

Freud, Sigmund. "The Unconscious." In *The Standard Edition of the Complete Psychological Works*, vol. 14. Edited and translated by James Strachey. London: Hogarth Press.

Gasché, Rodolphe. *Inventions of Difference: On Jacques Derrida*. Cambridge: Harvard University Press, 1994.

Herd, Harold. *Everybody's Guide to Punctuation*. London: Allen and Unwin, 1925.

McDermott, John. *Punctuation for Now*. London: Macmillan, 1990.

Meyer, Charles F. *A Descriptive Study of American Punctuation*. Ann Arbor, Mich.: University Microfilms International, 1983.

Nancy, Jean-Luc. *Etre singulier pluriel*. Paris: Galilée, 1996.

Nunberg, Geoffrey. *The Linguistics of Punctuation*. Stanford, Calif.: Center for the Study of Language and Information, 1990.

Partridge, Eric. *You Have a Point There: A Guide to Punctuation and Its Allies*. London: Hamish Hamilton, 1953.

Taylor, Mark C. *Tears*. Albany, N.Y.: SUNY Press, 1990.

Back
NICHOLAS ROYLE

Is "BACK" A TITLE? CAN IT BECOME ONE? "BACK" CARRIES, AT LEAST for me, the palimpsestuous desire and imprint of another title, of what I had also thought of calling this essay, namely "Coelacanth." What is happening when a title can be said to carry another on its back or lodged within itself? "Coelacanth" connotes the fish of very great antiquity, supposed to have been long extinct, till a living specimen was caught off the coast of East Africa in 1938, and now again, it is thought, threatened with extinction. To become extinct "again"? Is there a coelacanth among us? Are there coelacanths in what one reads? Would it be possible to feel a coelacanth, to experience it rush and come, passing between us at an unimaginable depth? What is the desire for the coelacanth? Or to put these questions in another form: might it be possible to conceive a coelacanthology, that is to say a study and anthology of the coelacanthine?

Let me take a step back. I would like to propose the following project or jetty: a kind of reading and writing that takes as its focus the openness of a sort of oceanic expanse in English, that corresponds to the kinds of thinking and feeling associated with the work of Jacques Derrida but that moves between or away from ports of call which one might provisionally describe as "belonging to the English language."[1] This would involve, by definition, a concern with the impossible and, in particular, with experiencing the impossible in one's body. I take this last phrase from Derrida who suggests that "the only thing that interests [him]" is the "impossibility" of "the mourning of mourning" [*le deuil du deuil*].[2] As he puts it: "I am trying to experience *in my body* an altogether other relation to the unbelievable 'thing which is not.'" Such an experience, he suggests, would be "something other than a consolation, a mourning, a new well-being [or] a reconciliation with death" (*Points*, 49). "It is," he says, "a terrible thing that I do not love but that I want to love"; it is "what bestows and withdraws [one's] idiom" (49). These remarks come in the interview published in English as "*Ja*, or the *faux-bond* II" and in the context of a discussion of Jonathan Swift's *Gulliver's Travels* and reading. This, for Derrida, is the pause-giving question: "what type of effect (of reading or non-reading) is absolutely *unanticipatable*, out of sight, structurally out of sight . . . ?" (41). He poses the question, he says, "blindly, mutely, deprived of a language in which to say 'the thing which is not' " (41).

One might, then, envisage this as one of the possible tasks of critical and theoretical work in English over the next few years: to turn back to the canonical texts (literary, philosophical, and other), in order to rethink their status as "great works of English" (starting off, it should perhaps be added, from Derrida's contention that one never reads or writes either in one's own language or in a foreign language),[3] and to make English as strange and disruptive to itself and to its institutions as Derrida's work makes French strange. This turning back would correspond to a rethinking of "English" in terms of what Nicolas Abraham named "anasemia." The jetty which I want to sketch here under the paradoxical heading of "Back" would concern the anasemic deconstruction of the English language.

"Anasemia" might be defined as literally "back-" (*ana-*) "meaning," except that it is precisely the conceptual poles of the "literal" or "metaphorical" that anasemia "originally" displaces. Abraham first introduced the term in 1968, in the essay published in English as "The Shell and the Kernel: The Scope and Originality of Freudian Psychoanalysis."[4] He speaks of a "scandalous antisemantics" whereby certain psychoanalytic terms, such as "Pleasure" or "Ego," come to "constitute new figures, absent from rhetorical treatises." Abraham writes:

> These figures of antisemantics, inasmuch as they signify no more than the action of moving up [or back] toward the source of their customary meaning, require a denomination properly indicative of their status and which—for want of something better—I shall propose to designate by the neologism *anasemia*. (85)

The most provocative elaboration of Abraham's neologism is perhaps Derrida's, in particular in the essay "Fors: The Anglish Words of Nicolas Abraham and Maria Torok."[5] In that strategy of ghostly paraphrase and displacement that is so characteristic of Derrida's idiom, the question of the anasemic becomes inextricable with that of the trace or cryptic structure of language in general. Abraham's questions become Derridean:

> How can we include in a discourse, *any* discourse that which, being the very condition of discourse, would by its very essence *escape* discourse? If non-presence, the core and ultimate reason behind all discourse, becomes speech, can it—or should it—make itself heard in and through self-presence? ("Fors," xxxii, citing Abraham)

Derrida follows Abraham in trying to attend to "this strange foreignness" ("Fors," xxxii) that inhabits words. After Derrida and Abraham, I would like to propose an exploration of English words in general as anasemic *effects*. Critical and philosophical analysis would open itself to another thinking of the "back" movement implied in the structure of the word "analysis" itself (*ana-*, "back," *lyein*, "to loose"). I am dreaming of a jetty that would immerse itself in the sensual but only on the basis of what may tentatively be termed the anasensual; a kind of writing, and thus reading, that would alter the very sensing of that hallucinatory realm to which we give the name "English"; a sensing of what is perhaps extremely ancient ("older" than English, or Anglo-Saxon, or Ancient Greek) and very new, the intimacy of the unknown and of the unanticipatable.

The "back" is sensual. Its sensuality is immediately intimated by the so-called materiality of the book and the metaphors through which it is enigmatically bodied. To look for a book in a bookshop or on library shelves is first of all to engage in spine-reading. To read a book is to have the spine hidden from you, resting on the table perhaps, or in your palms. Although Wallace Stevens once said that in order to read one ought to have eyes all around one's head, in fact we tend to believe we always face a book: to read, in this sense, is to become a beast with two backs. But the book is already such a beast itself: it has a spine and at least one other back. Figuratively (but what *is* a figure if it is not that which requires a back, however ignored such a prerequisite tain may traditionally have appeared to be?), we talk of the back of the book; but the phrase is perhaps undecidable. It can mean the back cover, the blurb on the back and so on, or it can mean the end of the text. To turn to the back of a book is not necessarily to know where to turn: "back," in its very uncertainty, indicates not so much the end as the closure of the book, not so much the enveloping balm of a happy anthropomorphism as the backbreaking force of a figure that is perhaps not a figure at all.

What is "back"? In "Fors" Derrida stresses that anasemia does not go back to the unveiling of origins or original meanings:

"While preserving the old word ['back'] in order to submit it to its singular conversion, the anasemic operation does not result in a growing explicitness, in the uninterrupted development of a virtual significance, in a regression towards the original meaning" (xxxiv). As he has noted elsewhere:

> The anasemic word has no meaning and does not belong to the semantic order; it is asemantic or presemantic. It is not really part of language in the sense in which the words of an intralingual transformation are all equally part of language [. . .] anasemia [involves] a kind of shift or departure from the everyday order of language which constantly dislocates the normal order of language.[6]

The jetty called "back" would only find its possibility in the anasemic. To present an account of "back" is, in this respect, to re-cite something that never happens. In his description of the movement of Abraham and Torok's *The Wolf Man's Magic Word* Derrida furnishes an analogous model:

> the account will have been called for *within* the concept, within the workings of the concept, *by the anasemic structure*. That structure describes a story or a fable *within* the concept; the story is described as a path followed backward by the structure in order to reach all the way back beyond the origin, which is nonetheless not in any way a proper, rightful, literal meaning. The concept is re-cited in the course of this journey. ("Fors," xxxiv)

The journey on which we are embarked passes back from Derrida and Abraham and Torok to the work of Beckett and Shakespeare. The example of what is apparently a single word, "back," comports two of the principal characteristics of the jetty: (1) as a deconstructive philology taking the form of a strange strategy without finality (a jetting) engaged with a transformation of the cultural, aesthetic, and ideological conceptions of "English"; and (2) complicit with this, the jetty as historically and temporally deconstructive, that is to say as a movement that is at once historical and radically *anachronistic*, attuned to a disruption of all linearity, teleology, calendricality, or movement forward and back.

To offer two epigraphs then, that ought to have been back at the beginning, two very brief, more or less aphoristic statements from Derrida. First, from *The Ear of the Other*, where the English translation has him say simply: "A text, I believe, does not come back" (156). Second, from *The Post Card*, where he declares: "In a word there will only be back (*du dos*), and even the word '*dos*', if you are willing to pay faithful attention to it and keep the memory."⁷ In *The Post Card* Derrida speaks of the back [*le dos*] nonstop, back to back; it is the truth of philosophy. As he indicates early on in a reference to Socrates and Plato, as depicted in Matthew Paris's fortunetelling postcard: "S. does not see P. who sees S., but (and here is the truth of philosophy) only *from the back*. There is only the *back*, seen from the back, in what is written, such is the final word. Everything is played out in *retro* and *a tergo*" (48). A question then, for us as for Derrida, of turning back. As he writes elsewhere in the "Envois": "Our great tropics: to turn the 'dos' in every sense, to all sides. The word 'dos' and all the families that swarm behind it, beginning with behind. There (*da*) is behind, behind the curtain . . . or behind oneself" (178). It may be evident especially from the last part of this quotation [in French: "Là (*da*) c'est derrière, derrière le rideau . . . ou derrière soi" (192)], that what is at stake in *The Post Card* is in part the question of the proper name, the signature, and idiom, the desire to inscribe a back there (*dos da, derrière da*), the call of the proper name. Let us, for a moment, put this call on hold.

"A text, I believe, does not come back." Or—to back this thought up with a related suggestion in *The Ear of the Other*— there is no "untouchable, virgin granny," no "intact kernel" (114) at the origin of a language or languages. One of the most obvious points about the Englishing or Anglishing of Derrida's French is the incursion or irruption of the word "back" at moments where, in French, the prefix "re-" is in operation. What in French is signified in the *re* of the *retrait* or *revenance*, for example, can appear in English as what draws back, what comes back and so on.

Is "back" a word? Is it a concept? As a title, for example, what would "Back" entitle? "Back" might just name the possibility of a title, the principle of the iterable that makes a title a title without, for all that, letting it lie still, at peace, on its "back." To put the word in quotation marks, as I have just done, is to testify to the ghostly work of iterability as a generalized movement of "putting in quotation marks," visible or not.⁸ Derrida's meditation on his "back" concerns, among other things, the thought of a sort of "back" logic linked to what Lewis Carroll calls "living backwards." As the Queen says in *Through the Looking Glass*:

> "That's the effect of living backwards . . . it always makes one a little giddy at first—"

"Living backwards!" Alice repeated in great astonishment. "I never heard of such a thing!"

"—but [the Queen adds] there's one great advantage in it, that one's memory works both ways."[9]

Derrida's work, in effect, breaks the back of history with at least two related moves: (1) by disturbing and deranging the linear logic according to which one event, one writer or one text comes after, behind or at the back of another. We might thus sense how, for example, the work of Derrida or the work of Beckett is "in" Shakespeare; and (2) by outlining a thought of what is at the back of any history, that trace or movement of alterity which belongs as much to "the opening of the future itself" as to a bizarre past, a past that was never present.[10]

"Back" would be both sensual and anasensual—the "implacable trace" (*P*, 48) that points to an experience in one's body, in one's own body and no one else's, but an experience that would be impossible, singularly impossible, anasemic, "this side of meaning" (*EO*, 109). The sensuality of the back is in a sort of double-bind with memory: to think back on the back is to be in another realm of the senses. In Shakespeare this motif of the sensuality of "back" as a memory is marked, for example, in Hamlet's memory of Yorick (we may think first of Yorick's skull perhaps, but it is at least as much a matter of remembering his back: "He hath bore me on his back a thousand times" [5.1. 185–86]) or in Cleopatra's dreaming memory of Antony ("His delights / Were dolphin-like, they show'd his back above / The element they liv'd in" [5.2. 88–90]). The back is linked to the sensual and amorous (as Derrida suggests in *The Post Card*, the amorousness of being behind cannot easily, as it were, be overlooked), but also to mourning and death, to the experience of the impossible.

This would be the hypothesis: that the work of Beckett and Shakespeare might be read through the strange figure and logic of "back," as a sort of uncanny program that would include a sense of finding Beckett's "back" already "in" Shakespeare's. A brief paragraph from "Stirrings Still" (1988) may offer a point of departure:

> Seen always from behind whithersoever he went. Same hat and coat as of old when he walked the roads. The back roads. Now as one in a strange place seeking the way out. In the dark. In a strange place blindly in the dark of night or day seeking the way out. A way out. To the roads. The back roads.[11]

Beckett's work is almost obsessively preoccupied with "back"—here with a sense of "back" which embraces various significations (the back of the body, being seen from the back, belonging to the past, seeking the back roads, the exit or way out, the little-known but intimate and familiar), but which at the same time seems to exceed or fall short of all sense. Above all I want to suggest that "back" in Beckett is the uncanny movement of return or repetition as such, the uncanniness of a calling back. It is, to deploy the terms of his poematic "Neither" (1962), the movement of being "beckoned back and forth," in which the voice itself comes to figure as "unspeakable home."[12] In "Neither" we may indeed feel the uneasy sonic rapport of a "beckoning" of "back" in "Beckett," the beckoning "back" as a sort of signature-effect. If so, it would only be in tracing a logic of going back "from impenetrable self to impenetrable unself by way of neither" (108). In other words it would be no more (and no less) than a testimony to the impossibility of answering to an identity, a beckoning into the abyss. If "back" beckons as a sort of signature-effect in Beckett's writing, we could say, it does so only by moving back, as if to a more removed ground. To recall for a moment the mad and deadly logic of the signature elaborated in Derrida's *Signsponge*, "back" would in some sense contain all of Beckett, be larger than his oeuvre as such.[13] It would not be clear whether "back" were "in" Beckett's writings or Beckett's writings an effect of "back." "Back" would be the ghostly mark of "what bestows and withdraws [one's] idiom" (in Derrida's phrase). Such an engulfment—the abyss and monument of "back"—is perhaps also the effect of trying to keep readerly company with Beckett's *Company* (1980), a rigorously "supine" text entailing an atopical scene in which "a voice tells of the past" to "one on his back in the dark" (8).[14] The voice that speaks of what is back in the past, and in the back of the mind of the one on his back in the dark, is a voice that comes back, one might say, without ever being present. It is a voice impossible to experience in one's body: "The fable of one fabling of one with you in the dark. . . . Alone" (89).

Difference within hearing-oneself-speak: *Krapp's Last Tape* (1958) bodies this forth in its astonishing conclusion:

> [*Pause.*] Perhaps my best years are gone. When there was a chance of happiness. But I wouldn't want them back. Not with the fire in me now. No, I wouldn't want them back.
> [KRAPP *motionless staring before him. The tape runs on in silence.*]
> CURTAIN[15]

"Back" is the last word of the last tape, the final playback, the last sound in Beckett's play. Krapp listens in silence to his own voice back in the past rejecting any desire to have that past back. The logic of "back" is always already doubled up. Even the affirmative "Not with the fire in me now" is back in the past. Here, perhaps, is a sense of the nihilism that Derrida seems to find difficult to work with in Beckett's writing; but here too is the cryptic concentration of a "remains," for example of "back" as strange remains and signature-effect, which Derrida so admires in Beckett's writing and which, like other distinguishing elements in his oeuvre, is perhaps finally so "decomposed" that it already contains in some sense anything that a deconstructive reading might seek to bear against or bring to it.[16] "Back" is a crypt in which, we might say, Beckett's play at once passes away and is still to come. Spoken not once but twice: "But I wouldn't want them back. . . . No, I wouldn't want them back." Or rather, not even spoken once, but always already a repetition: a speaking "back" that is possible only as a recording and as a recording of the impossible. Beckett's play is a playback or series of playbacks that bears witness, perhaps before anything else, to that principle of repetition that lets a voice be recognized and a word understood but that, at the same time, is the principle of the non-self-coincidence and ghostliness of word and voice. "Back," in all its singularity, begins in repetition. One cannot get back to the origin of the sounding or sense of "back." Like the "yes" (in Derrida's terms) or the "fire" (in Beckett's) that is the condition of the no ("No, I wouldn't want them back"), "back" never takes place, it does not have a place.[17] *Krapp's Last Tape* ends, without having begun, in an inaugural disjunction or backfiring of voice and sense: "back" in the abyss.

Let me try to trace this strange foreignness of "back" in a reading of Shakespeare and, in particular, of *Romeo and Juliet* (1595–96).[18] In its dramatization of the experience of a character listening to recordings of his own voice, *Krapp's Last Tape* presents a singularly "theatrical" and, we could say, *theoretically* explicit rendition of the condition of possibility of dramatic works, as Derrida describes it in his essay on *Romeo and Juliet*, "Aphorism Countertime":

> The survival of a theatrical work implies that, theatrically, it is saying something about theatre itself, about its essential possibility. And that it does so, theatrically, then, through the play of uniqueness and repetition, by giving rise every time to the chance of an ab-

solutely singular event as it does to the untranslatable idiom of a proper name, to its fatality (the "enemy" that "I hate"), to the fatality of a date and of a rendezvous.[19]

Every performance of *Krapp's Last Tape* stages itself as this "play of uniqueness and repetition," exposing itself, by necessity, to the possibility of the unanticipatable, while dramatizing the form of the dramatic work itself as the repetition of what is always already an uncanny "recording." Everything in *Romeo and Juliet*, in its tragic irony, its pathos, and what Derrida has called its "lunar" coldness, can be seen to configure and disfigure in the "back," and in particular in its elaboration of what it means to call back, to call oneself back.[20] Like *Krapp's Last Tape*, *Romeo and Juliet* is first and foremost a strange "playback." To follow the movements of "back" in Shakespeare's play permits us to add a sort of supplement to Derrida's reading of what he calls "the poisoned truth of this drama," namely "Non-coincidence and contretemps between my name and me, between the experience according to which I am named or hear myself named and my 'living present'" (423). "Back," in *Romeo and Juliet*, resembles a weird program. It appears repeatedly across the play in a movement of repetition or repetitiveness that concerns, first of all, a dividing and breaking up of sense within the word.[21] Thus in the opening scene of the play, in its very first appearance, "back" redoubles and divides. On the entrance of two Montague servingmen, the Capulet servant Sampson says to his fellow servant Gregory: "My naked weapon is out. Quarrel, I will back thee"; and Gregory retorts: "How, turn thy back and run?" (1.1. 34–35). Beyond any controlled polysemia of "back" (as though it were the equivalent of a sort of verbal "backgammon"), *Romeo and Juliet* seems to call for a calling back otherwise. At the start of act 2, Romeo enters alone and says: "Can I go forward when my heart is here? / Turn back, dull earth, and find thy centre out" (2.1. 1–2). He addresses himself, or rather he addresses his own body, as "dull earth," telling himself (or telling it) to turn back and fall towards its centre, in other words, to Juliet. This turning back, figured as the movement of gravity itself, would be for Romeo perhaps to experience the impossible in his body: the condition at once of desire and death.

"Back" haunts everything: its tropics are lethal. Derrida in his "Aphorism Countertime" has provided an extensive account of anachrony in Shakespeare's play, the anachrony of time itself and of the name: all of this, I would like to suggest, is inscribed in the effects of "back." Romeo and Juliet must come back to one another, but without understanding how or why. Romeo is (as the stage direction specifies) *"Retiring"* but Juliet comes back, once again, onto the balcony (the balcony scene is, above all, a scene of coming back): "Hist, Romeo, hist! O, for a falc'ner's voice, / To lure this tassel-gentle back again!" (2.2. 158–59). But then, once Romeo is called back, Juliet can only say: "I have forgot why I did call thee back" (170). To which he replies: "Let me stand here till thou remember it" (171). Even when Juliet finally "would have [Romeo] gone," it is only to desire "with a silken thread" to "pluck [him] back again" (2.2. 176–80.) To be called Romeo is to be called back, to call oneself back, to want to call oneself back. All this coming and going is enough to give at least one of the characters in the play a backache. As the Nurse, tired of taking and fetching messages, tells Juliet: "ah, my back, my back! / Beshrew your heart for sending me about / To catch my death with jauncing up and down!" (2.5. 50–52).

There would be no need for what Derrida calls Juliet's "implacable analysis" (427)—"O Romeo, Romeo, wherefore art thou Romeo? . . . What's in a name? . . ."—without these strange effects of being called back, of wanting to call oneself back. Shakespeare's play insists on the force of the name, in particular, as what cannot be called back. This is true not only of Romeo "himself" ("O be some other name"), but also of the act of naming that precipitates his banishment. Tybalt dies, and Romeo is consequently banished, because Tybalt refuses to retract when Romeo threatens him: "Now, Tybalt, take the 'villain' back again / That late thou gavest me" (3.1. 125–26). *Romeo and Juliet* suggests that, whether with the name or with tears, one cannot call them back, even as one calls them back. Such is Juliet's impossible imperative: "Back, foolish tears, back to your native spring" (3.2. 102).

At the back of this, there is the way out, the "back" roads, the arrival there (never on time) of that old, undiscovered country bus, Time's wingèd chariot "itself." The Friar may attempt to bless Romeo—"A pack of blessings light upon thy back" (3.3. 141)—but this back is in effect the place of death.[22] The "sight of death" (5.3. 206) itself, in the final scene of Shakespeare's play, is a curiously "empty" focus on Romeo's back. As Capulet exclaims: "O wife, look how our daughter bleeds! / This dagger hath mista'en, for lo his house / Is empty on the back of Montagu . . ." (5.3. 202–4). If the play finally calls back to the back itself as the place of death, however, it does this only in a sense by turning us away by turning its back, in particular by insisting on that celebrated Shakespearean-Derridean necessity according to which a letter can always not arrive at its destination. As Derrida's "Aphorism Countertime" suggests, this necessary possibility allows us to see Shakespeare's play as dramatizing "an anachrony of structure, the absolute interruption of history [*l'histoire*] as deployment of *a* temporality, of a single and organized temporality" (420). *Romeo and Juliet* is in a sense itself nothing other than "the irremediable detour of a letter" (420). In Friar Laurence's words: "he which bore my letter, Friar John, / Was stayed by accident, and yesternight / Return'd my letter back" (5.3. 250–52). The "back" here appears to be superfluous—a peculiar supplement to "Return'd" that indeed occurs only very rarely in Shakespeare's writings.[23] It is as if, according to the uncanny program, Shakespeare's play keeps back till the very end the most decisive and catastrophic turn of this figure—the "success" of returning back is death, the tragedy of Romeo and Juliet. "Back" is the ghostly return or *revenance* of writing as such.

"Back" names nothing. It would be the contretemps of the name itself, of voice and history. To attend with an Anglish ear, we might hear this in the English translation of Derrida's words about "the Anglish words of Nicolas Abraham and Maria Torok":

> To whom? To what does a name go back? But a *present* going back, a going back in the present, a bringing back to the present, to whatever kind of haunting return or *unheimlich* homecoming—isn't all that already the law of the name? ("Fors," xlviii)

To be angling for a coelacanth. . . . "Coelacanthology" (another word for the jetty I have tried to outline in this essay) would be a peculiar example of what is known in linguistics as a back-formation, that is to say of the making of a word from one that is taken to be derivative. "Coelacanth" would derive from "coelacanthology"—it would thus be a kind of spectro-cryptic word sharing its etymology with the more familiar word "coelacanth." "Coelacanth" is from the Greek *koilos*, "hollow"; *akantha*, "spine". In the *OED* it is given first as an adjective, in fact, and defined as "Having a hollow spine."

Notes

1. For the sense of the term "jetty," see Jacques Derrida, "Some Statements and Truisms about Neo-Logisms, Newisms, Postisms, Parasitisms, and other

Small Seismisms," trans. Anne Tomiche, in *The States of "Theory": History, Art, and Critical Discourse*, ed. David Carroll (New York: Columbia University Press, 1990), 63–95. Derrida defines a jetty as "the force of that *movement* which is not *subject, project,* or *object,* not even rejection, but in which takes place any production and any determination, which finds its possibility in the jetty" (65).

2. Jacques Derrida, "*Ja,* or the *faux-bond* II," trans. Peggy Kamuf, in *Points . . . Interviews, 1974–94* (London: Routledge, 1995), 30–77, here, 49. Further page references are to this edition, abbreviated *P* where appropriate. For the French text, see *Points de suspension: Entretiens,* choisis et présentés par Elisabeth Weber (Paris: Galilée, 1992), 37–81.

3. See Jacques Derrida, "Living On," trans. James Hulbert, in Harold Bloom et al., *Deconstruction and Criticism* (New York: Seabury Press, 1979), 101.

4. Nicolas Abraham, "The Shell and the Kernel: The Scope and Originality of Freudian Psychoanalysis," in Abraham and Maria Torok, *The Shell and the Kernel: Renewals of Psychoanalysis,* vol. 1, trans. Nicholas Rand (London and Chicago: Chicago University Press, 1994), 79–98. Further page references are to this edition.

5. Jacques Derrida, "Fors: The Anglish Words of Nicolas Abraham and Maria Torok," trans. Barbara Johnson, in Abraham and Torok, *The Wolf Man's Magic Word: A Cryptonymy,* trans. Nicholas Rand (Minneapolis: University of Minnesota Press, 1986), xi–xlviii. Further page references are to this edition.

6. Jacques Derrida, *The Ear of the Other: Otobiography, Transference, Translation,* trans. Peggy Kamuf, ed. Christie V. McDonald (New York: Schocken Books, 1985), 134. Further page references are to this edition, abbreviated *EO* where appropriate.

7. Jacques Derrida, *The Post Card: From Socrates to Freud and Beyond,* trans. Alan Bass (Chicago: Chicago University Press, 1987), 187. Further page references are to this edition, accompanied where appropriate by page references to the original French edition, *La Carte postale de Socrate à Freud et au-delà* (Paris: Flammarion, 1980).

8. For an account of deconstruction as a generalized "putting-into-quotation-marks," see "Some Statements and Truisms," in particular Derrida's argument that "There is . . . no attitude, let's say, in quotation marks, more historical, more "historian" (that is, pertaining to the specific work of the historian), more responsible in front of history (*Geschichte* or history) than that which puts into practice a vigilant but, in its very principle, a general *use* of quotation marks" (77).

9. Lewis Carroll, *Through the Looking-Glass* in *Alice's Adventures in Wonderland and Through the Looking-Glass* (New York: Signet, 1960), 172.

10. See, for example, Jacques Derrida, "Afterw.rds: or, at least, less than a letter about a letter less," trans. Geoffrey Bennington, in *Afterwords,* ed. Nicholas Royle (Tampere, Finland: Outside Books, 1992), 200; and *Of Grammatology,* trans. Gayatri Chakravorty Spivak (Baltimore: Johns Hopkins University Press, 1976), 66.

11. Samuel Beckett, "Stirrings Still," in *As the Story Was Told: Uncollected and Late Prose* (London: John Calder, 1990), 116–17.

12. Samuel Beckett, "Neither," in *As the Story Was Told,* 108–9. Further page references are to this edition.

13. See Jacques Derrida, *Signéponge/Signsponge,* trans. Richard Rand (New York: Columbia University Press, 1984).

14. What is "supine" in Beckett's text would at the same time be inextricable from the motif of lying or saying "the thing which was not": "Supine now you resume your fable where the act of lying cut it short . . ." (87).

15. Samuel Beckett, *Krapp's Last Tape*, in *The Complete Dramatic Works* (London: Faber and Faber, 1986), 223.

16. I am thinking here of Derrida's remarks on why he has not been able to write about Beckett's work: see "This Strange Institution Called Literature," trans. Geoffrey Bennington and Rachel Bowlby, in *Acts of Literature*, ed. Derek Attridge (London and New York: Routledge, 1992), 33–75. Permit me to refer here to the chapter "On Not Reading: Derrida and Beckett," in my book *After Derrida* (Manchester: Manchester University Press, 1995), 159–74, where I consider at greater length the question of Derrida's "avoidance" of writing about Beckett.

17. Cf. Jacques Derrida, "Ulysses Gramophone: Hear Say Yes in Joyce," trans. Tina Kendall and Shari Benstock in *Acts of Literature*, ed. Derek Attridge (London and New York: Routledge, 1992), 256–309, esp. 298.

18. All references to Shakespeare are to *The Riverside Shakespeare*, ed. G. Blakemore Evans et al. (Boston: Houghton Mifflin, 1974).

19. Jacques Derrida, "Aphorism Countertime," trans. Nicholas Royle, in *Acts of Literature*, 414–33: see 419. Further page references are to this edition.

20. On the lunar, see "Aphorism Countertime," 431.

21. I should perhaps emphasize here that the question "Did Shakespeare intend to generate these 'back'-effects when he was writing this play?" is a question that is perhaps inevitable but at the same time disqualified by the logic of "back" itself. The same of course applies for "back" in Beckett.

22. This is already ominously implied in Juliet's characterization of her estranged lover in the preceding scene: "Come, night, come, Romeo, come, thou day in night, / For thou wilt lie upon the wings of night, / Whiter than new snow upon a raven's back" (3.2. 17–19).

23. The only other instances that I have been able to trace are *Richard II*, 1.3. 119–20 ("Let them lay by their helmets and their spears, / And both return back to their chairs again") and *King Lear*, 1.1. 95–97 ("Good my lord, / You have begot me, bred me, lov'd me: I / Return those duties back as are right fit"). The phrase "back return'd" occurs once, in *Troilus and Cressida* (2.2. 186).

Works Cited

Abraham, Nicholas, and Maria Torok. *The Shell and the Kernel: Renewals of Psychoanalysis*, vol. 1. Translated by Nicholas Rand. London and Chicago: Chicago University Press, 1994.

Attridge, Derek, ed. *Acts of Literature*. London and New York: Routledge, 1992.

Beckett, Samuel. *Krapp's Last Tape*. In *The Complete Dramatic Works*. London: Faber and Faber, 1986.

———. "Stirrings Still." In *As the Story Was Told: Uncollected and Late Prose*. London: John Calder, 1990.

Carroll, Lewis. *Through the Looking-Glass* in *Alice's Adventures in Wonderland and Through the Looking-Glass*. New York: Signet, 1960.

Derrida, Jacques. "Afterw.rds: or, at least, less than a letter about a letter less." Translated by Geoffrey Bennington. In *Afterwords*. Edited by Nicholas Royle. Tampere, Finland: Outside Books, 1992.

———. *The Ear of the Other: Otobiography, Transference, Translation*. Translated by Peggy Kamuf. Edited by Christie V. McDonald. New York: Schocken Books, 1985.

———. "Fors: The Anglish Words of Nicolas Abraham and Maria Torok." Translated by Barbara Johnson. In Abraham and Torok, *The Wolf Man's Magic Word: A Cryptonymy*. Translated by Nicholas Rand. Minneapolis: University of Minnesota Press, 1986.

———. *Of Grammatology*. Translated by Gayatri Chakravorty Spivak. Baltimore: Johns Hopkins University Press, 1976.

———. "Ja, or the *faux-bond* II." Translated by Peggy Kamuf. In *Points . . . Interviews, 1974–94*. London: Routledge, 1995, 30–77.

———. "Living On." Translated by James Hulbert. In Harold Bloom et al. *Deconstruction and Criticism*. New York: Seabury Press, 1979.

———. *The Post Card: From Socrates to Freud and Beyond*. Translated by Alan Bass. Chicago: Chicago University Press, 1987.

———. *Signéponge/Signsponge*. Translated by Richard Rand. New York: Columbia University Press, 1984.

———. "Some Statements and Truisms about Neo-Logisms, Newisms, Post-isms, Parasitisms, and other Small Seismisms." Translated by Anne Tomiche. In *The States of "Theory": History, Art, and Critical Discourse*. Edited by David Carroll. New York: Columbia University Press, 1990.

Royle, Nicholas. *After Derrida*. Manchester: Manchester University Press, 1995.

Shakespeare, William. *The Riverside Shakespeare*. Edited by G. Blakemore Evans et al. Boston: Houghton Mifflin, 1974.

Contributors

DAVE BOOTHROYD studied philosophy at the universities of Essex and Warwick and is senior lecturer and course leader for cultural studies at the University of Teesside, UK. He is a founding coeditor of the international electronic journal *Culture Machine* and is currently completing a monograph, *Culture on Drugs: Narco-cultural Studies of High Modernity*, for Manchester University Press.

SCOTT BREWSTER is lecturer in English at the University of Central Lancashire. He is author of *Crossing Borders: Northern Irish Poetry* (Sheffield Academic Press, forthcoming 2001), and coeditor of *Inhuman Reflections: Thinking the Limits of the Human* (Manchester University Press, 2000) and *Proximities: Studies in Irish Culture* (Routledge, 1999). He has also published articles on Irish poetry and fiction, D. H. Lawrence and Gothic fiction.

JO CROFT is a lecturer in literature and cultural history at Liverpool John Moores University. She has published articles on adolescence and psychoanalysis, and youth culture. She is currently writing a book on borderline identitities.

KNUT OVE ELIASSEN is associate professor in comparative literature in the Department of Scandinavian Studies and Comparative Literature, University of Trondheim, Norway. He has published articles on aesthetics, contemporary French philosophy (Foucault, Lyotard, Deleuze, Baudrillard), Thomas Bernhard, and Marivaux. He is currently writing a book on the French eighteenth-century novel.

CHARLES FORSDICK is a lecturer in French at the University of Glasgow. He has published articles on exoticism, contemporary travel writing, and postcolonial literature in French. He is the author of *Victor Segalen and the Aesthetics of Diversity*.

RACHEL JONES completed a doctorate in philosophy and literature at the University of Warwick and now teaches in the Department of Philosophy at the University of Dundee. Her research interests include: Kant and post-Kantian philosophies of the self; aesthetics, especially the sublime; feminist philosophy; German Expressionism; German women philosophers of the twentieth century.

PEGGY KAMUF is professor of French and comparative literature at the University of Southern California. She is the translator of several works by Derrida and editor of *A Derrida Reader* (Columbia University Press, 1998). Her own books include *Fictions of Feminine Desire*, *Signature Pieces* (Cornell University Press, 1988), and *The Division of Literature, or The University in Deconstruction.* (University of Chicago Press, 1997).

PETER KRAPP maintains theory websites in Minneapolis (Minnesota) and Santa Barbara (California); he has published in English and German on the alleged convergence of theory and hypermedia, on deconstruction, and on the history of the voice. He is a doctoral candidate in the programme in theory of literature and communication at Konstanz University, and also a Ph.D. candidate in German at the University of California, Santa Barbara.

IAN MACLACHLAN is lecturer in French at the University of Aberdeen, having previously taught at the Universities of Oxford and Leicester. He has written on Blanchot, Derrida, Jabès, and Laporte, and has translated texts by Blanchot and Laporte. His book *Roger Laporte: The Orphic Text* is forthcoming in the *Legenda* series published by Oxford's European Humanities Research Centre. He is currently preparing a book on time and literary value in contemporary French literature and philosophy.

LAURENT MILESI is a lecturer in English/American literature and critical theory at Cardiff University, and a member of the ITEM Research Group on Joyce's manuscripts in the C.N.R.S. (Paris). His essays are mainly on Joyce and related aspects of modernism, twentieth-century American poetry, postmodernism and poststructuralism (Lacan and Derrida). He is currently completing *The "Litteral" of Language in Finnegans Wake* and *Post-Effects: Literature, Criticism, and the Future Perfect*. He is also editing a collection of essays on Joyce, language, and theory for Cambridge University Press.

JACQUELINE RATTRAY has recently completed her Ph.D., *The Surrealist Visuality of José Maria Hinojosa: A Sight for Sore Eyes*, at the University of Aberdeen. She has published on Hinojosa in relation to French surrealism and the visual arts, most recently in *Romance Studies*. She is currently working on the politics of madness in surrealism.

NICHOLAS ROYLE is professor of English at the University of Sussex. He is editor of the *Oxford Literary Review*, author of *Telepathy and Literature: Essays on the Reading Mind* (Blackwell,1991), *After Derrida* (Manchester University Press, 1995), *E. M. Forster* (Mississippi, 1999), coauthor (with Andrew Bennett) of *Elizabeth Bowen and the Dissolution of the Novel* (Macmillan Press, 1995) and *An Introduction to Literature, Criticism and Theory* (Prentice Hall, 2d ed, 1999). He has recently edited a book entitled *Deconstructions: A User's Guide* and is currently completing a study entitled *The Uncanny*.

NAOMI SEGAL is professor of French studies at the University of Reading, where she founded the interdisciplinary M.A. on The Body and Representation in 1994. She researches mainly on nineteenth- and twentieth-century French and comparative literature, gender, and sexuality. She is the author of eight books, including *The Adulteress's Child* (Polity Press, 1992), *Scarlet Letters* (Macmillan Press, 1996, with Nicholas White), *Coming Out of Feminism?* (Blackwell Publishers, 1998, with Mandy Merck and Elizabeth Wright) and *André Gide: Pederasty and Pedagogy* (1998). She is currently completing an edited collection in French, *Le désir à l'oeuvre: André Gide à Cambridge 1918, 1998* (forthcoming 2000) and an interdisciplinary coedition, *In/determinate Bodies* (forthcoming 2001).

MICHAEL SHERINGHAM is professor of French at Royal Holloway, University of London, associate director of the Institute of Romance Studies, editor of Cambridge Studies in French, and a regular contributor to the *Times Literary Supplement*. He has written extensively on André Breton and surrealism, on modern and contemporary French poetry, and on autobiography and related genres. Current publications include essays on memory and the archive, autobiography, and women's writing, and new forms of biography. He is currently completing a book on theories and practices of "The everyday." His publications include *French Autobiography: Devices and Desires* (Oxford University Press, 1993) and *Parisian Fields* (ed.), (Reaktion Books, 1996).

PAUL SUTTON is a lecturer in film studies at the Bolton Institute. He has published a number of articles on European cinema and film theory, as well as an interview with, and essay on, Jean Baudrillard. Forthcoming publications include a translation of Félix Guattari's *The Three Ecologies* (Athlone, 2000).

MICHAEL SYROTINSKI is reader in French at the University of Aberdeen, cofounder of the Aberdeen Critical Theory Seminar, and of the Scottish Forum for Francophone Studies. He has written many articles on contemporary French and Francophone literature, literary theory, psychoanalysis, and translation. He has translated, with Christine Laennec, a selection of Jean Paulhan's *récits* (Nebraska, 1994), and recently published *Defying Gravity: Jean Paulhan's Interventions in Twentieth-Century French Intellectual History* (Albany: SUNY Press, 1998). He is currently completing a book entitled *Reinscribing Francophone African Subjectivity*.

ALEXIS TADIÉ is *maître de conférences* at the University of Paris-Nanterre. He has written on the English eighteenth century and on Salman Rushdie.

JANE WALLING is a lecturer in French at the University of Durham. Her main research interests are nineteenth- and twentieth-century French prose fiction, the history of ideas, and comparative literature

Index

Abraham, Karl, 214
Abraham, Nicolas, 328–29, 330, 337
acinema, 159
Addison, Joseph, 113
Adorno, Theodor W., 250, 252, 253, 254, 256
adultery, 31
aesthetics, 18, 21, 30, 89, 129, 142, 179, 183, 184, 188, 193, 198, 205–6 n. 25, 250, 251, 255, 265–68, 283; of ambiguity, 22; of gastronomy, 186, 191–92, 205–6 n. 25, 215, 219, 222, 282; of the miniature, 19
aesthetic theory, 7, 132, 193
amnesia, 199
anachrony, 62–63, 197, 208 n. 37, 330, 335, 337
anaesthetics, 10, 248, 251, 252, 254, 263, 265, 266, 268
anagnoresis: as truth, 198
analepsis, 202
analogy, 208 n. 37
anamnesis, 10, 179, 193, 195, 197, 198–203, 251, 306
anasemia, 328–29, 330, 332
anasensual, 10, 11, 329, 332
anthropomorphism, 9, 75
antipictorialism, 114
Anzieu, Didier, 11, 28–30
Aragon, Louis, 166
Aristotle, 7, 166–67, 276
Auerbach, Eric, 260, 261
aura, 296, 303
Austin, Gilbert, 114–15
autobiography, 71, 145, 315

back, 20, 21, 327–37
Baldwin, James, 25
Balzac, Honoré de, 272
Barthes, Roland, 80, 128, 133, 156–57, 160–61, 162, 186, 198

Battersby, Christine, 83, 86, 101–2, 103 n. 20
Batteux, Charles, 7
Baudelaire, Charles, 12, 130, 131, 204 n. 9, 252–68, 272
Baudrillard, Jean, 128
Beckett, Samuel, 206 n. 27, 330, 332, 333, 334
Benjamin, Walter, 252, 253, 259, 265, 266, 303
Bergson, Henri, 83
Berkeley, George, 7
Bersani, Leo, 286
Bick, Esther, 28
Binet, Alfred, 237–38
Blair, Hugh, 113
Blanchot, Maurice, 78, 129, 194, 196–97, 252
Bleuler, Josef, 214
blindness, 41, 73, 78, 230
Bloom, Harold, 73
body, 327; and eating, 220–21; language, 112, 115; technological, 304, 305; textualized, 153, 304
bodymorph, 40, 49–50
Bokor, Miklos, 44
Bonnefoy, Yves, 139–45, 147, 150
Botticelli, Sandro, 148
Breton, André, 166, 168
Breuer, Josef, 158
Brooks, Peter, 154, 157, 158–59
Burke, Edmund, 114
Byzantine art, 132

Cabanès, Auguste, 229–30
Campion, Jane (director, *The Piano*), 30–35
Carroll, Lewis, 331–32
Cavell, Stanley, 129
Celan, Paul, 318, 319
Certeau, Michel de, 108, 109, 117, 129

345

Cézanne, Paul, 132, 134
Chamfort, Sébastien-Roch Nicolas, 27
christianity, 250, 255
Clark, Timothy, 70
Classen, Constance, 10
cogito, 88
Coleridge, Samuel, 70, 75–77, 167
Collard, Cyril, 25–26
colonization, 31, 34, 181, 191
color, 127–51, 186, 240, 279, 282; as stable phenomenon, 8, 130, 151; as language system, 8, 130, 141, 144, 150–51; symbolism, 127, 133, 151
Condillac, Etienne Bonnot de, 7
consensuality, 10, 30
Constable, John, 139
consubstantiality, 58
conversation, 110–12
Cook, Eleanor, 78
Corbin, Alain, 244 n. 24
Cordonnier, Noël, 237
Corvin, Michel, 133
criticism, as echo-chamber, 69–70, 72
cybernetics, 12
Cytowic, Richard, 235

Dalí, Salvador, 168–69
Dante, 148, 255
David, Christian, 132
deafness, 313–14
degenerationism, 232–35
Delacroix, Eugène, 140
Deleuze, Gilles, 101, 194, 195, 202, 206 n. 27
Democritus, 7
Derrida, Jacques, 43, 57, 59–64, 70–72, 77, 252, 302, 304, 318–20, 327–29, 330–31, 332, 333, 334, 335, 336, 337
Descartes, René, 88, 235, 237, 273, 275, 276, 287
desire, 17, 18, 94, 95, 285, 286; contrasted with need, 47; gay, 26, 35 n. 36; and love, 27, 30
destinerrance, 70
Deville, Michel (director, *La Lectrice*), 153–63
Diderot, Denis, 7, 9, 27, 83, 106, 113
difference: and sameness, 45–46, 50–51, 101

disgust, 188–89, 214, 222, 238
Duthuit, George, 132, 140

echoes, 9, 69, 102
Eco, Umberto, 129
Edison, Thomas, 299, 300
Eliot, T. S., 202
embodiment, 92, 93, 100, 101, 183, 279
empiricism, 7
Enlightenment, 7, 8, 87, 88
eroticism, 21, 25, 27–35, 156; and aesthetics, 285; and ethics, 39, 53; and exegesis, 52; and violence, 34
esemplastic power, 167
Esquivel, Laura, 183–85
ethnography, 230, 238–42
everyday, the, 127–51
exoticism, 229, 231–32, 238
expressionism, German, 84
eyes, 107–8, 112, 135–36, 167; inner, 73, 78

Fanon, Franz, 26
fauves, 132
feeling, 108, 134, 232
feminism, 43, 46, 54 n. 11, 72, 75, 83, 102, 217
fermate, 96–97, 100
fetishism, 31–32, 154, 156, 157, 158
food: as architecture, 186–87; and writing, 192, 205 n. 25, 216
Foucault, Michel, 8, 24, 83, 175 n. 24
Freud, Sigmund, 28, 30, 158–59, 161–62, 217, 219–20, 221, 251, 254, 300, 318
futurity, 62, 71, 74–75, 77, 79, 194–203, 302, 332

Gadamer, Hans Georg, 295–96
Gage, John, 128
Gagnebin, Muriel, 132
Galen, 8
Garache, Claude, 140
Garrick, David, 106–7
Gasché, Rodolphe, 318–20
Gautier, Théophile, 19–20, 24
gaze, the, 20, 85, 89, 93, 95–97, 155, 156, 157
gender, 10, 11, 24, 27, 40, 75, 85, 86, 104 n. 28, 162, 216

INDEX

Genette, Gérard, 206 n. 27, 208 n. 37, 209 n. 51
Gerber, Marjorie, 24
gesture, 112–13, 116, 295
Giacometti, Alberto, 139
Gide, André, 25–26, 231
Goll, Claire, 83–84, 93–102
Goll, Yvon, 84
Grass, Günter, 210 n. 54
Gray, Margaret E., 208 n. 43
Greenaway, Peter, 157
Greuze, Jean-Baptiste, 108
Grosz, Elisabeth, 27

Haddon, Alfred, 239–41
Hall, Stanley, 217, 220–21
Halperin, David, 26
Harrison, Joyce, 24–25, 26
Hartman, Geoffrey, 69, 73
Hawthorne, Nathaniel, 31
hearing, 18, 29, 69, 107–8, 110, 118, 209 n. 45, 230, 231, 241, 279, 311–15, 324, 333; colored, 11, 237; with the 'ear of the other', 70–72, 75
Hegel, G. W. F., 7, 43
Heidegger, Martin, 8, 43, 320–32, 323
Hinojosa, José María, 169–73
Hoffmansthal, Hugo von, 22
Hogarth, William, 106
Hölderlin, Friedrich, 148
Hume, David, 7
Husserl, Edmund, 8
Huysmans, Joris Karl, 12, 188, 190, 204 n. 9, 235–36
hyphenation, 9, 10, 315–24
hypnoid state, 158, 161–62

idealism, 276
imagination, 8, 88, 89, 94, 139
immanence, 40, 91, 132
impressionism, 132
incorporation, 214–15, 223
invisibility, 134, 137, 300, 324
Irigaray, Luce, 39–54, 83, 84, 85–86, 87, 98, 100, 101

Jaccottet, Philippe, 9, 145–50
Jay, Martin, 11, 167
Jean, Raymond, 153
Joyce, James, 108, 179, 181, 182, 190, 201, 305

Jünger, Ernst, 131
Jürgenson, Friedrich, 301

Kandinsky, Vasily, 130–31, 132
Kant, Immanuel, 7, 83–91, 94, 98, 100, 101, 103 n. 15, n. 20, 249, 253, 254, 260–62
Kasack, Hermann, 86–87, 103 n. 13
Keats, John, 70, 77–79
Kierkegaard, Soren, 83, 101, 300
Kittler, Friedrich, 301
Kristeva, Julia, 203 n. 3, 206 n. 27

Lacan, Jacques, 159, 160, 196, 308 n. 29
Lanchester, John, 188–91, 203 n. 2
Large, Duncan, 207 n. 31, 208 n. 37
Lefebvre, Henri, 128, 129
Lessing, Gotthold Ephraim, 114
Levinas, Emmanuel, 27, 39–54
Lévi-Strauss, Claude, 19, 128
Lille, Alain de, 271
Lingis, Alphonso, 27
listening, 9, 18, 111
literacy, 108
Locke, John, 7, 113
Ludwig, Paula, 9, 83–93, 100–102
Lukács, Georg, 254
Luria, A. L., 298–99, 304
Lury, Celia, 160–61
Lyne, Adrian (director, *Fatal Attraction*), 30–31, 32, 34–35
Lyotard, Jean-François, 78, 159, 197, 202, 207–8 n. 37, 251, 252, 253, 267

MacLane, Mary, 213–23
magical realism, 198, 201, 208 n. 39
Magritte, René, 173
Man, de, Paul, 12, 250, 284, 290 n. 35
Mapplethorpe, Robert, 21, 26
Marquez, Gabriel Garcia, 198
Marshall, Donald, 69–70
masculinism, 11, 43, 50, 51, 54, 85–6, 157, 158, 160
materiality, 88, 92, 94, 100, 101, 134; of act of reading, 306; of the book, 329; of color, 130; of flesh, 49; of food, 194, 202; of word, 110, 112, 115
Matheson, Richard, 301
Matisse, Henri, 132

Maupassant, Guy de, 154, 158
medecine, and literature, 229, 233
memory, 102, 193, 194–203, 249, 265, 281, 298, 302–4, 305, 306, 307 n. 14, 332
Mercer, Kobena, 26
Merleau-Ponty, Maurice, 8, 9, 43, 47–51, 133–38, 146, 150–51
Meyer, Conrad Ferdinand, 18–19, 20
Michelangelo, 18
mimesis, 160, 161, 166, 251
modernism, 179, 188, 190, 202, 205 n. 23, 250, 265
Mondrian, Piet, 139
mothers, 29, 72, 300; mother-daughter relationship, 31–33, 49, 311–15; mother tongue, 73, 77, 312
Mozart, Wolfgang Amadeus, 48
music, 70, 73, 85–93, 94, 96–102, 109, 131

Nancy, Jean-Luc, 57, 58, 62, 320–24
narcissism, 23, 221–23
neurophysiology, 8
Newton, Isaac, 129
Nietzsche, Friedrich, 18, 43, 71–72, 76, 79, 83, 266–67
Nordau, Max, 233–35
noumenal, 11, 88
Novalis, 272
Nyman, Michael, 109

ocularcentrism, 11, 47, 167, 174 n. 5
Ong, Walter, 10, 111, 117, 230–31
ontology, 64
orality, 108, 119, 214
orientalism, 26, 37 n. 34
Orlan, 23–24
otobiography, 71

painting, 114, 132, 134, 138, 142–45, 147, 173, 284
palimpsest, 196, 209 n. 51, 327
paranoia-critique, 168–69, 174 n. 14
Partridge, Eric, 316–17
patriarchy, 42, 47, 53, 72, 79, 85
Perec, Georges, 129
phallocentrism, 50
phenomenal, 11, 88, 89, 275, 306. *See also* noumenal
phenomenology, 8, 9, 39–54, 150

Plato, 84, 87, 94–95, 98, 100, 101, 251, 331
poetry: and color, 138–51; and metaphor, 166–67; as sculpture, 19; and sensual experience, 249, 252, 253; symbolist, 250; and telephony, 70
politics, 192, 198, 202–3
polymorphous perversity, 158, 160, 169
Pope, Alexander, 115
pornography, 21
postcolonialism, 180, 198
postmodernism, 10, 180, 197, 202, 209 n. 23
Poulet, Georges, 8, 195
Poulsen, Vlademar, 299
Poussin, Nicolas, 139
prephenomenology, 44
Priestley, John, 107–8
printing, 115–17
promnesia, 179, 180, 199–203
prosthetic culture, 160–61
Proust, Marcel, 7, 8, 22–23, 179, 180, 184, 186–88, 190, 193, 194–99, 201, 202, 203, 249, 271–88, 298
psychoanalysis, 8, 132, 158–60, 161–62, 300, 328

Queneau, Raymond, 129

Rand, Richard A., 77
Rathenau, Walter, 301
Raudive, Konstantin, 301
reading, 9, 12; aloud, 117, 120 n. 10, 153, 163 n.1; in the Book of Nature, 271–88; and eating, 218; as forepleasure, 158; as hybrid experience, 107; as performance, 153, 156; in Proust, 276–77; silently, 117
Réda, Jacques, 129
Renaissance, 129
Reni, Guido, 114
repetition, 295–97, 301, 302, 303, 305, 306 n. 3, 315, 318, 319, 324, 331, 334, 335
resonance, 83, 90, 91, 97, 99, 101, 102
Reverdy, Pierre, 166, 167
Richard, Jean-Pierre, 8, 179, 194, 271
Richardson, Samuel, 113
Richter, Jean-Paul, 272
Rickels, Laurence, 300

Riffaterre, Michael, 168
Rilke, Rainer Maria, 20–21, 23
Rimbaud, Arthur, 12, 243 n. 17
Rodin, Auguste, 18, 20–21
Romanticism, 9, 94, 114, 129, 131, 233, 249, 272
Romantic poetry, 69–80, 249, 250, 254, 272
Rousseau, Jean-Jacques, 7
Rousset, Jean, 207 n. 31, 209 n. 48
Royle, Nicholas, 70, 300
Rubens, Peter Paul, 140
Rushdie, Salman, 10, 106, 179–84, 193, 194, 196, 197–203, 203–4 n. 8, 210 n. 53

Sade, Marquis de, 34
sadism, 31, 214
Sainte-Beuve, Charles Augustin, 272
Sartre, Jean-Paul, 17, 20, 27
Scheherazade, 193
Schelling, Friedrich von, 276, 277, 281
Schiller, Friedrich, 7
Segalen, Victor, 10, 229–42
senses: cultural specificity of, 10; hierarchy of, 10, 18, 47, 230, 235; higher, 10, 18, 230; immediacy of, 89, 132, 140; lower, 11, 18, 230, 265; number of, 11; sixth sense, 11. *See also* hearing; sight; smell; taste; touching
senselessness, 9, 249, 260, 265, 298, 311, 314
sensorium, 10, 70, 230, 231, 235, 241, 243 n. 8, 255, 324
sensory impressions, 88–89
sensualist philosophy, 7, 229
sensual reading, 7, 8, 42, 51, 53, 153, 159, 161, 162–63, 271–76, 279–81, 286–88, 302, 315, 323, 329
sensus communis, 9, 253, 264
sexual difference, 85, 101; and ethics, 8, 42, 49
Shakespeare, William, 10, 57–66, 330, 332, 334–37
Shattuck, Roger, 206 n. 27, 209 n. 43
Shaviro, Steven, 159–60
Shaw, George Bernard, 233
Shelley, Percy Bysshe, 77
Sherman, Allan, 17, 28

sight, 18, 29, 107–8, 113, 230, 231, 233, 241; and reading, 116, 118, 120 n. 32, 285; second, 11; and seer/seen distinction, 50, 298; as touch, 43, 44, 135, 147; visionary, 73, 272
singularity, 11, 102, 135, 137–38, 303, 315, 317–24, 334
skin, 17–37, 58, 92, 216, 217, 230; ego (*le moi-peau*), 11, 28–30; and racial difference, 22, 24–27
smell, 10, 18, 29, 108, 209 n. 45, 230, 231, 232, 233, 235, 259, 264, 265, 279
Socrates, 331
Sollers, Philippe, 108
soul, 91–92, 100, 151, 233, 254, 255–57, 273, 277, 287, 302, 305
soundscapes, 109, 111
Staiger, Emil, 249
Sterne, Laurence, 9, 106–22, 182
Stoker, Bram, 305
Stoller, Robert, 156
subjectivity and senses, 8, 9, 11, 41, 43, 44, 45, 48, 60, 70, 71, 74, 83, 85, 87, 88–94, 98, 101, 129, 134–38, 146, 149–50, 154, 159, 160, 162, 215, 217, 221, 223, 232, 233, 249, 250, 251, 256, 258, 262, 263, 266, 280–81
sublime (Kantian), 89, 94, 132, 260–62, 265, 268
surface: and depth, 22–24
surrealism, 129, 166–69, 171
Swedenborg, Emanuel, 12, 272
Swift, Jonathan, 328
synaesthesia, 9, 11–12, 30, 78, 93, 100, 179, 197, 203, 205 n. 25, 209 n. 45, 229, 232–35, 236, 241, 264, 279, 298
syncategorems, 321
syncategoremical imperative, 10, 323

tactility, 9
taste, 18, 29, 108, 186, 209 n. 45, 216, 235, 240, 254–55, 258; and eating, 213–14
telepathy, 10, 11, 69, 300, 301
telephony, 79–80, 296, 298–99, 301, 305
teletechnology, 9, 69, 76, 77, 295, 296, 298–304

theology, 55 n. 27
Theroux, Alexander, 128
Titian, 140
Torok, Maria, 328, 330, 337
touching, 17, 29, 33, 39, 99, 230, 235, 241, 287; interrupted, 58; of the other, 40, 57–58; passive versus active sense, 17–18; and power relations, 27; self-, 41, 47, 48, 57–58; and tact, 59; sound as, 92
transcendentality, 41, 91, 94, 139
typography, 118

uncanny, the, 232

Valéry, Paul, 24
Van Gogh, Vincent, 140
Van Velde, Bram, 142–43
Verlaine, Paul, 148, 233

Vinaver, Michel, 129
virtual reality, 12
visible, the, 19–20, 47–48, 134, 275, 278; and language, 135, 138
visuality, 112–15, 117–19, 156, 160, 167–72, 238, 241–42, 265
voice, 87, 99, 108, 109, 154, 156, 295, 296, 298–99, 300–302, 305, 306, 333
voyeurism, 285, 290 n. 40

Warhol, Andy, 12, 295–306
Wittgenstein, Ludwig, 133, 167, 168
Wordsworth, William, 69, 70, 72–75, 79

Yeats, W. B., 142–43

Zola, Emile, 235